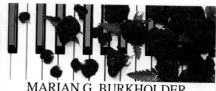

Supermarket Remedies

Cass Ingram, D.O.
with Judy Kay Gray, M.S.

Knowledge House
Buffalo Grove, Illinois 60089

Printed in the United States of America
First Edition

ISBN 0911119647

Disclaimer: This book is not intended as a substitute for medical diagnosis or treatment. Anyone who has a serious disease should consult a physician before initiating any change in treatment or before beginning any new treatment.

For ordering information call (800) 243-5242

Published by:
Knowledge House
212 Willow Pkwy.
Buffalo Grove, Illinois 60089

Table of Contents

Introduction

Today, the definition of medicine is changing dramatically. Medicines should enhance health. They should be relatively safe to use. Certainly, their side effects shouldn't be worse than the illness itself. Yet, this isn't the case with many of the drugs, as well as medical procedures, used today. This is why the medicines of nature, such as food, herbs, spices, vitamins, and minerals, are becoming increasingly popular. While pharmaceutical medicines have side effects which are dangerous or even life threatening, natural medicines may be curative while being entirely free of side effects.

Medicines should help us feel better. They should be useful in the treatment, cure, and/or prevention of disease. By this definition food is medicine. This is because it nourishes the body, providing it with the nutrients necessary to maintain health. It is medicine, because it gives the body strength and energy. It is medicine, because it supplies the body with basic constituents needed to ward off disease. Finally, it is medicine, because it can be used specifically to cure certain symptoms, illnesses, and diseases.

While synthetic drugs are the most commonly utilized types of medicines in America today, this has not always been the case. As little as 50 years ago natural medicines were the primary treatment dispensed by physicians in Europe as well as the United States. Currently, in some parts of the world natural medicines are essentially the only treatment modality. In the Western world the use of such medicines is resurging, and it is likely that eventually natural substances, such as herbs, vitamins, minerals, and food, will displace synthetics as the primary type of medicine dispensed and consumed in the United States as well as the rest of the world.

1

What a realization it is that ordinary food which is available in the supermarket can be used to improve health and even treat illness. To achieve this, all that is required is to simply understand which foods should be consumed for a given health complaint and perhaps how much of the food to consume.

Anyone can become an expert concerning the health benefits of food. This is because food is the safest type of health aid. If you wish to stay as healthy as possible while expending the least amount of time, energy, and money, learn how to use common foods for everyday complaints.

Food has been utilized as medicine by the human race for untold thousands of years. Unfortunately, in much of the Western world the formerly premier status of food as medicine has been utterly neglected, that is until recently. After decades of indifference by the medical profession, as well as the researchers, the incontestably valuable attributes of medicinal foods are resurfacing. This resurgence is largely because of the immense interest of the American public in preventive and natural medicine. The fact that currently a greater number of individuals visit alternative care practitioners, such as chiropractors, osteopathic physicians, acupuncturists, herbalists, etc, than orthodox physicians is a glaring statistic that mainstream medicine would like to ignore. However, the ratio is nearly two alternative visits for every orthodox visit.

This unprecedented interest in natural medicine makes good sense. For instance, the fact that ordinary food or perhaps an herb or spice could be used to prevent or ameliorate disease is of immense value as well as being highly practical. Imagine knowing the right food to eat or avoid in the event of an illness. Consider the value of comprehending which food(s) prevent the scourges of modern civilization: cancer, , Alzheimer's disease, diabetes, asthma, infectious diseases, osteoporosis, arthritis, prostatitis, cataracts, and glaucoma. Imagine the importance of knowing which foods help avert sudden health disasters, in other words, which foods help cure illnesses such as colds, flu, sore throat, headache, backache, muscle cramps, nausea, indigestion, joint pain, constipation and diarrhea. Virtually every individual endures some sort of potentially disastrous illness and, yet, has no idea what to do to resolve it. He/she has no clue as to which remedy to take and no idea that something could be done immediately to eradicate the problem not at the doctor's office or pharmacy but at the nearest grocery store.

Food has always been medicine. That's the way it has been since the beginning of humankind. Undoubtedly, it was the sole medicine of primitive man. Natural medicines, that is food and herbs, were the medicines of the ancient Egyptians. In ancient Greece food and herbs were the exclusive medicines. Hippocrates described dozens of foods as cures. The Greek pharmacopoeia (i.e. catalogue of medicines) primarily contained references to foods and herbs. For instance, Greek physicians frequently dispensed garlic and onions as disease-fighting medicines. In fact, they listed some 100 diseases in which they were effective. While the Romans added little to Greek knowledge, they did adhere to many of the Greek prescriptions. Plus, they loved using food as a remedy, and their favorites included grapes, garlic, olives, and olive oil. Galen, Rome's most famous physician, relied heavily upon the Greek herbs as medicines. Yet, food as a cure has an even more ancient and profound history than the Greeks and Romans. Abraham was a proponent of natural medicines, and it is believed that he knew of the health benefits of foods such as yogurt and honey. Jesus used food and herbs as cures, and the Bible is replete with references regarding the immense value of food. Muhammad propounded the benefits of numerous foods and herbs. His medical prescriptions are widely written. Honey was one of his favorite dispensations, and he used it successfully for intestinal complaints, particularly diarrhea. He also promoted the health benefits of medicinal herbs as well as protein rich foods such as fresh meat, fish, and unprocessed goat's milk. The fact is every prophet of ancient times promoted food as medicine.

Greek knowledge in natural medicine was expanded immensely during the Middle Ages by the scientists of Islam. A 14th century herbal catalogue written by Ibn Baytar contained over 1400 entries for foods and herbs, with proof of their efficacy as well as a description of how to prepare them. History records that during the entire extent of the Islamic Empire, which ranged from the 8th through 15th centuries, food and herbs were the primary medicines dispensed. In fact, as early as the 9th century A.D. Baghdad, the capital of the Empire, housed some 60 pharmacies, staffed by pharmacists who dispensed natural medicines by prescription. Incredibly, the use of natural medicines by Islamic physicians spanned fully 700 hundred years. In contrast, modern medicine, as practiced in the United States and Europe with its emphasis on synthetic drugs, is a mere 100 years old

In the innumerable civilizations of the Orient, past and present, natural medicines were/are the only types of medicines. The Chinese possess a 4,000 year plus history of using various foods and herbs for treating disease. All native American civilizations—the mainland tribes, the Incas, and the Mayans—relied upon natural medicines for curing disease. They mastered the precise use of hundreds of plants, foods, and herbs as medicines. In short, all ancient civilizations learned the use of foods and herbs for treating and preventing disease. This means that natural medicine is infinitely older than modern medicine. Furthermore, it is time tested, in other words, it has endured a greater degree of research than modern medicine and, thus, holds the status of being the most thoroughly proven of all types of medicine.

Natural doesn't necessarily imply total safety. After all, mercury, platinum, silver, cyanide, and lead are natural, but they are inedible and toxic. Therefore, because a substance is natural doesn't mean it is safe, nor does it mean it has positive medicinal actions. For instance, in China dried lizards are used as "medicine." The Chinese grind the lizards and add them as an active ingredient in specific concoctions. No doubt, ground lizard is natural, but it is not a documented medicine and may do more harm than good.

Historically, primitive societies always used foods and plants as medicines. Even today, numerous primitive societies depend exclusively on the plants of their locale for preventing and treating health complaints. Amazingly, drug companies are relying heavily upon the primitives in their quest for future drugs. They are spending untold millions of dollars in the attempt to "discover" new, profitable cures.

Nutrition as a science is generally separate from herbal medicine. Nutrition is the science of what we eat. In the science of herbs while some plants may be used as medicines, they are never eaten for their food value. For instance, an individual might take black cohosh or valerian herbal capsules but would never eat these herbs. Even so, numerous herbs, such as ginger root, garlic, fennel, oregano, coriander, basil, and onion, are equally valuable if not more valuable for their curative powers as are the more obscure medicinal herbs. Plus, the "food herbs" are entirely safe and can be consumed in large quantities. In contrast, the non-food herbs may cause toxicity. For instance, certain herbs, such as chapparal, comfrey, and Melaluca, contain chemicals which can poison

4

the liver. Licorice root in large amounts may cause reversable high blood pressure. Ginseng may cause hirsutism, that is abnormal hair growth, and other hormonal disturbances. Usually, these ill effects occur only if the herb is consumed in large amounts over prolonged periods. However, some herbs possess toxicity to the extent that they should never be given to pregnant women or babies. These facts underscore the immense value of foods which possess herbal and medicinal powers, since food is safe even in relatively large amounts. In fact, with food-like herbs, such as garlic, onions, radishes, oregano, basil, fennel, sage, etc., large amounts are usually well tolerated with insignificant side effects if any. In fact, the higher dosages actually accelerate the cure. Don't worry about consuming natural foods and chemicals. In other words, an individual is not going to get sick or suffer any "permanent" damage from eating edible substances, even powerful ones like oregano, basil, garlic, fennel, cumin, etc. In contrast, alcohol causes millions of cases of liver poisoning every year, including thousands of fatalities, but we rarely give this fact much thought. However, the medical profession would like us to believe that there is significant toxicity in herbs, even in food-grade herbs, and this is simply not the case.

Food benefits the body by providing it with the building blocks it needs. These building blocks—proteins, amino acids, fatty acids, steroids, phospholipids, vitamins, coenzymes, and minerals—are used to create the basis of human existence: living cells. The body contains some 70 trillion of these complex microscopic beings, and they must be nourished to survive. Now it is known that what we eat directly effects the chemistry and function of our cells and influences the cellular environment towards either health or disease. Simply put, what we eat determines how healthy or how sick the cells are in the body. What we eat may also determine how quickly we can recover from an illness and how well we can enhance our abilities to prevent the onslaught of disease. Yet, what is perhaps even more fascinating is the fact that each food contains a unique array of disease-fighting chemicals, and it is now possible to use the food or food extract to combat specific illnesses. For instance, let's review the health value of fish. At one time mothers knew that fish was good for an individual and called it "brain food." Whether instinctive or by chance, mother was entirely correct. Researchers now know that a certain oil in fish, particularly fatty fish, such as salmon,

5

mackerel, and herring, is required by the brain for optimal function and may be regarded as essential for normal brain development. The oil is needed by the brain for the conduction of nerve impulses. This oil is more than brain food. Thousands of articles are published every year about how EPA and DHA (*eicosapentanoic acid and docosahexanoic acid*) block a variety of disease processes. In particular, researchers are fascinated by fish oil's peculiar powers for fighting inflammation. Incredibly, the oil fights any type of inflammation in any region of the body. This means that eating fatty fish may be an ideal remedy for all types of inflammatory diseases, including arthritis, lupus, asthma, bronchitis, irritable bowel syndrome, bursitis, tendonitis, migraine, sinusitis, vasculitis, gastritis, and esophagitis. A simple rule is that any illness which ends with "itis" is a candidate for the fish oil prescription.

Food may be a detriment to the body. Certainly, processed foods cause more harm than good. For instance, let's evaluate the typical American fare: a lunch of a hot dog and French fries with ketchup, mustard, and relish. The beverage is the standard cola drink. Such a meal is a kind of nutritional suicide. The hot dog provides protein, but the nitrates and dyes in it destroy the body's protein and amino acids, plus these chemicals destroy vitamins C and B_6, both of which are required for protein digestion and metabolism. The bun and French fries provide starch calories, but they are "empty calories," meaning they provide no significant nutrients such as vitamins, minerals, natural fatty acids, or coenzymes. The oil (the more correct terminology would be grease) in which the fries are cooked destroys vitamins and provides none. Obviously, the cola provides nothing but sugar calories plus some dubious chemicals. The refined sugar depletes vitamins and minerals, particularly vitamin B complex, vitamin C, potassium, magnesium, and zinc. The ketchup and relish contain sugar, usually in the form of corn syrup, and this aggravates the nutritional deficit. As far as vitamin and mineral content in this all-American meal, whatever it provides is entirely overwhelmed by the losses it creates. In other words, you are on the minus side as a result of eating processed foods.

Food can poison the individual in yet another way: food allergy. A food might be all-natural, it might provide immense health benefits, but, if an individual is allergic to that food, it can make him/her sick. It is a paradox that a food could come to the aid of one person and make yet another person sick. Why this occurs is difficult to explain. However, let us review some examples. One of my patients suffered from mind-bending migraines occurring as often as three times per week. She had a habit that seemed perfectly healthy; she squeezed a wedge of lemon or lime in her V-8 or tomato juice every morning. However, I determined that she is deathly allergic to lemons and limes, which was documented by blood allergy testing. When the lemons and limes were eliminated from the diet, the headaches disappeared. Another patient was on a macrobiotic diet, which was prescribed to combat her cancer. While on the diet she had lost some 40 pounds, and she definitely didn't need to lose the weight. When I first saw her she was essentially skin and bones. I tested her for food toxicity and found that she was highly allergic to legumes, rice, and grains, the primary constituents of the macrobiotic diet. After changing her diet she gradually regained her normal weight and is today in excellent health. For further information regarding the role of food allergy in disease see *How to Eat Right and Live Longer* (formerly *Eat Right to Live Long*), chapters 9 and 10.

What is in Food?

Food consists of chemicals. Carbohydrates, protein, fat, vitamins, and minerals are all chemicals. Yet, these are natural chemicals. Food may also contain synthetic chemicals, which are added by food processors. However, the primary concern is this: What are the essential elements of food which account for its health giving attributes? Let's review each of the major categories of chemicals found in food to get an idea of what is really in it.

Carbohydrates: these consist of sugar molecules either in the form of a single sugar, two sugars (i.e. *disaccharides*) or as starches. Chemically, a starch is merely a string of sugar molecules held together via molecular bonds. Carbohydrates are utilized by the body almost exclusively as fuel.

Proteins: these are nitrogen based substances, which consist primarily of nitrogen, carbon, and oxygen. Proteins may also contain sulfur. All proteins are made up of building blocks called amino acids. Every cell in our bodies is synthesized primarily from amino acids.

Some amino acids can be synthesized in the body. However, a number of them cannot be synthesized and must be obtained from the diet. A deficiency of any of these *essential amino acids* leads to detrimental effects upon cellular function, structure, and reproduction.

Fats: primarily a source of fuel, fats consist almost exclusively of carbon and hydrogen. They are also important for the body as a source of stored fuel. Certain fats, such as linoleic and linolenic acids, as well as phospholipids, are required for maintaining the structure and function of cells. Such fats are absolutely essential for our existence. Without them, the cells and organs of our bodies degenerate. We would literally shrivel up and die.

Vitamins: vitamins are defined as substances which are so essential that life fails to exist without them. They are relatively complex molecules, which combine some of the chemistry of sugars, amino acids, and fatty acids. They function primarily as catalysts, controlling the rate and efficiency of the molecular activities within our cells. Vitamins help our bodies make use of the food and fuel we consume.

Minerals: minerals may be defined as atomic catalysts required for initiating cellular reactions. Certain minerals, such as calcium, are used primarily for structural functions. However, the majority of the minerals are the catalyzing agents for enzymatic reactions. Certain minerals are essential for human existence; for instance, if levels of calcium, magnesium, sodium, or potassium drop precipitously, death may rapidly ensue.

Flavonoids: there has been much news regarding the healthful properties of various chemicals in food besides vitamins and minerals. The majority of these chemicals belong to a class of compounds known as flavonoids. These substances are complex drug-like molecules, which exhibit a wide range of functions. The number of flavonoids is so vast that it would take all of the researchers globally to quantify and classify them, and even this effort would be insufficient. Suffice it to say that a lack of dietary flavonoids increases the risks for a variety of diseases, especially lung disease, arthritis, diabetes, and cancer.

Just Another Radio Show

After appearing on 2,000 plus radio interviews telling the public what foods to eat, as well as which ones to avoid, writing this book is like performing another radio show. For those who are unfamiliar, I am a guest expert on hundreds of radio stations every year. Many interviews are unannounced so you will possibly miss them. This illustrates the importance of utilizing this book. By reading and studying it, in a sense, it is as if you are listening to me whenever you want to. While on the air I have repeatedly discussed the health benefits of natural substances and how they can be used for medicinal purposes. These might be foods or herbs that your grandparents or great grandparents knew of and used as medicines, perhaps unconsciously. Now you read about it. You learn what is in the food or beverage. Hopefully, you will understand to some degree how these natural substances work. You find out which illnesses a certain food aids, which symptoms it resolves, and why it performs its unique functions.

Food is the safest type of medicine to consume. Certain foods, like ginger root, oregano, and garlic, act more like medicines than foods. How fantastic it is to enjoy pleasurable tastes, while gaining the medicinal benefits. Individuals with serious diseases are in the greatest need of medicinal foods, and such foods are safe to consume for those who are taking traditional drugs.

The supermarket is the first stop for vitamins and minerals, not the local vitamin shop. Pills cannot sustain life, but food will readily sustain it. In other words, even though a one-a-day vitamin contains all of the vitamins and minerals necessary for survival, try living on vitamin pills plus water—you won't last long. Yet, if you ate nothing but eggs and water, meat and water, milk and water, or many of the other foods that people eat everyday, you could survive and thrive (along with at least some fruits and vegetables). This is despite the fact that the vitamin pill technically contains a greater array of vitamins and minerals and in larger quantities than any of the foods mentioned. Everyone knows these facts instinctively, but how often do people give it thought? Yet, in this era it is common for individuals to attempt to consume their vitamins and minerals from pills rather than from the food they eat. The exception is if the pills/formulae are themselves produced from unprocessed natural foods such as algae, rice bran, herbs, etc. Then, they would be utilized by the body nutritionally like food.

Chapter One

Doctor, What Should I Eat?

Are you confused about what you should be eating? Do you feel helpless because of the innumerable opinions about what is eating right? Do you feel, after listening to all of the opinions, that there is nothing left to eat? In other words, are you unsure about what to believe?

One of the reasons for the confusion is there is a great deal of misinformation in the field of nutrition. Plus, there are dozens of opinions, and the experts seem to change their views constantly.

When it comes to diet and health most individuals are gullible. Thus, they tend to believe anything found in newspapers, magazines, and books as gospel. They may even trust it over common sense. This has lead to mass paranoia.

These issues are serious problems. Incredibly, despite all of the sophistication of modern times, the average person simply doesn't know what to eat. If you are one of the many confused, don't give up hope yet. Through the information in this book the confusion will be eliminated.

With nutrition we shouldn't blindly follow whatever we read. Yet, we do follow unquestioningly the orthodox advice. We avoid fresh red meat, eggs, whole fat milk, butter, and salt. Despite the fact that no one has ever provided sufficient proof that such natural foods are harmful, we have changed decades old eating patterns because of what we hear and read.

Health is a sacred commodity. No one can afford to make mistakes which could put his/her body at risk. Thus, the individual must give nutritional information careful thought. He/she must determine whether or not a particular dictum makes sense before embarking upon wholesale dietary changes. The point is it is reasonable to utilize common sense as the determinant regarding what is eating right.

It is unwise to adhere to any extreme approach regarding diet. For example, cutting out all of the fat is extreme. Erasing every trace of cholesterol is extreme. Eating a strict meat-free diet, that is attempting to exist upon fruits, vegetables, beans, and grains, is extreme. Eating mostly pasta is extreme. None of these diets are nutritionally balanced. For instance, strict vegetarianism leads to widespread deficiencies of essential amino acids, as well as certain trace minerals, such as calcium, zinc, selenium, sulfur, and copper. Diets heavy in pasta may also cause trace mineral deficiencies and are insufficient in protein and essential fatty acids. However, the low fat diet is the one that most individuals feel a necessity to follow, because fat has been universally "blamed" as the primary dietary culprit in the cause of disease. Yet, the low fat diet is perhaps the most nutritionally insufficient if not outright dangerous type of diet known.

Conflicting information is constantly disseminated regarding the fat issue. One minute we are informed that fat is bad, and then we are told we cannot live without it. For instance, we are told that extra virgin olive oil, which is 100% fat, is an essential component of the diet. Ironically, while fat is deemed harmful, salmon, which is 50% fat, is regarded as a health food. We are reminded that nuts and seeds, which are 80% fat, are healthy and help block diseases, such as heart disease and cancer, and yet we are seduced to reduce dietary fat to as little as 20%, a feat which is impossible if an individual regularly eats nuts and seeds.

Certain low fat diet guru's, such as Dean Ornish, M.D. and John McDougal, M.D., recommend the reduction of dietary fat to as little as 10%. This is a dangerously low level of intake, because fatty acids are critical for the function of all organ systems. Essential fatty acids, saturated fat, and cholesterol all perform critical functions within the cells of our bodies. All of these fatty acids are required for the functional integrity of human cell membranes. Additionally, critical nutrients needed for the basic maintenance of organ function, such as carnitine, vitamin A, and vitamin D, are absolutely lacking in a low fat diet. The brain, which controls the function of the entire body, requires a daily supply of fatty acids. The fact is adherence to extreme low fat diets may lead to cellular damage in a wide range of organs, including the brain, liver, kidneys, heart, stomach, sinuses, bone marrow, lymph glands, adrenal glands, thyroid gland, ovaries, uterus, and skin.

We have become paranoid about eating. For instance, we are told to hold the butter, but now it is known that margarine is the harmful spread and butter is the acceptable and even healthy addition. Protein is supposedly harmful, even relatively moderate amounts, and, yet, it is certain that we cannot live without it. Salt is supposedly taboo, but it is absolutely necessary for survival. Non-fat foods are proclaimed to be the mainstay, yet, this means an individual must avoid fresh meat, milk products, eggs, avocados, nuts, and seeds, which are among the most nutritionally rich of all foods.

One easy way to carve through the maze of nutritional confusion is to rely on common sense. Food should be viewed as a source of nourishment. Its purpose is to support life and enhance health. An individual must eat *real food* in a balanced ratio to survive. If a substance is truly a food, it should assist health and certainly not detract from it. Food is made by the natural powers of the universe. Scientists have never been able to produce it from scratch in a laboratory. Therefore, real food should be defined as edible substances produced by Nature, which contain both fuel value and nutrients. The fuel consists of either primarily protein, (for example, meat), fat, (for example, an olive), or carbohydrate, (for example, an orange). The content of protein, fat, carbohydrates, vitamins, and minerals is what makes it a food, and these substances must be regarded as the useful or "good" parts. That is the simplest definition of diet and nutrition. Another way to comprehend this is that if it is not made by Nature, it cannot be a food. By these definitions eggs are a food but fake eggs are not, whole milk is a food but coffee creamer is not, real cheese is a food, while synthetic cheese is not, avocado is a food, while synthetic fat additives are not, real meat is a food but soy or wheat burgers are not, an ear of corn is a food, while frosted corn flakes are not, pure honey is a food but corn syrup is not. While it is true that some of these compounds are edible, they have been so thoroughly processed that they fail to resemble, physically and nutritionally, the original whole food.

It is ludicrous, as well as unscientific, to judge a substance negatively just because it is high in fat or protein. Some foods are mostly fat, some mostly protein, and some mostly carbohydrate, but they are all foods. The point is that protein foods, fatty foods, and carbohydrate foods are all a part of a healthy diet, because they provide valuable fuel and nutrients in a natural form.

It is important to realize that food impacts our health in a major way. The quality of our health is directly related to the food we eat. We literally become a sort of living soup consisting of whatever we ingest. In other words, the food that we eat is precisely of what our organs and cells are made. Graphically, if we eat an orange, our cells will be partially made of that orange, and if we eat a hot dog, our cells will partly consist of the elements in it. If we eat food which contains synthetic chemicals, our cells will house those chemicals, and this will be detrimental. Obviously, the human body operates at top efficiency when supplied with natural chemicals. Conversely, it will malfunction if it is contaminated with synthetic chemicals. We should only consume foods which support cellular function, not those which contaminate our cells. Eat real protein, such as that found in fresh meat, fish, eggs, milk products, nuts, and whole grains, because our cells need protein. Avoid processed meats, which contain various synthetic chemicals such as nitrates, artificial flavors, and food dyes. Eat natural fats, the fats that God makes in Nature, and avoid all processed and adulterated fats such as margarine, refined vegetable oils, and deep frying oils. Eat natural sources of sugar, such as fresh fruit and vegetables, and eliminate refined sugar and synthetic sweeteners. Eat fresh real vegetables instead of canned, processed, or chemically/genetically altered vegetables. Eat fresh fruit instead of canned, sugar-laden varieties.

These are easy rules to follow. Obviously, anyone can eat right by following these principles. Every individual should eat right, since the benefits are immense. Better health, increased strength and stamina, plus a more vibrant, attractive appearance are all consequences of smart and healthy eating. Could anything be superior to that?

Chapter Two

Top 12 Diseases and their Supermarket Remedies

For over a century America has led the world in manufacturing, industry, science, and technology. Yet, since the 1970s America's leadership and share of the world market has declined precipitously. Of even greater concern is the fact that the health of Americans is also declining, since the United States leads the world in degenerative diseases. These diseases are also known as *diseases of civilization*. Is it possible that the decline in American industry and productivity is related to the decline in health? It is certainly a reasonable premise which requires further study.

Degenerative disease is essentially a modern plague, and millions of individuals in North America suffer from some element of it. Here are the disconcerting statistics. In the United States heart disease, which is a degenerative condition, remains the number one cause of death despite all of the advances of modern medicine. Alzheimer's disease, which is a type of degeneration of the brain, is the fourth leading cause of death. Cancer, the second leading killer, is on the rise. Since the early 1900s the cancer rate has skyrocketed, and, astonishingly, nearly one third of all Americans will succumb to it at some period during their life-times. By the year 2000 it is estimated that as many as one of two people will be stricken with cancer. The fact is modern medicine simply cannot keep pace with the vast numbers of individuals stricken with this killer. The types of cancer which are rising in incidence exponentially include skin cancer, particularly melanoma, leukemia, lymphoma, lung cancer, testicular cancer, breast cancer, and liver cancer. Modern medicine has entirely failed to halt the onslaught of this killer.

Lung disease is another major killer. It has reached epidemic proportions, with tens of millions of individuals crippled by emphysema, asthma, and chronic lung infections. The list of debilitating lung infections which are on the rise includes tuberculosis, bronchitis, histoplasmosis, candidiasis, and pneumonia.

Digestive disorders are incredibly common, and the primary afflictions include irritable bowel syndrome, ulcerative colitis, celiac disease, gastritis, hiatal hernia, gastric or duodenal ulcer, diverticulitis, Crohn's disease, and pancreatitis. All of these digestive syndromes are directly related to our living and eating habits, that is what we eat, drink, smoke, or chew.

The skin is an organ, and, if it fails to receive the nutrients it requires, it degenerates. Thus, poor diet and nutritional deficiency may lead to dry or oily skin, dermatitis, eczema, psoriasis, lupus, and skin infections as well as accelerated aging of the skin.

The modern way of living creates a number of rather bizarre diseases. Dozens of diseases which are commonplace today were rarely or never seen before in civilization. These diseases include chronic fatigue syndrome, irritable bowel syndrome, polymyositis, lupus, multiple sclerosis, muscular dystrophy, ALS, AIDS, scleroderma, sarcoidosis, and fibromyalgia. Even coronary artery disease was relatively rare until the mid-20th century. There are also the currently in vogue mental illnesses, which were largely unknown until recently, including obsessive compulsive syndrome, attention deficit disorder, SAD (seasonal affective disorder), bulimia, anorexia, and panic attacks. There are the infectious disorders, some modern day—hepatitis C, Epstein-Barr, meningitis, E. coli, Hantavirus, Lyme disease, candidiasis, Ebola, Cryptosporidium, and Ehrlichiosis. There are also the commonly known infectious diseases— colds, flu, hepatitis A and B, strep, staph, Salmonella, and herpes. There are the parasites—Giardia, tapeworms, pinworms, hookworms, flukes, trichomonas, and amebas.

Regarding the fight against infection progress has been minimal. Like the defunct cancer war, medicine has failed miserably in the war against germs. Despite the advent of antibiotics, with all their supposed power and promise, the microorganisms are winning. This is because the microbes are mutating, rendering the antibiotics ineffective. A recent article (1996) published in *Hippocrates* magazine pointed to the alarmingly high rate of infection in hospitals due to drug resistant microbes. The editors warned that despite aggressive medical treatment a minimum of 130,000 individuals die every year from infections caused by antibiotic resistant organisms. Howard S. Gold wrote in the *New England Journal of Medicine* (1996) that there is little hope that the pharmaceutical firms can keep pace with the raging mutants. Yet, there is an even more ominous statistic. According to an article in the *Journal of the American Medical Association*, published in July, 1997, fully one half million Americans develop blood poisoning in hospitals every year. As many as 50% die. What a catastrophe this is and what a dreadful shame, since most of these infections are preventable.

The drug resistant microbes, which permeate hospitals and contaminate medical instruments, cause millions of cases of catastrophic illnesses every year. Tens of thousands of deaths result. Obviously, medicine has not only lost the war against microbes but has gone backwards. Bacteria, fungi, and parasites all have developed resistance to drugs.

Despite all of the technological advances of modern medicine degenerative disease remains the number one killer. The extent of these dilemma can be readily comprehended by simply entering a hospital or nursing home. These institutions are filled with individuals suffering from poor health, who are incapable of functioning in any respectable fashion. Many of these individuals are entirely dependent upon society. Some are so weak that if they were left to the elements, they couldn't survive. This is because degenerative disease, as well as infectious disease, has crippled them physically, mentally, and emotionally as well as financially.

Being chronically ill is the worst possible thing that can happen to an individual. Without good health the quality of life is dramatically diminished. Unfortunately, poor health is common in America; tens of millions of individuals are afflicted with severe degenerative illnesses, which compromise lifestyle as well as life span.

There are thousands of diseases which afflict the human race, many of which have been known since ancient times; many are relatively new. Whether new or ancient all diseases have a common root: disruption of the normal function of the cells and organs of the body. The existence of disease is evidence of the loss of the natural balance within the body. Thus, disease represents a sort of internal or cellular chaos.

Food can come to the rescue by helping the body restore balance. Some foods aggravate illness, and these must be rigorously avoided.

17

However, there are a great number of health enhancing foods, which should be incorporated into the diet on a regular basis.

The good news is that the healing processes of the body are enhanced by eating certain foods. The body needs the nutrients in food to heal itself. Plus, some foods contain natural chemicals, such as flavonoids, sulfones, indoles, organic acids, and antioxidants, which have special actions on certain organs and should be eaten frequently in case such organs are diseased.

There is one word of caution: food heals, if it is pure and free of harmful chemicals. Thus, the advice in this book refers to chemical-free and nutrient-dense foods. These are the foods which possess the greatest healing potential.

The following is a list of common diseases along with their supermarket cures. Now you will learn how to use food as medicine, right out of the grocery store.

Heart Disease

Heart disease represents a category of illnesses afflicting the heart muscle as well as the arteries and veins. This anatomical group is collectively known as the circulatory system. The circulatory system is responsible for delivering blood to every organ and cell of the body. Our health is utterly dependent upon its proper function, since blood is the carrier of nutrients, that is protein, fatty acids, vitamins, minerals, and oxygen, required for cellular survival. If circulation is compromised, so is nutrition, and, thus, our health may fail.

Modern medicine has attempted to cure heart disease, but the results have been dubious. The fact is heart disease remains the number one killer and is rising in incidence world-wide despite the use of high-tech and aggressive medical treatment. This means that common treatments, such as by-pass surgery, angioplasty, blood thinners, and potent drugs, have done little if anything to alter the course of this disease. This is because the medical profession often neglects to address the fact that heart disease is directly related to diet as well as alcohol consumption and cigarette smoking. Stress is also a significant factor. In other words, heart disease is caused primarily by the way we live, and diet is the number one factor.

18

Recently, alcoholic beverages have become in vogue as sort of a cure for heart disease. This philosophy has been promoted heavily by the industry as well as the medical establishment. Yet, there is not a shred of evidence proving curative effects. However, the idea is based upon the fact that in Europe, where much wine is drunk, there is a lower incidence of heart disease. Indeed, alcohol causes a variety of heart disorders, including coronary artery disease, atherosclerosis (hardening of the arteries), cardiac arrhythmia, and cardiomyopathy, the latter being described as degeneration of the heart muscle. Call it what you want, alcohol is not a health food.

Currently, doctors disseminate the wine prescription as if there is proven dietary need for it. It is as if doctors believe that heart disease is due to a deficiency of wine. This attitude is ludicrous, as there is no known "vitamin-like" function of alcohol for the heart or any other organ. In fact, alcoholic beverages destroy a wide range of vitamins, notably thiamine, riboflavin, niacin, pantothenic acid, pyridoxine, folic acid, cobalamin, vitamin K, vitamin E, and vitamin C. Ironically, heart disease is caused by a deficiency of these and other nutrients. For instance, minerals, particularly magnesium, potassium, manganese, copper, selenium, and zinc, are required for normal cardiac function. Alcohol, an aggressive diuretic, induces mineral loss, and virtually all alcoholics are severely deficient in trace minerals.

Think about it. The European diet is different than the standard American fare. However, the wine consumption isn't entirely novel; Americans drink it too. Certainly, the main issue is that the European diet is drastically different than ours. Europeans eat primarily fresh foods, and processed foods form only a minimal portion of the diet. For Europe's country folk the entire diet may consist of fresh foods; in other words, fast foods, candy bars, and soda pop are not commonly on the menu. Europeans eat for sustenance, and food represents a cultural experience. They take pride in creating healthy menus and are accustomed to taking the time to do so. Furthermore, the food is raised in an entirely different manner than the American method. Europeans use more natural methods of cultivating and minimize the use of synthetic fertilizers, pesticides, and herbicides. They also tend to eat food as fresh as possible, often directly after harvesting, whether from farm or garden.

Recently, researchers determined a fact that likely accounts for the decreased incidence in cardiovascular disease in Europe: the European diet is richer in vitamin E than is the American diet. Researchers have documented how high dietary intakes of vitamin E protect against heart disease, reducing heart attack risk by as much as 75%. That is a more logical reason for cardioprotection than alcohol. Ironically, vitamin E rich foods are fatty, such as eggs, liver, fatty fish, nuts, butter, and oils, and these are precisely the foods which Americans are told to avoid. Yet, Europeans continue to eat such foods in liberal quantities, without any apparent harm. It is obvious from the European experience that what an individual eats or drinks has a greater bearing upon the health of his/her heart than any other factor. Improper diet and nutritional deficiency is the number one cause of heart disease.

Lately, emphasis has been placed by researchers on the protective effects of antioxidants upon the cardiovascular system. After more than thirty years of intensive research scientists have essentially proven that a wide range of antioxidant vitamins and minerals, particularly vitamin C, beta carotene, vitamin E, folic acid, vitamin B_{12}, pyridoxine, manganese, magnesium, and selenium, block the development of cardiovascular disease. The research provides invincible proof that heart disease is directly related to diet and can be cured by altering the diet and by selectively consuming nutritional supplements. For instance, the Nurses Health Study published in *Circulation* showed a 50% reduction in heart attack risk for women just by taking vitamin E supplements for over two years. Other researchers have found that supplementing the diet with trace minerals decreases heart attack risks by over 100%. Similar results have been found as a result of the regular intake of vitamin C, pantothenic acid, thiamine, vitamin D, vitamin B_{12}, and beta carotene. An editorial in the *New England Journal of Medicine* published in 1995 suggests that a high intake of folic acid, pyridoxine, and vitamin B_{12} could decrease the heart attack incidence in men by as much as 300%.

Heart disease patients shouldn't be afraid to include fat in the diet. Fat is a necessary nutrient, and a reasonable amount must be included in the diet every day. The heart actually depends upon the inclusion of a certain amount of fat in the diet on a daily basis and will malfunction if that fat is unavailable. This is because the heart desires primarily fatty acids, preferring them over proteins and carbohydrates. According to Guyton's textbook of human physiology fat is the favorite cardiac fuel, and the heart always utilizes it aggressively, using glucose only as a last resort. Cardiac textbooks note that up to 90% of all fuel consumed by the heart comes from fat. However, be sure to eat only the natural unprocessed fats, while avoiding the synthetic ones. Simply put, eat the "good" fats, and avoid the "bad" fats. Good fats are those found in Nature which are not processed. Examples include butter, extra virgin olive oil, nut/seed oils, and coconut fat. Bad fats include hydrogenated or partially hydrogenated oils and refined liquid vegetable oils. The point is that heart disease patients don't have to live on the tasteless, disheartening low fat diet typically prescribed by cardiologists. Fat can be included safely in the diet. In fact, if it is too rigidly avoided, damage will be done.

There is another reason to eat fat: carnitine. This nutrient, which is found primarily in the juice of red meat, meat fat, skin of poultry, milk fat, avocado, and fatty fish, is described by amino acid expert Dr. Eric Braverman in *The Healing Nutrients Within* as a "heart tonic." Carnitine is a rather rare amino acid, because it is only found in a few foods, and the reason it is rare is because these foods are precisely the ones Americans are taught to avoid. *The Physician's Desk Reference* proclaims that carnitine is indicated for the treatment of heart disease and that a deficiency leads to, among other things, muscle failure, including degeneration of the heart muscle.

Carnitine is a critical nutrient needed for the function of the internal organs, particularly the liver, kidney, muscles, and heart. It's primary metabolic role is to transport fuel in the form of fat into the cells so it can be burned as energy. Some researchers find it of such value that they deem it a vitamin. The fact is carnitine must be a component in the diet for optimal health of the heart.

Top Twelve Supermarket Remedies

Top 12 Remedies	Curative Factors
almonds	magnesium, vitamin E, fatty acids
avocados	fatty acids for fuel, carnitine, vitamin E
beef	carnitine, fuel fats, B vitamins
broccoli	calcium, magnesium, beta carotene, vitamin C
filberts	vitamin E; potassium
garlic	thins blood; provides sulfur and selenium

Top 12 Remedies	Curative Factors
olives and olive oil	improves HDL cholesterol; provides fuel
onions	thins the blood; vitamin C
grape (sour grape)	strengthens arteries/heart muscle
rice bran	normalizes cholesterol; B vitamins
sardines	fish oils, carnitine, calcium
vinegar	potassium, flavonoids, acetic acid

Cancer

This is unquestionably the dread of humanity. Despite all efforts in attempting to curb this epidemic and untold billions of dollars spent, cancer has become virtually the number one cause of death in America. A horrifying disease, it literally consumes the individual, organ by organ and cell by cell.

Cancer is largely preventable. Furthermore, certain natural substances have been shown to be useful in cancer treatment. Yet, the key is to prevent cancer from striking, because it is often difficult to cure once it is established.

Certain foods fight cancer, if they are consumed regularly. Cruciferous vegetables are one of the most highly touted cancer preventives. According to research performed in major medical centers throughout the world the cruciferous vegetables, a category which includes broccoli, cabbage, Brussels sprouts, kale, kohlrabi, watercress, and cauliflower, contain a variety of cancer fighting chemicals. One of these chemicals, *sulforaphane*, activates the body's anti-cancer defenses by accelerating the synthesis of cancer-fighting enzymes. Cruciferous vegetables are also rich in *indoles*, which may exert direct toxicity against cancer cells. They are also high in anti-cancer nutrients such as vitamin C, beta carotene, riboflavin, folic acid, and selenium.

Vegetables of the lily family (or garlic family), notably garlic, leeks, shallots, and onions, boost cancer defenses through a variety of mechanisms. They improve circulation, thus improving the rate of oxygen delivery to the cells. Cancer develops readily when cellular levels of oxygen decline. The fact is oxygen is a poison to cancer cells.

The garlic family also helps promote the synthesis of sulfated proteins in the body, such as enzymes and structural proteins, because these vegetables are incredibly rich in sulfur. Enzymes are needed to help digest cancerous cells. Other enzymes, notably *glutathione peroxidase* and *superoxide dismutase*, inactivate toxic chemicals before they can initiate cancerous changes. Glutathione is the cells' front line defender against toxic chemicals. High levels of glutathione are an insurance against genetic damage from poisons such as heavy metals, pesticides, herbicides, chlorinated hydrocarbons, and nuclear irradiation. The regular consumption of sulfur-bearing vegetables, particularly garlic, onions, leeks, shallots, broccoli, cauliflower, celery, turnips, and watercress, increases glutathione levels.

Sulfur bearing vegetables also bolster the body's defenses against toxic chemicals, largely by increasing the synthesis of glutathione peroxidase. Synthetic chemicals and pollutants are a primary cause of cancer, and, thus, it is crucial to include anti-cancer vegetables regularly in the diet. In particular, garlic possess tremendous powers for inactivating cancer causing chemicals. Dozens of studies prove that it blocks the cancer promoting action of potent carcinogens such as aflatoxin, nitrosamines, pesticides, and chlorinated hydrocarbons. In some of these studies the administration of garlic was found to halt the growth of chemically induced cancers.

Garlic's blood thinning action accounts for another anti-cancer effect. Thick blood aids cancer spread. By thinning the blood garlic impedes the ability of cancer cells to spread throughout the body.

Currently, it is in vogue to follow a vegetarian style diet in the event of cancer. However, this type of diet is often nutritionally insufficient. The problem is that cancer patients need protein, especially sulfur-bearing proteins, to maintain optimal health, and vegetarian diets are notoriously low in protein. Furthermore, cancer patients often suffer from impaired digestion. Vegetable proteins, such as the type found in grains, beans, and soy, are among the most difficult of all types of protein to digest and absorb. For instance, the absorption of protein from milk may be as high as 80%. With eggs, protein absorption may be as high as 90%, while the absorption of protein from soy or wheat may be as low as 20%. Furthermore, milk and eggs are exceptionally rich in sulfur-bearing proteins, whereas the standard vegetable protein sources such as soy, corn, wheat, barley, rye, and beans, are relatively low. Protein is needed to build healthy cells and, therefore, to maintain the health of the anti-cancer defenses. For instance, the white blood cells, the number one anti-cancer defense, are made primarily from protein. For cancer patients this underscores the value of eating protein rich foods on a regular basis such as whole milk, eggs, yogurt, almonds, and organic meats.

Cancer patients must consume foods rich in complete protein, that is foods which contain the eight essential amino acids, if they are to achieve optimal protection against the disease. All eight amino acids must be available in the blood before the reconstruction of critical immune cells, such as white blood cells, liver cells, and lymph cells, can occur. In fact, these eight essential amino acids are the limiting factor for the synthesis of all immune cells. In other words, cellular protein synthesis, in fact, the very synthesis of the cells themselves, halts in the event of a deficiency of one or more of the essential amino acids. Furthermore, protein forms the building blocks for structural components of all cells, which give inner strength to all cells and organs. Structural proteins strengthen the body's defenses against cancer and help impede the spread of the disease. These facts alone raise serious concerns regarding the safety of a strict vegetarian diet. Only foods of animal origin, such as milk, cheese, yogurt, eggs, meat, poultry, seafood, and fish, contain all eight amino acids. If the individual stringently avoids such foods, the development of an imbalance in amino acids is virtually guaranteed. The result will be lowered energy, impaired mental function, and decreased resistance against disease. In other words, if you have cancer, don't attempt to live on fruits, grains, and vegetables alone.

A strict low fat diet is also an erroneous approach to cancer treatment. This is because such a diet leads to a deficiency of fat soluble vitamins, all of which are crucial anti-cancer substances. These vitamins, particularly vitamins A, D, E, and beta carotene, have been proven to block the DNA damage that precedes the development of cancer. True, it is important to eliminate the noxious fats, such as margarine and refined vegetable oils, from the diet. However, there is no proof that natural fats, such as those found in, for instance, an egg, olive, almond, avocado, milk, or even a steak, cause cancer. If beef or milk fat are a cause of cancer, the Masai, an African tribe which subsists almost exclusively on cow products, would be riddled with tumors, but the fact is there is no cancer in this tribe. The Eskimos, while consuming vast amounts of fat, were cancer free until they adopted a Western diet.

24

The low fat diet is dangerous, because it is deficient in the fat soluble vitamins. Vitamin A is a well known anti-cancer substance, and it occurs naturally only in a few foods, notably fresh meats, organ meats, fatty fish, crab, and butter. All of these foods are eliminated on the low fat diet. Vitamin D is a potent cancer blocker, which has been shown to be instrumental in the prevention of cancers of the bowel, breasts, and prostate. The most recent research, described by Dr. Michael Holick, professor of dermatology at Boston University Medical School in the February 1st, 1996, edition of *Family Practice News*, indicates that vitamin D may even prevent melanoma. There is no vitamin D in vegetation, not even a molecule. It is only found in animal foods, such as liver, fish liver oil, salmon, the skin of poultry, fresh meat, herring, sardines, whole fat milk products, and butter, all of which are removed with great precision in a low fat diet. Vitamin E is found in vegetation, but it is found in the greatest amounts in vegetation with a high fat content such as avocados, peanuts, almonds, filberts, and soy beans. Most of these foods are eliminated on a low fat diet. Furthermore, the absorption of fat soluble vitamins, such as vitamin E and vitamin A, is dependent upon the consumption of fat, since fat provokes the synthesis of bile and fat-splitting pancreatic enzymes. Thus, a low fat diet usurps the body's needs for fat soluble vitamins both by reducing the total dietary intake and impeding absorption.

The body cannot absorb fat soluble vitamins from food without the secretion of bile and pancreatic enzymes, both of which are elaborated as a result of a fatty bolus. The fact is the secretion of bile and pancreatic lipase is stingy in the event of a low fat meal. This is because the body perceives no need to secrete fat digesting chemicals unless it receives a message of need, that message being when the individual consumes sufficient amounts of fat. The message fails to be sent when taking a vitamin A, D, and/or E supplement alone, because there is not enough fat in the pill to provoke bile flow.

Certain vitamins are highly active against cancer. These vitamins include riboflavin, niacin, folic acid, beta carotene, vitamin A, and vitamin D. Minerals which possess the greatest anti-cancer effects include selenium, magnesium, calcium, manganese, and zinc. Beta carotene and vitamin A are notable, because only the dietary forms, not the synthetic, have been shown to be effective against cancer. Recent evidence indicates that synthetic vitamin A may cause side effects, which could be due to its interfering with the utilization or absorption of natural vitamin A. Obviously, the point is to receive vitamin A from food and natural-source nutritional supplements such as cod liver oil and/or halibut liver oil.

Cancer must be understood, but it must not be feared. The body can heal cancer. For decades it has been known that cancer can be reversed even without medical therapy. This is known as spontaneous remission. Autopsies reveal that many undiagnosed cancers were halted exclusively by the body's immune system. It is common for an individual to die from diseases other than cancer, but when autopsies are performed pathologists often see evidence of cancer. However, when pathologists explore the tumor site, they often discover that all that is left is a cavity filled with scar tissue and dead cancer cells. The point is cancer can be defeated.

Top Twelve Supermarket Remedies

Top 12 Remedies	Curative Factors
almonds	anti-cancer cyanogenetic glycosides; vitamin E
broccoli	anti-cancer chemicals such as indoles
cabbage and sauerkraut	anti-cancer chemicals
garlic	kills parasites/cancer cells and enhances immunity
horseradish	kills cancer cells
papaya	anti-cancer enzymes
cumin	anti-cancer chemicals (cuminaldehyde; limonene),
sweet potatoes	beta carotene; vitamin E
tomatoes	lycopene; beta carotene
turnips	anti-cancer chemicals
rosemary	anti-cancer chemicals and antioxidants
yogurt	healthy bacteria are anti-cancer; protein, vitamin D

Diabetes

This disease has reached epidemic proportions, afflicting tens of millions of Americans. It is exclusively a dietary induced disease. The dietary connection is easy to comprehend. The fact is diabetes is caused primarily by the excessive consumption of sugar, that is refined sugar. The name "sugar diabetes" certainly implies that fact. Innumerable researchers, including the scholarly Professor Yudkin of London, England, have thoroughly documented the connection between increased carbohydrate consumption and increased incidence of diabetes. Such research clearly shows that as a society's consumption of refined carbohydrates rises so increases the occurrence of diabetes, and this is a parallel rise.

While usually considered a disease of the pancreas only, diabetes is a disease of all digestive organs. It is also a disease of the hormonal system. In other words, diabetics suffer from dysfunction of virtually all major organ systems. In diabetes the body is unable to digest, process, assimilate, and metabolize sugar. Organs which are primarily afflicted include the pancreas, liver, intestinal tract, cardiovascular system, adrenal glands, and thyroid gland.

Since diabetes is a systemic disease, treatment with insulin alone fails to curtail the aberrant physiology. The fact is diabetes is caused largely by nutritional deficiency, and, thus, nutritional support through correct diet, vitamins, minerals, enzymes, essential fatty acids, and amino acids, offers the greatest potential for cure. The nutrients most commonly deficient in diabetics include chromium, magnesium, manganese, potassium, copper, zinc, vitamin A, vitamin D, vitamin E, vitamin C, essential fatty acids, and all of the B vitamins. Carnitine, an amino acid, is also lacking. This amino acid is invaluable for aiding fat metabolism and for preventing ketosis, a metabolic condition which plagues diabetics.

One of the cardinal features of this disease is disrupted metabolism of carbohydrates and fuel in general. However, the greatest disruption occurs in the metabolism of sugar, particularly refined types such as white sugar and corn syrup. Furthermore, diabetics are unable to properly metabolize even natural unrefined sugars such as pure honey, maple syrup, and molasses. Even fruit, with its naturally high sugar content, poses a problem.

While sugar intolerance in diabetics is well known, few people realize that fats and proteins are actually well tolerated by diabetics and serve as a superior source of fuel calories. In general, the ideal diabetic diet would constitute strict avoidance of sugar and starch with heavy reliance upon fat and protein. The dietary approach found in *How to Eat Right and Live Longer* (formerly *Eat Right to Live Long*) the newest edition of my primary book, is perfect for diabetics.

It seems incredible that the majority of individuals are unaware that disease is largely the result of dietary practices. Diabetics are certainly aware that if they fail to adhere to a rather strict diet, they become ill and often place their lives at risk. Diabetes was one of the first diseases in modern times which was treated exclusively with diet, and it is the ideal example of a diet-induced disease. The fact is diabetes only occurs in civilizations wherein there is massive consumption of refined sugar. The disease was unheard of in native Eskimos, whose diet was entirely sugar free. It is non-existent in the Masai tribesmen, who subsist primarily on a diet of milk, butter, and meat. The people of various Mediterranean islands, including Crete, Sicily, and Sardinia, whose diets are rich in fat from foods such as olives, olive oil, cheese, milk, and meat, are free of diabetes. The mountain dwellers of Switzerland are entirely free of heart disease and diabetes despite eating a diet that is heavy in fat. Yet, when individuals from these civilizations migrate to Westernized countries and adopt the typical diet, they eventually succumb to diabetes/heart disease at the same rate as do Westerners. Sugar consumption is the major dietary change; the total intake of fat is little different.

Diabetics are highly vulnerable to developing a wide range of illnesses, including chronic infections (particularly fungal infections), heart disease, hardening of the arteries, high blood pressure, kidney failure, osteoporosis, skin diseases, ulcerations, and cataracts. This is a further indication of the existence of wholesale nutritional deficiencies in diabetics. It is also an indication of the toxicity of sugar, which disrupts all of their bodily functions.

Diabetics must change their diets drastically if significant improvement is to occur. The diet must be sugar-free. Furthermore, complex carbohydrates, such as cereals, breads, pasta, potatoes, and beans, should be restricted. This is readily accomplished by adhering to the diet in *How to Eat Right and Live Longer*.

Top Twelve Supermarket Remedies

Top 12 Remedies	Curative Factors
artichokes	contain inulin, a natural type of insulin
avocados	carbohydrate-free fuel; carnitine
beef	carnitine, B vitamins, protein
broccoli	magnesium, calcium, folic acid, riboflavin
cilantro	potassium; magnesium
cumin	enhances liver/pancreatic function
eggs	lecithin, vitamin E, vitamin D
garlic	improves circulation; insulin-like action
oregano	potent anti-fungal, chlorophyll, minerals
rice bran	provides natural B vitamins (use Nutri-Sense)
salmon	fish oils improve the effectiveness of insulin
sardines	fish oils; RNA/DNA

Arthritis

Arthritis is one of the most feared of all diseases. This is because it not only causes severe pain, but it can also cripple and disfigure the individual.

Any condition in which the bones or joints become inflamed, sore, or swollen may be deemed arthritis, since this term is defined as "inflammation and/or pain" in the joints. There are numerous types of arthritis, and each has different symptoms and causes. However, in all cases there is a common thread; pain and inflammation.

Infection is a major cause of joint inflammation. Researchers have determined that infection may be the primary cause in both osteoarthritis and rheumatoid arthritis. Causative organisms include parasites and fungi as well as bacteria such as Salmonella, Klebsiella, Proteus, strep, staph, and numerous others.

Nutritional deficiencies are widespread in arthritics. They are routinely deficient in B vitamins and usually have a severe deficiency of vitamin C, vitamin A, vitamin D, vitamin K, and bioflavonoids. Mineral deficiencies are also exceedingly common, the primary ones being magnesium, manganese, potassium, copper, zinc, silicon, boron, and calcium.

Few people realize that diet plays a major role in the cause of arthritis. The fact is food can either cause or cure arthritis. Foods which cause or aggravate arthritis do so through the phenomenon known as food allergy. Dairy products, grains, citrus fruit, and legumes are among the most common provocative foods. The allergic reaction is far from obvious— don't expect to see a rash, wheezing, or some other acute symptom. Rather, food allergy reactions afflict arthritics in a more insidious fashion. The suspect food causes a toxic reaction in the body and, more specifically, in the joints, and this results in pain and inflammation. In other words, there are chemicals in the food, whether natural or synthetic, which may poison the joints. On the other hand, certain foods contain substances which block inflammation. Furthermore, foods may contain chemicals which act as pain killers. For instance, almonds contain an aspirin-like compound. Amazingly, a large handful of almonds contains greater pain killing potency than an aspirin pill.

Arthritics are often placed on low fat, low salt diets, but this is an erroneous approach. Low fat diets induce a deficiency of fat soluble vitamins, which are critical for maintaining the health of the joints. Furthermore, salt is needed to boost the function of the adrenal cortex, which is of tantamount importance in the prevention of arthritis. The adrenal glands produce steroid hormones, which block inflammation and swelling in the joints, a common consequence of allergic reactions. Thus, proper adrenal function is required to prevent allergy-induced joint damage.

Because food allergies are a major factor in the cause of arthritis, it is important to diagnose precisely which foods are involved. Allergies may be determined through blood testing. However, the majority of food allergy tests, particularly ELISA, RAST, and scratch tests, are inaccurate and incomplete. Often, the results are confusing if not misleading. A specialized test known as the *Food Intolerance Test* performed by Biotrition Laboratory yields predictable, accurate results. This has been the most valuable of all methods I have used for discovering an individual's food allergies. Certainly, my health improved dramatically after discovering my own food allergies with this test. For instance, I was deathly allergic to wheat, rye, cheddar cheese, asparagus, raspberries, and even bananas. Wheat made me feel tired, and bananas gave me headaches. My co-author's allergies include barley, cocoa, cashews, peaches, eggs, beans, lemons, limes, and spearmint. Every individual has his/her own unique pattern. For more information contact Biotrition at (847) 640-1377.

Top Twelve Supermarket Remedies

Top 12 Remedies	Curative Factors
almonds	natural pain killers; magnesium
cilantro	natural pain killers; potassium
horseradish	potent antiinflammatory enzymes
kiwi	antiinflammatory enzymes; vitamin C
oregano oil	antiinflammatory; anti-pain
papaya	rich in enzymes; improves digestion/fights inflammation
parsley	magnesium, calcium, folic acid
grape/sour grape	bioflavonoids (resveratrol/Pycnogenol)
salmon	fish oils reduce inflammation
salt	boosts adrenal function
sardines	fish oils reduce inflammation
watercress	sulfur, folic acid, vitamin C

Alzheimer's Disease

One hundred years ago this disease was virtually unknown. Currently, it is the fourth leading cause of death in America. Alzheimer's disease is manifested by progressive degeneration of the brain and nervous system, and the primary affliction is loss of the thinking ability of the brain. In other words, victims of this disease are no longer able to use their mental capacities for normal living. Everyday tasks become impossible, and the individual essentially becomes a living mental cripple, requiring help for such mundane tasks as using the rest room, dressing, and eating.

Alzheimer's disease may be difficult to diagnose in its early stages and may be confused with rather benign mental disorders. The early signs include memory loss, decreased productivity, difficulty performing simple tasks, speech impediment, disorientation, confusion, irritability, agitation, mood swings, personality changes, and apathy. If several of

31

these symptoms exist, Alzheimer's disease should be suspected. However, all of these symptoms are also warning signs of nutritional deficiencies, particularly deficiencies of vitamin B_2, B_5, B_6, folic acid, B_{12}, magnesium, and vitamin E.

Like all other degenerative diseases Alzheimer's disease is directly related to erroneous diet. It is a neglected fact that the brain is an organ and, like any other organ, it requires good nutrition. The fact is the brain has massive demands for nutrients, and, if the needed substances are not supplied, dysfunction or, ultimately, degeneration is likely to occur. Nutrients required for optimal brain function include thiamine, riboflavin, niacin, folic acid, vitamin B_{12}, choline, inositol, biotin, pantothenic acid, pyridoxine, vitamin C, magnesium, calcium, potassium, manganese, cobalt, selenium, amino acids, vitamin E, beta carotene, glucose, and essential fatty acids. Can you think of a major nutrient that has not been named? The brain needs a steady supply of virtually every major nutrient. Diets deficient in any of these nutrients will lead to mental symptoms and, ultimately, mental diseases.

The excessive consumption of refined sugar is the most common dietary intolerance in Alzheimer's patients. Usually, these individuals are extreme sugar addicts and have a history of "always eating their desserts." Sugar destroys B vitamins and depletes minerals. Thus, it induces a deficiency of nutrients which are critical for the brain.

In Alzheimer's disease the brain is damaged through a process known as oxidation. Sugar accelerates the oxidation of brain tissue. In other words, it prematurely ages the brain. How this occurs was first discovered in the 1970s by Dr. Anthony Cerami, a researcher at Rockefeller University in New York. Dr. Cerami found that when excessive amounts of sugar are consumed protein molecules, which are found in all cells, including brain cells, are suddenly damaged. The sugar, in a sense, corrodes the protein, altering it from its normally flexible nature to a stiff, sticky substance. Obviously, as a result of the sugar-induced damage, the biological function of these proteins is severely disrupted. In other words, sugar damages the structure and function of cellular proteins irreparably. The greatest amount of damage occurs when the blood sugar level rises suddenly and massively, as would occur from eating rich sweets such as cakes, pies, sweet rolls, and candy. The researchers also found that even natural sugar, such as that found in orange or apple juice, damaged protein. For Alzheimer's disease the solution is a reduced sugar diet, a plan for which is found in *How to Eat Right and Live Longer.*

Top Twelve Supermarket Remedies

Top 12 Remedies	Curative Factors
almonds	vitamin E, calcium, magnesium
artichokes	insulin-like action; trace minerals
beef	amino acids, carnitine, B vitamins
broccoli	folic acid; vitamin C
cilantro	potassium; magnesium
cumin	phospholipids; antioxidants
eggs	choline, B vitamins amino acids
rice bran	B vitamins, gamma oryzanol, magnesium
rosemary	potent fat-soluble antioxidants
sardines	RNA/DNA; vitamin A
vinegar	acetic acid; potassium
yogurt	amino acids; B vitamins

Attention Deficit Disorder

ADD, or whatever label is currently being applied to this insidious syndrome, is an unnecessary disease. That is because it is 100% due to erroneous diet.

Children are fed perhaps the worst diets upon the planet. These unassuming individuals have no clue how badly they are being poisoned by the plethora of junk and processed foods they consume. They eat every manner of chemically infested and nutritionally depleted food known to the human race. Their taste buds are contaminated with massive amounts of refined sugar, flour, and rice products. Children eat their weight in a year or so in various food additives, their bodies living or, perhaps, more correctly, dying, in a chemical soup of food dyes, MSG, artificial flavors, caffeine, BHT, BHA, propylene glycol (antifreeze), sulfites, and artificial sweeteners. Tens of thousands of synthetic chemicals are "legally" added to the foods and beverages. No wonder childrens' nervous systems are misfiring. No wonder that as many as one third of all children in grade school are taking Ritalin. No wonder millions of youngsters are taking mood altering drugs such as Prozac and Xanax. It is no surprise that they are plagued with an assortment of serious illnesses, including blood sugar disturbances, asthma, arthritis, viral syndromes, intestinal disorders, skin infections, and high cholesterol.

Attention deficit disorder is a rather ludicrous term. The disorder should be called *Food Poisoning of the Mind Syndrome*. Processed, chemically-infested foods fail to nourish the brain and can only exert negative effects. In other words, the only reason that the child is unable to maintain a studious or attentive posture is that his/her brain is receiving the wrong chemicals, substances which negatively affect the child's mental function and behavior. Instead of brain-building fat soluble vitamins and fatty acids, the child's brain is poisoned by deep fried oils or margarine, which destroy the fat soluble vitamins. Instead of B vitamins for natural mental energy, the brain is contaminated with refined sugar, which depletes B vitamins directly from the brain. Instead of receiving from the diet mood controlling and intellect boosting amino acids, the brain is polluted by MSG, sulfites, food dyes, artificial flavors, and preservatives, which disrupt the function of the neurons. For instance, B vitamins nourish nerve cells, while MSG and food dyes destroy B vitamins as well as nerve cells. Obviously, the bodies and brains of our children are bombarded with massive amounts of chemicals just from the food additives and pesticide residues alone. Does it make sense, then, to further contaminate the brain with potent medicines? In fact, the only sensible approach is to radically change the child's diet and to supply as many brain-nourishing nutrients as possible. This should be the sole approach for eradicating attention deficit disorder.

Children with attention deficit disorder suffer from a wide range of vitamin and mineral deficiencies. Routinely, they lack vitamins A, D, E, and K, virtually all of the B vitamins as well as vitamin C. The fact is a deficiency of fat soluble vitamins, particularly vitamins A and D, is largely responsible for attention deficit disorder. Deficiencies of calcium, magnesium, potassium, selenium, zinc, and manganese also play a major role.

Essential fatty acid deficiency plays perhaps the most critical role in causing attention deficit disorder. The essential fatty acids are required for normal brain development, and the growing brains of children are especially in need of these critical nutrients. The deficiency is caused by

34

eating processed food, which is not only devoid of these fatty acids but also contains substances which interfere with their metabolism. American children who adhere to the modern diet, especially the low fat diet, suffer from some degree of the deficiency. Rich dietary sources of essential fatty acids include nuts, seeds, wild game, soybeans, rice germ, seed oils, avocados, and flax. Obviously, these foods are rarely on childrens' menus today.

Top Twelve Supermarket Remedies

Top 12 Remedies	Curative Factors
almonds	magnesium; vitamin E
avocados	fuel calories, blood sugar control, fatty acids
beef	fuel calories, B vitamins, amino acids
cantaloupe	folic acid, potassium, pyridoxine
peanuts	fuel calories, B vitamins, potassium
broccoli	B vitamins, vitamin K, minerals
filberts	fuel calories, calcium, vitamin E
rice bran	B vitamins, vitamin E, essential fatty acids, and minerals (use Nutri-Sense)
salmon	vitamin D and E; fish oils for the brain
sweet potato/squash	vitamin A; minerals
watercress	vitamin C; calcium
yogurt	calcium, amino acids, vitamin D

Asthma

It seems that medicine has been unable to discern just what causes this disease. Yet, the cause of asthma is not so elusive. The fact is diet plays a greater role in causing this illness than any other factor.

There is no need to search for some esoteric cause of asthma. All the further that usually needs to be investigated is what is on the dinner table, that is what is the daily menu, and this is especially true for children.

There is no doubt that environmental pollutants play a major role in causing lung diseases, including asthma. Yet, the greatest pollution is the result of eating poisonous foods. The fact is the number one cause of asthma attacks in the United States is a chemical found in commercial food: yellow dye #5. Also known as *tartrazine*, this dye is found in hundreds of processed foods, notably pickles, pickle relish, canned fruit, cheese, pudding, cake, cookies, cereals, candy, ice cream, gelatin, wine coolers, soft drinks, drugs, and multiple vitamins. Refined vegetable oils are another major cause. This is because refined vegetable oils promote inflammation within the lung tissues. This was recently delineated by an article published in Australia; researchers from Sidney's Institute of Respiratory Medicine determined that various commercial vegetable oils "increased the prevalence of childhood asthma." When studying various societies the researchers found that as the consumption of commercial vegetable oil rises so does the incidence of asthma increase. Furthermore, they determined that in societies where butter or olive oil are the primary dietary oils, the incidence of asthma is low. What this means is that saturated and monounsaturated fats protect against asthma, while polyunsaturates aggravate it and may even cause the disease.

Food itself may provoke asthmatic attacks, even normal healthy food. This occurs through the phenomenon known as food allergy. Foods most likely to induce asthma include citrus fruit, beans, peanuts, wheat, rye, malt, pork, seafood, eggs, tea, and cow's milk.

Asthmatics are commonly deficient in a wide range of nutrients. In particular, they require significant amounts of vitamin C, B vitamins (especially riboflavin, folic acid, vitamin B 12, and pantothenic acid), vitamin E, vitamin D, and vitamin A. Mineral deficiency is also common. Minerals which have been shown in scientific studies to help reverse asthma include magnesium, calcium, and selenium.

Top Twelve Supermarket Remedies

Top 12 Remedies	Curative Factors
beef	amino acids; saturated fats
ginger	antiinflammatory compounds
grapes/sour grape	bioflavonoids; antiinflammatory compounds
horseradish	volatile oils; vitamin C
kiwi	antiinflammatory enzymes; vitamin C
olives and olive oil	monounsaturated fatty acids; vitamin E
oregano	volatile oils, calcium, chlorophyll

Top 12 Remedies	Curative Factors
rice bran	B vitamins, magnesium, chromium
rosemary	fights spasticity and secretions; antioxidants
salmon	antiinflammatory fish oils; pantothenic acid
salt	increases adrenal steroid synthesis; iodine
sweet potatoes	beta carotene; potassium

Candidiasis

This is an infection caused by a yeast known as *Candida albicans*. This parasite belongs to a category of microbes collectively know as fungi (plural of fungus). Candida albicans is ubiquitous, meaning it is found everywhere: in the soil, water, food, and in us. While it is not regarded as a normal inhabitant, Candida is commonly found in humans in the mouth, bowel, and vagina as well as on the skin. In the appropriate numbers they cause no harm. Their growth is checked by the presence of the naturally occurring healthy bacteria, that is the Lactobacilli. If the balance between the Lactobacilli and the yeasts is upset, the yeasts overgrow. Such an imbalance greatly upsets the chemistry of the body, ultimately leading to disease.

Candidiasis has become ultra common in today's world, largely as a result of the overuse of antibiotics. Antibiotics destroy inhibitory bacteria, giving the yeasts an opportunity to invade the tissues. Nuclear irradiation also increases the invasiveness of yeasts.

Fungal infections are readily transmitted between humans. These opportunists are known for their ability to aggressively invade the body, particularly in people who are debilitated. Individuals suffering from chronic illnesses, nursing home residents, the immunocompromised, individuals on multiple drugs, and hospitalized patients are the most vulnerable. In particular, individuals suffering from low white counts, known medically as *neutropenia*, are highly likely to develop internal fungal infections.

According to Hagan and Klotx there has been an immense increase in fungal infections in hospitalized patients. Dr. Hagan notes that many of these infections begin when patients' bodies are "seeded" with the fungus through contaminated medical instruments. He describes how some thirty patients were infected with an unusual fungus known as R. rubra, one that usually doesn't infect humans, via contaminated instruments used to examine the lungs (i.e. bronchoscopes). This means the infections were medically induced, which is technically known as nosocomial (hospital acquired) infections. The fungus obviously originated from a single patient's lung tissue and was directly implanted into dozens of non-infected individuals.

Obviously, if medical instruments are heavily contaminated, infections will spread in hospitals like wild fires. This happens in thousands of medical facilities every day. Individuals who have undergone invasive diagnostic procedures, whether in the lungs, stomach, prostate, heart, bladder, kidney, or colon, have a high likelihood of developing a fungal infection. This is especially true for those who have undergone multiple procedures. Aggressive strains of Candida are commonly seeded through contaminated medical instruments. Currently, hospital acquired fungal infections have superseded bacterial infections as a cause of complications, that is they are an utter epidemic.

Various factors predispose the individual to the development of fungal infection. They include high sugar intake, stress, antibiotics, chemotherapy, birth control pills, pregnancy, radiation exposure, and invasive medical procedures. The excessive use of antibiotics is perhaps the primary cause of Candida infection. However, other drugs, notably cortisone, aspirin, Indocin, Clinoril, Voltarin, Prozac, and Motrin, may depress the immune system to such a degree as to induce fungal infection.

If infection by Candida albicans becomes chronic, ill health will result. Dr. Iwata of Tokyo, Japan discovered decades ago that Candida albicans produces toxins which depress immune function. Iwata extracted the suspect chemical and appropriately coined it "Canditoxin." He determined that this toxin was so powerful that if it was injected into laboratory animals, it immediately caused disease. The fact is most of the injected animals died within 48 hours. As reported in *JAMA* in 1977 even local infections by Candida lead to depressed immunity. The researchers discovered that vaginal Candida infections induced systemic immune dysfunction. Interestingly, once the yeasts were killed, the entire immune system was liberated, and a complete cure was achieved. Oil of oregano is the top remedy for killing yeasts (see Oregano section).

The symptoms of chronic fungal infection are vague, and this may explain why the condition is so difficult to diagnose. Symptoms include indigestion, bloating, gas, diarrhea, constipation, irritable bladder, loss of bladder control, chronic kidney/bladder infections, urinary urgency, fatigue, muscular weakness, itching, dry skin, eczema, dermatitis, psoriasis, prostate problems, sinus problems, mouth sores, loss of libido, vaginal itching, cravings for sweets, chemical sensitivity, hives, irritable bowel, PMS, depression, mood swings, mental confusion, irritability, bizarre behavior, chronic pelvic or abdominal pain, and infertility. Patients with chronic candidiasis usually visit numerous doctors, perhaps over a period of years, often to no avail. A vague diagnosis may be suggested, such as chronic fatigue syndrome, fibromyalgia, or chemical sensitivity, but no deliberate treatment or cure is offered. Often, patients are told that their complaints are due to stress or mental aberrations, and, thus, mood altering drugs, such as Xanax or Prozac, are prescribed. Thus, the diagnosis is missed, and the patient remains ill or may even worsen in condition.

Candida can infect virtually any part of the body. Internally, it commonly infects the mucous membranes, including the membranes of the mouth, tongue, sinuses, lungs, esophagus, intestines, vagina, and urethra. The organism may also invade the surface tissues, particularly the skin folds, the skin surrounding the nails, the fingernails, the toenails, and the scalp. Candida albicans has a preference for moist regions, and, thus, the skin folds are common sites of infestation. So are the sinuses, bronchial tubes, and mouth. In infants, Candida albicans is the most common cause of diaper rash and may also cause cradle cap.

If infection by Candida exists, it must be regarded seriously. Aggressive action must be taken to destroy the organism, hopefully without destroying the body. This illustrates the value of natural anti-fungal substances, which are harmless to human cells and organs but which are toxic against the yeast.

Top Twelve Supermarket Remedies

Top 12 Remedies	Curative Factors
avocado	antifungal fatty acids; sugar free food
basil	antifungal volatile oils
beef	sugar free food, selenium, amino acids
chicken/chicken soup	sugar free food; delivers garlic broth

Top 12 Remedies	Curative Factors
cumin	antifungal essential oils
garlic	natural antifungal agent
ginger root	antiseptic enzymes and oils
horseradish	antiseptic enzymes and oils
onion	antifungal and provides sulfur
oregano	potent antifungal activity due to its antimicrobial volatile oils
radishes	selenium, sulfur, antibiotics
yogurt	yeast-fighting Lactobacilli

Irritable Bowel Syndrome

This is yet another disease due to errant diet. Stress is a major cause, as is infection. The most common infective causes are intestinal parasites and yeast.

Irritable bowel syndrome is manifested by severe digestive distress affecting the entire digestive tract, although the colon bears the brunt of the damage. Colonic symptoms include cramps, spasticity, diarrhea, constipation, mucousy stools, hemorrhoids, and bloody stools. If untreated, irritable bowel may lead to more serious syndromes such as Crohn's disease and ulcerative colitis.

Diseases of the colon are readily treated by dietary manipulation. Of greatest import is the food allergy connection. Food allergies are the prominent cause of irritable bowel syndrome. In other words, certain foods, even the additive-free all natural ones, are so toxic to the individual that they provoke digestive distress and colonic attacks. Breneman proved this in his book *Basics of Food Allergy*. He inserted extracts of suspect foods into the colons of irritable bowel patients and observed the reaction via fiberoptics, that is via a colonoscope. Invariably, when the food extract was placed upon the colon wall, an irritable bowel attack was induced, as represented by severe cramps, mucous formation, diarrhea, and spasticity.

As a result of this severe intestinal distress malabsorption of nutrients is widespread. Severe deficiencies of folic acid, thiamine, vitamin A, vitamin K, selenium, magnesium, and zinc are common. In particular, researchers document how the addition of folic acid leads to an improvement in symptoms. This is because folic acid is needed for the regeneration of the bowel lining. Foods rich in this vitamin include fresh red meat, eggs, and dark green leafy vegetables.

Irritable bowel syndrome is manifested by severe inflammation of the intestinal tract. This inflammation may be the result of toxic food reactions, food allergy, parasites, and/or infection. Thus, foods which fight inflammation, infestation, and infection are invaluable.

Pancreatic insufficiency is common in colonic disease, as is adrenal insufficiency. For a weak pancreas eat large quantities of enzyme rich foods such as papaya, kiwi, ginger, and horseradish. Adrenal weakness greatly increases the vulnerability for colitis attacks. Foods high in protein and natural fats, such as avocados, almonds, pine nuts, rice bran, salmon, and sardines, help strengthen adrenal function. Plus, these foods are rich in pantothenic acid, the key vitamin for enhancing adrenal function. Also, certain herbs/spices, particularly rosemary, cumin, sage, fennel, and oregano, strengthen adrenal function. The edible Oil of Rosemary from North American Herb & Spice is particularly valuable for regenerating those glands. Oil of fennel is also useful, because, in addition to boosting adrenal function, it combats spasticity, gas, and bloating. Salmon and sardines are high in fish oils, which reduce inflammation within the digestive tract.

Top Twelve Supermarket Remedies

Top 12 Remedies	Curative Factors
avocado	fuel fats; essential fats
artichoke	blood sugar regulation; folic acid
ginger	antiinflammatory compounds; enzymes
honey	antiseptic action; digestive aid
horseradish	antiinflammatory enzymes
kiwi	enzymes; vitamin C
papaya	enzymes; vitamin C; seeds are anti-parasitic
oregano	natural antibiotic; soothes digestive tract
rosemary	balances adrenal function; anti-spasmodic
salmon/sardines	fish oils, vitamin A, vitamin D
fennel	blocks spasticity; strengthens adrenal glands
wild rice	starch, fiber, B vitamins

Panic Attacks

Panic attacks are sort of the "in vogue" mental disease. Millions of North Americans suffer from them. Yet, it is inappropriate to classify panic attacks as a disease. Rather, they are merely symptoms.

Panic attacks occur as a result of the inability of the body to tolerate stress, whether physical, mental, or emotional. In other words, when an individual cannot physiologically tolerate a perceived or real stress, he/she has an attack. Thus, virtually any individual could suffer from such an attack. However, for an individual with the disorder, even everyday events or stresses may trigger an attack. These attacks are a sign of adrenal failure, that is the adrenal glands, the coping mechanism of the body, have lost their capacity to neutralize stress.

Diet is directly related to the genesis of this condition. Sugar consumption is the greatest player. Currently, in America the average consumption of refined sugar exceeds a whopping 150 pounds per person per year. High sugar consumption greatly stresses the adrenal glands, depleting their ability to synthesize anti-stress hormones. High sugar intake causes this damage, largely because it induces widespread nutritional deficiencies. Nutrients, such as pantothenic acid, vitamin C, magnesium, and potassium, all are needed by the adrenal glands for proper function; all are depleted by refined sugar. With prolonged consumption, the glands become so weakened that the body's ability to mount an anti-stress response becomes virtually impossible. Thus, relatively insignificant stresses may provoke a massive attack.

If the adrenal glands are strengthened, the panic attacks will be diminished and, ultimately, cured. Yet, refined sugar is only one of the culprits. Diets high in carbohydrates, even complex carbohydrates, increase the need for steroids, and this may lead to a depletion of the anti-stress hormones. This means that the typical low fat diet, rich in pasta, breads, beans, rice, and similar starches, may induce adrenal exhaustion. In order to rebuild the glands the diet must be exceptionally low in carbohydrates and rich in protein and fat. If you have panic attacks, it is advisable to avoid sugar-rich foods for at least two weeks. Follow a meat and vegetable diet. For snacks, eat salted nuts such as almonds, filberts, Brazil nuts, pecans, and pistachios; after about sixty days add starches to tolerance.

Top 12 Remedies	Curative Factors
almonds	calcium, magnesium, fatty acids
filberts	calcium, magnesium, fatty acids
beef	protein; fuel calories
chicken	protein; B vitamins
cumin	strengthens adrenals/pancreas
eggs	amino acids, B vitamins, choline
fennel seed/oil	strengthens adrenal glands; improves digestion
peanuts and peanut butter	protein; B vitamins
royal jelly	improves coping mechanism; B vitamins
salt	improves adrenal reserve
vinegar	potassium; acetic acid
yogurt	amino acids; B vitamins

Anemia

Anemia is defined as a reduction in the total amount of red blood cells in the body. It may also indicate the existence of abnormal types of red blood cells. While anemia is regarded as a disease of the blood, it is almost always related to disordered digestion as well as poor diet. In fact, according to *Taber's Medical Dictionary* anemia is not a disease but is merely a symptom of disease. It is a warning of internal dysfunction and/or malnutrition. The key to curing it is through discovering the exact cause.

There are dozens of types of anemias. Some types may be due to serious illnesses such as cancer, rheumatoid arthritis, lead poisoning, arsenic poisoning, severe trauma, and toxic chemical exposure. Others may be the result of heredity: for instance, sickle cell anemia and thalassemia. Digestive disorders may result in anemia, notably poor stomach acid secretion (known as hypochlorhydria and achlorhydria), liver disease (particularly hepatitis), ulcerative colitis, and malabsorption. Infectious diseases are yet another cause, and the most common culprits are intestinal parasites, particularly hookworms, flukes, and tapeworms. In women uterine bleeding due to a fibroid uterus is another major cause.

For the individual with anemia a careful evaluation by a physician is often required. Blood tests are helpful in delineating the cause. This is especially true when anemia occurs suddenly in the elderly. It is important to rule out the more serious illnesses such as cancer and lead poisoning. In other words, it is crucial to determine precisely what is causing the anemia. However, in the vast majority of cases the cause is nutritional, and the cure is accomplished through improved diet and nutritional supplementation. In other words, the red cells, which number in the tens of billions, are literally starving to death for lack of certain nutrients. Thus, the cure is to rebuild them nutritionally. Key nutrients needed to rebuild red blood cells include amino acids, essential fatty acids, phospholipids (for instance, lecithin), riboflavin, niacin, pyridoxine, folic acid, vitamin A, vitamin E, B_{12}, vitamin C, copper, iron, and zinc.

A high protein diet is mandatory. Obviously, red blood cells consist mainly of protein. Proudfit notes in *Normal and Therapeutic Nutrition* that protein should be derived from foods of the highest biological value, particularly milk, eggs, meat, and cheese; 100 to 200 grams daily is recommended. This means that an anti-anemic meal might include a 16 ounce steak, twelve ounces of liver, or a tub of cottage cheese instead of the typically skimpy protein portions of the "modern" diet.

Top Twelve Supermarket Remedies

Top 12 Remedies	Curative Factors
apricots	vitamin A; iron
beef	iron, folic acid, riboflavin, B_{12}, copper
beets	iron; betaine
cumin	trace minerals (iron); phospholipids
eggs	iron, folic acid, B_{12}, riboflavin, copper
filberts	vitamin E; phospholipids
rice bran	use Nutri-Sense; trace minerals, lecithin, niacin
spinach	iron, vitamin C, amino acids
oregano	iron; chlorophyll
watercress	contains blood building factors; vitamin C
wild rice	amino acids; minerals
yogurt	amino acids; B vitamins

Chronic Fatigue Syndrome and Fibromyalgia

These syndromes are more correctly described as symptoms of diseases rather than diseases themselves. In fact, both chronic fatigue syndrome and fibromyalgia were coined by the medical profession as a sort of garbage can diagnoses. For instance, there is no such thing as a syndrome of fatigue. Fatigue is merely a symptom, a warning that the function of the human body has gone awry.

The key to curing fatigue, as well as the chronic fatigue syndrome, is to determine the precise cause of the fatigue or associated symptoms. When the cause is treated appropriately, the condition is readily resolved.

What is chronic fatigue, anyway? It is merely a lack of energy in the body, organs, and cells. A lack of energy, whether physical or mental, can only be due to a deficiency, and the only substances which our bodies could be deficient in are nutrients. Alternatively, the body can be poisoned, and that will cause fatigue. Even so, poisoning causes fatigue by inducing nutritional deficiency.

The primary cause of chronic fatigue is adrenal insufficiency. The result of this condition is that the adrenal glands fail to produce sufficient quantities of critical steroid hormones. In the extreme adrenal insufficiency may lead to a potentially fatal condition known as *Addison's disease.*

Chronic fatigue is also a warning sign of yet another potentially dangerous condition: chronic infection. Adrenal insufficiency leaves the body vulnerable to the development of a wide range of infections. In other words, when the adrenal glands fail, the immune system becomes dysfunctional. Yeast and other fungal infections are particularly common. Parasitic infection may also take its toll, and individuals with the syndrome are readily infected by organisms such as Giardia, Cryptosporidium, flukes, tapeworm, and amebas. The problem is when the adrenally weakened individual is exposed to a noxious microbe, the microbe easily evades the immune defenses and gains a foothold in the body, leading to persistent infection. In other words, the organism readily finds a home in the individual with weak adrenal glands. These microbes sap the individual of all energy reserves. Obviously, the infective organism must be destroyed before the fatigue can be eliminated.

Chronic fatigue may also be caused by nutritional deficiencies.

45

Carnitine deficiency is common. This highly specialized amino acid is responsible for the delivery of fatty acids into cells so they can be utilized as fuel. A deficiency of carnitine results in a defect in energy metabolism, leading to fatigue, weak muscles, muscle soreness, and exhaustion.

Carnitine deficiency leads to exercise intolerance, plus, individuals with the deficiency recover poorly after exercise. Numerous scientific studies delineate how a deficiency of carnitine results in the extreme muscular/physical exhaustion typical of chronic fatigue. For instance, researchers in Japan, publishing in the *Clinical Infectious Diseases,* found that all of the chronic fatigue patients tested had a deficiency of carnitine in the blood. As the carnitine levels increased, the fatigue improved dramatically. Carnitine is found primarily in the juice and flesh of red meat, poultry, eggs, and whole milk products. Avocados are the only significant vegetable source, although peanut butter contains a fair amount. Because of the emphasis on consuming a low fat diet carnitine deficiency is epidemic, and the deficiency is particularly common in vegetarians.

Recently, researchers discovered a connection between salt and chronic fatigue. They routinely measured a deficiency of sodium and chloride in the blood of individuals suffering with the syndrome. When salt was administered the patients' symptoms, which included fatigue, muscular weakness, mental disturbances, lightheadedness, and low blood pressure, improved dramatically.

Low blood pressure was perhaps the most dramatic symptom in the chronic fatigue patients. This symptom is directly caused by a lack of sodium, since this is the major electrolyte in the body. Sodium and chloride are the key substances responsible for maintaining the correct volume of fluids in the bloodstream. According to research published in the *Journal of the American Medical Association* (1995) the low blood pressure in chronic fatigue patients has a simple cause: salt deficiency. Of the 19 patients evaluated all improved; half saw their symptoms virtually vanish as a result of the salt therapy.

This lack of sodium in chronic fatigue patients is merely a warning of the failure of adrenal glandular function. These glands conserve sodium, preventing its loss in the urine. When the glands are weak, and, therefore, their hormone output is compromised, sodium and chloride are dumped into the urine. Regardless of intake, the individual becomes deficient.

Ironically, the sodium deficiency in chronic fatigue patients becomes exceedingly critical, perhaps life-threatening, because the majority of the individuals are on a low salt diet. However, the correct approach is the unlimited use of salt. In fact, salty snacks are recommended between meals to boost salt levels and balance adrenal function. Healthy salty snacks include home made jerky (i.e. without the nitrates), almonds/pecans, salted roasted nuts, seaweed, pickles, olives, peanut butter, and whole grain crackers or chips free of hydrogenated oils.

Top Twelve Supermarket Remedies

Top 12 Remedies	Curative Factors
avocados	fatty acids; carnitine
beef	amino acids; carnitine
chicken	amino acids; B vitamins
cumin	phospholipids, antioxidants
garlic	antimicrobial; sulfur
grape/sour grape	flavonoids; tartaric acid
oregano	antimicrobial, calcium, magnesium
peanuts	amino acids; carnitine
salt	boosts adrenal function
salmon	pantothenic acid; amino acids
shrimp	amino acids; iodine
yogurt	amino acids, vitamin D, calcium

Fibromyalgia is another garbage can diagnosis, and the term really means very little. Technically, fibromyalgia means soreness of the muscles (*myalgia*) and other soft tissues (*fibro*, i.e. for "fibrous"). Physicians categorize individuals under this heading when they don't know what else to do.

Fibromyalgia is a curable disease, because the causes can be determined. Poor diet is the number one cause. In this respect, food allergy is the major culprit. Patients with fibromyalgia are commonly allergic to grains, legumes, citrus, yeast, MSG, sulfites, cocoa, and milk products. There may be other provocative foods, including nuts, fruit, vegetables, eggs, and meats. To determine precisely what are an individual's food allergies blood testing may be necessary. The Food Intolerance Test, performed by Biotrition of Rolling Meadows, Illinois is ideal for determining these allergies, because it is simple to perform, plus it is thorough, and it is more accurate than any other type of food allergy test available (ph: 847-640-1377). Test results are invaluable for individuals with both fibromyalgia and chronic fatigue as well as irritable bowel syndrome. For greater details on high grade food allergy testing see *How to Eat Right and Live Longer* (formerly *Eat Right to Live Long),* chapters 9 and 10. Other major causes include chemical toxicity, heavy metal poisoning, yeast infection, bowel toxicity, and parasitic infestation.

Top Twelve Supermarket Remedies

Top 12 Remedies	Curative Factors
almonds	magnesium; salicylates
beef	protein; fuel calories
broccoli	B vitamins, bioflavonoids, vitamin C
cantaloupe	potassium, folic acid, vitamin C
dill	magnesium; potassium
filberts	calcium; vitamin E
ginger root	antiinflammatory enzymes; natural antibiotics
grapes/sour grape	flavonoids, tartaric acid, malic acid
kiwi fruit	antiinflammatory enzymes; vitamin C
oregano	antiinflammatory essential oils; trace minerals
salmon	fish oils, vitamin E, vitamin D
watercress	volatile oils; vitamin C

Chapter Three
Supermarket Remedies

Almonds

The use of almonds as a natural medicine parallels the time of Abraham and even earlier. Mentioned in the Old Testament, the almond tree almost assuredly was first cultivated in North Africa and the Middle East, where it has been utilized for untold centuries as both food and medicine. Contrary to popular belief, the almond is a fruit rather than a nut.

Almonds are a nutritional treasure chest and are, in fact, one of the most nutrient dense foods known. They contain more calcium than any other "nut" and are one of the richest known sources of vitamin E. They are exceptionally rich in iron, folic acid, copper, magnesium, phosphorus, potassium, zinc, and riboflavin. This plethora of nutrients makes them so nourishing that you could virtually live for prolonged periods on almonds alone.

Almonds are one of the richest sources of protein of any food, containing a whopping 24 grams per 5 ounces. This means they are richer by weight in protein than meat or eggs. In fact, almonds are so dense in protein that an individual can achieve the minimal daily requirement just by snacking on a bunch of almonds. However, despite the immense supply of protein the primary constituent of almonds is fat in the form of almond oil. By weight, fat accounts for some 55% of the total, while the protein content is approximately 19%. The carbohydrate content is low at about 20%.

Because of the oil content, almonds are a tremendous source of cellular fuel. The oil, once digested and assimilated, readily enters human cells, where it is combusted into energy.

Almonds contain various types of fat, including saturated, monounsaturated, and polyunsaturated fatty acids. However, like all vegetable sources of fat, they are devoid of cholesterol. All of these fats are valuable nutritionally. The saturated fats are used primarily as fuel. The monounsaturates are useful fuel sources and are also beneficial because of their protective effects upon the circulatory system. They aid in normalizing blood cholesterol levels, plus they increase the levels of HDL cholesterol, the type necessary for preventing fat deposits within the bloodstream. In fact, studies have shown that simply eating a handful of almonds per day can lower abnormally high cholesterol levels by as much as 15%, the same degree of reduction expected from consuming olive oil.

The polyunsaturates in almond oil include the essential fatty acids, so named because they are essential to life itself. Without them the organs and cells of our bodies degenerate. There are two essential fatty acids: linoleic and linoleic acids. Almonds provide primarily the former.

Essential fatty acids are needed to maintain the health of every tissue in the body, and they are particularly required for the health of the hair, skin, and nails. It is no wonder that the warning signs of essential fatty acid deficiency include dry skin, acne, brittle nails/hair, slow growing nails, hair loss, enlarged facial pores, excessive sebum (oily skin), dryness or scaling behind the ears, excess ear wax production, dry eyes, scaly patches of skin, and dry mucous membranes. If the deficiency becomes extreme, a variety of skin disorders may result, including dermatitis, eczema, psoriasis, and acne. Ill effects of the deficiency upon the internal organs may be manifested as poor resistance to infection, recurrent skin infections, mental disturbances, PMS, joint pain, prostatitis, hormonal disorders, including thyroid, adrenal, and ovarian dysfunction, and, in children, delayed development (mental or physical). The hormonal system is particularly vulnerable to degeneration as a result of essential fatty acid deficiency, and the function of all glands progressively declines in the event of the deficiency. Thus, disorders of the thyroid, adrenal, ovarian, prostate, testicular, and pituitary glands may be directly related to essential fatty acid deficiency.

Almonds are also rich in fiber, containing a greater amount by weight than most vegetables. Much of the fiber is found in the brown outer coating, so blanched or slivered almonds contain less.

Eating almonds is tantamount to consuming a trace mineral supplement, since they contain vital amounts of minerals, particularly calcium, magnesium, potassium, phosphorus, and boron. Amazingly, a cup of almonds, which amounts to a double handful, contains as much as 1000 mg of potassium, 370 mg of magnesium, 7 mg of iron, and 4 mg of zinc. The calcium content is even more impressive; a large snack of almonds, about 5 ounces, contains some 50% of the RDA for this mineral.

Boron, a mineral which is found in significant amounts in almonds, has recently become of interest, largely because of its role in calcium metabolism. Apparently, dietary boron, a mineral known to few Americans, prevents calcium loss from the bones. Boron is found naturally in food and water, but only a few foods contain a dense supply of it. Almonds are one of the richest sources. Studies performed in North Dakota determined that women, particularly postmenopausal women, need boron to retain calcium and magnesium in the bones. The researchers found that adding this mineral to the diet led to a rise in estrogen synthesis. In fact, the estrogen levels doubled. Estrogen is regarded as crucial for preventing bone loss in women, and boron may be useful for naturally raising estrogen levels.

There are numerous less obscure trace minerals which are needed to prevent bone loss. They include manganese, copper, sulfur, and zinc. In fact, all of the known trace minerals help increase the strength and density of bones. Vitamins required for preventing bone loss include vitamins C, A, D, K, B_2, B_5, B_6, and folic acid. Vitamins B_2, B_5, and B_6 influence estrogen production by normalizing its metabolism in the liver. Thus, estrogen excess may be prevented by the regular intake of these vitamins.

Almonds contain a litany of vitamins. In fact, they are so rich that they may be regarded as a sort of natural vitamin supplement. The vitamin E content is most significant. A daily ration of almonds, the amount you might eat as a snack, serves as a tasty and convenient vitamin E supplement. This vitamin E content largely explains the positive benefits of almonds upon circulation. Numerous scientific studies have shown how vitamin E helps normalize blood cholesterol by boosting levels of HDL (good) cholesterol. The vitamin E content of almonds is so considerable that a double handful per day provides at least the minimum daily requirement.

Normally, nutritionists regard milk as a top source of riboflavin. However, one cup of almonds contains as much riboflavin as three cups of milk. Few people realize that almonds are extremely rich in folic acid, containing a greater amount of this vitamin than highly touted sources such as eggs, cauliflower, beans, broccoli, and turnip greens. Their immense supply of niacin rivals that contained in meat, the richest common source. Chicken, whole grains, spinach, and cheese are traditionally regarded as top sources of biotin, but almonds supercede them all. Both niacin and biotin are required for fat and carbohydrate metabolism. Perhaps this explains why almonds are so valuable for combating diseases due to sugar intolerance, including cardiac disease, hypoglycemia, diabetes, attention deficit disorder, and obesity.

Top Almond Tips

1.Whenever possible, buy almonds in the shell. Shells keep them fresh by diminishing exposure to oxygen, and, therefore, preventing the oil from oxidizing. They have a sweeter taste and are also more nourishing. Prolonged storage may cause almonds to become rancid. Rancid oils cause free radical damage, meaning that the oils are so toxic that they destroy the cells in the body.
2. Don't eat only raw almonds. Cooked almonds are also good for you. Furthermore, raw almonds contain several compounds which, if consumed in excess, may upset the body's chemistry. For instance, raw almonds contain goitrogens, which interfere with thyroid function. If you have a thyroid problem, eat roasted almonds. Almonds also contain a substance called protease inhibitor. This is an enzyme inhibitor, which is so powerful that it can stop the pancreas from producing protein-digesting enzymes.
   Cyanide is another compound in raw almonds, but it is usually found only in the bitter variety. Don't get too scared, since cyanide occurs in minute amounts. Millions of individuals have consumed bitter almonds over the centuries, with little or no harm done. In fact, epidemiological evidence points to the consumption of almonds, whether bitter or sweet, as dramatically decreasing the risk for cancer. This anti-cancer effect is likely a consequence of the direct toxicity of cyanide against cancer cells. Ancient civilizations ate bitter almonds as a cancer preventive, and today's researchers are aware that in societies where almonds are a regular part of the diet the populace remains relatively free of cancer. However, if almonds are bitter, do not eat large amounts of them. The rule

is that if an almond is so bitter that it offends the taste, don't eat it. If you have cancer, it will suffice to eat regular almonds on a daily basis. On the other hand, almonds which are only slightly bitter are harmless.

3. Make your own roasted almonds. Roast fresh raw almonds in a mixture of salt and heavy oil. The best oils for roasting are coconut, extra virgin olive oil, almond oil, hazelnut oil, and clarified butter. Heavy oils are more stable and less likely to turn rancid from heating. They are the safest types to use, and the roasting should be conducted at a low temperature, around 250 degrees for about one hour. Stir frequently.

4. Check your grocer for dry roasted almonds. Blue Diamond produces an excellent dry roasted almond product, containing only almonds and salt. If this brand is unavailable, ask your grocer to stock it. Or, dry roast your own. Soak the almonds in saltwater for a couple of hours or overnight if you prefer a salty taste, then allow them to dry. Roast at a low temperature (250 degrees); stir frequently. Do not overcook, since this will make them unpalatable and less nourishing.

5. Use almonds in cooking. Add slivered almonds to rice recipes and/or stir fry. Sprinkle slivered or sliced almonds over sweet potatoes, squash, and other vegetables. Use chopped almonds in fresh fruit cocktails.

6. When buying shelled almonds be sure to smell the almonds after opening. If they have an overpowering odor, they are probably rancid. Taste the almonds; if they are sweet, they are acceptable for consumption, but, if they taste bitter, stale, or sour, they may be rancid. Return them and try another brand.

7. Chew almonds well. They are extremely fibrous, and chewing helps liberate the nutrients so that they can be more readily assimilated. Digestion begins in the mouth, so to get the most out of any food, always chew thoroughly.

8. Almond milk is an invigorating and tasty beverage. Because almonds are high in fat and protein, they can be blended into a sort of milk substitute. It may be strained to remove the fibrous texture, but it is more nutritious to leave it unaltered. You can use almond milk in cooking; flavor it with high quality natural fruit flavorings or vanilla. Also, combine it with fruit, coconut milk, and/or a high grade of chocolate and make luscious smoothies. This is an especially valuable drink for those allergic to cow's and goat's milk, since almonds are exceptionally nutrient dense and are especially high in calcium.

Top Almond Cures

1. If you are constantly tired, almonds are an ideal snack. Their impressive concentration of vitamins, minerals, protein, and fat helps the body create immediate energy. To combat fatigue try eating a handful of almonds; most likely, you will notice an immediate energy boost, especially if they are salted.

2. If you have a family history of cancer or if you have contracted cancer, eat almonds every day. Consume at least one handful daily. Cancer patients should consume almonds raw. Raw almonds contain cyanogenetic glycosides and protease inhibitors, both of which have been found to combat cancer.

3. If you can't sleep at night, eat a handful of almonds before retiring. Almonds are one of Nature's richest sources of calcium and magnesium, both of which are sedatives. The protein in almonds helps stabilize blood sugar levels. This remedy works best if the almonds are salted. Salt strengthens adrenal function, and this aids in the regulation of blood sugar levels.

4. If you have poor circulation, eat almonds regularly as a snack, condiment, or combined with other food. Since they are exceptionally rich in vitamin E, calcium, and magnesium, almonds provide much needed nutrient power for assisting cardiac function. All of these nutrients strengthen the ability of the heart to pump blood. Magnesium and vitamin E exert direct actions upon the arteries. Magnesium increases blood flow by preventing arterial spasms and, thus, helps keep the arteries open. Spasms of the coronary arteries are a major cause of angina as well as heart attacks. Vitamin E also helps prevent arterial spasms by increasing the oxygen content of the blood. As an antioxidant it helps prevent hardening or degeneration of the arteries, a condition known medically as *atherosclerosis*. Thus, vitamin E helps keep the arteries youthful by sustaining them in their normal flexible state. Blood clots are another major cause of heart attacks. Vitamin E and magnesium help prevent the formation of clots within the arteries or veins.

5. If you have a headache, almonds might rid you of the pain. They contain salicyclic acid, which is essentially natural aspirin. A small handful of almonds contains as much pain killing power as a tablet of aspirin. There is a word of caution: some individuals are allergic to

salicylates, whether synthetic or natural, and, in this case, consuming almonds might aggravate the headache.

6. If you have a backache, almonds may be a superior choice versus pain killing drugs. This curative effect is largely due to their naturally occurring aspirin content but is also a result of the rich supply of calcium and magnesium. These minerals decrease spasticity of back muscles and also aid in building healthy bones and joints. With almond therapy, the pain should improve within one to two weeks after eating at least one half cup on a daily basis. As with all ailments if no improvement is evident, seek medical help.

7. If you cannot control your weight, almonds should be a regular part of the diet. By eating almonds, especially raw almonds, you will likely lose weight immediately. Almonds contain rich supplies of nutrients which help the body burn fat, including niacin, choline, inositol, biotin, thiamine, and magnesium.

8. Brittle or slow growing nails indicate the existence of nutritional deficiency and are primarily associated with deficiencies of minerals, essential fats, and protein. Since almonds contain all of these nutrients in rich quantities, they are the ideal "fingernail food." If the health of your nails is poor, eat almonds on a daily basis, at least 5 ounces per day.

Apricots

The apricot apparently originated in China, where the first recorded evidence is found in a Chinese manuscript dated prior to 2000 B.C. Alexander the Great brought apricot seeds from the Orient to the West; within decades the trees flourished throughout Greece and the fertile crescent. The current variety was developed by Arabic-speaking merchants during the Middle Ages, who spread it throughout the Western world. By the 17th century this versatile tree could be found growing in Europe virtually everywhere, even in the harsh climate of England.

Apricots are exceptionally rich in vitamin A (in the form of beta carotene), and are perhaps richer in this nutrient than any other fruit. They are also a top source of iron and contain a considerable amount of protein. Dried apricots are a nutrient dense snack, and a small handful provides well over the RDA for vitamin A and a good portion of the RDA for iron.

A large serving of dried apricots provides as much as one half the RDA for this mineral. Furthermore, they are the only fruit listed by Ensminger in her top 20 sources of vitamin A (i.e. as beta carotene). Dried apricots contain a whopping 14,000 I.U. per 100 grams, an amount which is easily consumed in one sitting.

Apricots received their fame as a health food primarily as a result of publicity about the Hunzas—that long lived remote society of the Himalayas. For centuries the Hunzas have eaten apricots, as well as apricot pits and oil, as a staple food. On average they live some 20 years longer than Americans. Furthermore, they are apparently entirely free of heart disease and cancer. Researchers believe that apricots, apricot pits, and apricot oil are largely responsible for the Hunzas' longevity. Perhaps the inordinately rich beta carotene content of apricots contributes towards the reduced risk of degenerative disease. Or, possibly some unknown chemical in apricots or apricot pits prolongs life and fights disease. Yet, there are other numerous factors: fresh mountain air, pure water, lack of stress, chemical free foods, etc. Thus, the Hunza lifestyle is entirely different than the one led by modern humans. Undoubtedly, diet is the major factor accounting for their longevity.

Apricots are easy to digest, and the nutrients within them are readily absorbed. Pediatricians often recommend apricots for infants with sensitive stomachs. They are an ideal fruit for individuals suffering from food allergies, since allergy to apricots is rare.

Top Apricot Tips

1. Don't buy apricots preserved with sulfites. Sulfites are oxidizing agents, which commonly cause allergic reactions. Essentially, sulfites are a type of food bleach. It is easy to tell which apricots are preserved with sulfites: they are bright yellowish-orange in color, possessing a brighter color of yellow than even the fresh fruit.

Why this chemical is added to food is difficult to comprehend, since dried fruit has an indefinite shelf life. Sulfites do brighten the color of dried or preserved foods, so perhaps it is a cosmetic addition. Unfortunately, sulfites diminish the health value of dried fruit. When apricots are dried naturally, they, like raisins, assume a darker color than the fresh fruit. Naturally dried, sulfite-free apricots are dark orange, almost reddish in color. Ask your grocer to stock sun dried apricots. These sulfite-free apricots are available from specialty food distributors, and supermarkets may carry them upon demand.

2. Keep fresh apricots refrigerated in a brown paper bag. This is because plastic bags contain hydrocarbons, which may damage nutrients such as vitamin C, vitamin E, and beta carotene. Ask your grocer to bag the apricots in a small brown paper bag or the new "breathable" cellophane or plastic bags.

3. Apricots and cream is a nutritionally correct recipe. The cream liberates the fat soluble beta carotene, while aiding in its absorption. If you tolerate milk products, fresh apricots drizzled with cream or half and half is a readily digested and highly nutritious dessert.

4. Stewed fresh apricots is an excellent food. However, don't add sugar. Instead, use raw honey and whole milk or stew them in their own juice. What could be better for taste and nutrition than stewed apricots in hot milk and honey on a cold wintery day? Yet, today, such a recipe is rarely consumed, although it was once one of America's most popular recipes.

5. For sweetening cereal try adding chopped apricots instead of sugar. When added to cooked cereal, apricots offer luscious flavor and plenty of sweetness.

6. Keep dried apricots on hand when fresh apricots are out of season. Shred the apricots, and use them on fruit and vegetable salads. Add chopped dried apricots to nut mixes. They provide valuable amounts of potassium and vitamin A (as beta carotene), both of which are needed for maintaining organ function during the cold season. Dried apricots can be reconstituted with water. Immerse dried apricots in a small amount of water. Cook in a covered pan on low heat only until tender. These apricots are sweet, tender, and tasty. Learn to eat foods without added sweetener. In time, the natural sweetness of food will become desirable, and added sugar will seem foreign.

7. Remember that dried fruit, including apricots, is mostly sugar. If you are sensitive to sugar, you may need to consume dried apricots sparingly despite their immense nutritional value.

8. If unsulfured apricots are unavailable, buy Turkish apricots. These apricots are sun ripened and are less likely to be contaminated with pesticides than American grown apricots. Turkish apricots are nutrient

rich, since they are grown on virgin mountainous soil; they may even be organic, although no such distinction appears on the label. Remember, the rule is chemical-free apricots are dark orange in color.

9. Try apricot/almond milk for a nourishing and tasty beverage. The almonds provide protein, and the apricots provide vitamin A (as beta carotene). In a blender add blanched almonds, fresh or dried apricots, and water. Blend until smooth; add water to achieve desired thickness.

Top Apricot Cures

1. If you have sensitive skin or suffer from a skin disorder, eat apricots regularly. Sensitive skin, as well as dry skin, may signal beta carotene deficiency. Another signal of deficiency is skin which is ultra sensitive to sunlight. The rich beta carotene content of apricots aids in healing skin and diminishing sensitivity. Beta carotene blocks the toxicity of ultraviolet rays, which makes it particularly valuable for individuals who work outdoors or who sunburn easily. Remember, the beta carotene in apricots is more readily absorbed if the apricots are eaten with fat, which stimulates beta carotene absorption. Fat is a key link for the absorption of fat soluble vitamins, and it must be included in the diet for optimal assimilation of these vitamins. Beta carotene can do its beneficial work only if it is absorbed into the blood and deposited in the skin. Fat, as well as protein, is required for this process to proceed optimally. You also need a healthy liver. The liver makes bile, which is required for efficient absorption of fat and fat soluble vitamins. So, eat apricots along with foods high in naturally occurring fats such as milk, cream, or avocados; you will receive a greater nutritional punch for the effort.

Apricots contain a special protein, which speeds the healing of damaged skin. To get enough of this protein, try eating a handful of dried apricots daily. You will almost certainly notice an improvement in the health of the skin, probably within a month.

2. If you have acne, eat lots of apricots. Beta carotene fights acne, and apricots are rich in this vitamin. The combination of special skin healing proteins and beta carotene makes apricots ideal for reversing this distressing ailment. Eat apricot pits, the richest source of the skin protein. Only small amounts, like an ounce daily, are needed.

3. Anemic individuals must eat apricots to boost the intake of naturally occurring iron. Dried apricots offer a more concentrated iron supply than fresh apricots; the natural iron is non-toxic, whereas synthetic iron can poison the internal organs.

4. For constipation, eat dried apricots on a daily basis. Not only do they provide fiber, but they also contain a mild natural laxative. Plus, they are less harsh as a laxative than prunes.

5. Apricots are soothing for a sensitive stomach. They are one of the easiest of all fruits to digest and rarely cause allergic reactions. Both fresh and dried apricots are well tolerated and are recommended by allergists as an ideal food for individuals plagued with digestive problems, sensitive stomach, or food allergy.

6. Eating fresh apricots after each meal may help ease indigestion or heartburn. Pit the apricots, and serve them in whole milk if you tolerate milk or heavy cream. Add a teaspoon of raw honey. The heartburn/indigestion will usually improve immediately, and this remedy is also useful for a nervous or upset stomach.

7. Anyone with cancer or with a strong family history of cancer should eat apricots as often as possible. The minimum prescription is two apricots per day. Break open the seeds and eat the pits. The pits contain anti-cancer chemicals called *cyanogenetic glycosides*. Only an ounce per day or less is necessary. There is no harm in eating small amounts of apricot pits. They certainly don't hurt the Hunzas, who eat them on a daily basis.

8. No one should smoke. However, if you are exposed to cigarette smoke, eat apricots on a daily basis. The rich content of beta carotene helps prevent smoke-induced lung degeneration.

Artichokes

Ancient history records artichokes as a food of immense powers. Grecian scholars praised them, listing artichokes as the favorite vegetable. Artichokes first reached the Western world in the Middle Ages. They were brought to Europe by Islamic traders during the 10th century. The name artichoke is of Arabic origin.

As with many of our vegetables, artichokes were brought to America by Spanish and French colonists. If you have never eaten artichokes, it is no surprise. This vegetable is a newcomer to the American palate, becoming popular only since the latter part of the 20th century.

As early as the 18th century European physicians knew of artichoke's curative powers. Dr. Meyrick noted in 1740 that the juice of artichoke leaves is a powerful diuretic and listed it as an effective cure for kidney ailments as well as heart failure. European doctors used artichokes for ameliorating yellow jaundice and found them useful for treating arthritis. Current research describes how artichokes help stimulate digestive secretions, increase urine flow, and normalize blood sugar.

Rather than being a vegetable, the artichoke is strictly a flower or, more precisely, an unopened flower bud. Only certain parts of the plant are edible, particularly the heart, which is, in reality, a flower part known as a *receptacle*. The receptacle is the central part of the plant. The outer part, that is the leaves, contains mostly indigestible fiber, but there is a small edible portion at the end of each leaf.

Artichokes grow proficiently only in temperate climates near oceans or seas. They thrive on soils rich in salt, since iodine is a critical nutrient for their growth. In fact, artichokes are one of the richest plant sources of this valuable element. The majority of the artichokes available in grocery stores come from Mediterranean countries, notably Italy and Spain, although a fair amount is grown in California.

The artichoke is exceptionally nutritious. Most vegetables contain only a small percentage of nutrients and are mostly water, fiber, and carbohydrate. Artichokes are far from rabbit food. A large helping provides as much as 50% of the RDA for folic acid, a feat accomplished by few foods. Artichokes contain small amounts of niacin, riboflavin, and biotin. Since they are ground hugging plants, artichokes are rich in minerals, particularly iron, calcium, phosphorus, manganese, iodine, magnesium, and potassium. A large artichoke contains 90 mg of magnesium, which is 30% of the RDA. Two artichokes give about a milligram of manganese, which is about half of the daily minimum.

Approximately one third of the edible weight of artichoke hearts consists of a valuable carbohydrate known as *inulin*. Inulin's immense value is a consequence of its ability to enhance the action of insulin. Other carbohydrates, such as the starch in wheat or the sugar in corn, agitate pancreatic function, leading to the massive release of insulin. Insulin is needed to normalize blood sugar levels and does so by catalyzing the entry of sugar into the cells. However, excessive insulin secretion, which typically occurs after a high carbohydrate meal, ultimately causes the blood sugar to drop, and this leads to a variety of symptoms, including fatigue, depression, dizziness, irritability, anxiety, moodiness, apathy, blurry vision, headache, insomnia, and tremors. Diets high in sugar or starch create tremendous stress upon the pancreas' ability to produce insulin. Eventually, the insulin is depleted and diabetes may result. Inulin, the carbohydrate found in artichokes, is the only carbohydrate which acts in exactly the opposite manner. It decreases the need for insulin, thus reducing the strain on the pancreas from a carbohydrate load. Inulin improves blood sugar tolerance by acting metabolically as a sort of food-borne insulin.

Artichokes, particularly the leaves, contain yet another novel chemical: *cynarin*. The name of this chemical is a derivation of the plant's botanical name: *Cynara scolymus*. Scientific studies show that cynarin boosts liver function. It is so effective that it even helps the liver cells regenerate after they are destroyed by toxicity. Cynarin works largely by stimulating the production of bile, but it also protects liver cells from toxic damage. The ability to increase bile flow is probably the reason artichokes are useful for lowering excessively high cholesterol levels. Artichokes also help lower triglyceride levels.

Top Artichoke Tips

1. Never buy fresh artichokes that appear brownish or woody; this means they are too fibrous and past their nutritional prime. Another sign of their being inedible is if the artichoke is opened.
2. Avoid buying artichoke hearts packed in oil. The oils are refined and/or hydrogenated. Instead, purchase water packed or fresh artichokes.
3. It is perfectly fine to serve fresh artichokes with a fat-containing dip such as garlic butter. Fat helps improve the absorption of beta carotene, a fat soluble substance. Mayonnaise is a popular fatty dip for artichokes. Unfortunately, commercial mayonnaise is made with hydrogenated oil and refined vegetable oil. The superior option is to make your own

mayonnaise from pure extra virgin olive oil, fresh egg yolks, and vinegar. The recipe for this luscious and nutritious dip is found in *How to Eat Right and Live Longer*.

4. Avoid boiling fresh artichokes for prolonged periods. Excessive boiling may reduce the vitamin content to nil.

5. If you buy canned artichokes, purchase only the hearts. Artichoke bottoms should be used for garnish only; they are mostly fiber and are indigestible.

6. Eat artichokes with meat dishes. Artichokes provide significant amounts of folic acid, and meat provides a rich amount of B_{12} as well as extra folic acid. The two nutrients work as a team; there is no B_{12} in vegetation.

7. Artichokes should be added to soups. They greatly enrich the nutrient content of soups and broths, plus they enhance the taste. Cooking helps liberate the trace minerals from the fibrous parts of the plant.

8. If buying artichokes in the can, be aware that there are small, medium, and large ones. Purchase the smallest variety available, since they are more tasty, tender, and nutritious than the larger sizes.

Top Artichoke Cures

1. If you crave sweets and/or if your appetite for sweets is beyond control, eat artichokes with meals. Have a tossed salad topped with two or three artichoke hearts, or eat fresh steamed artichokes. If you do this regularly for one month, the uncontrollable urge for sweets will be diminished. This beneficial effect is largely due to the rich content of thiamine, folic acid, magnesium, cynarin, and inulin.

2. If you suffer from diabetes and/or hypoglycemia, eat artichokes every day. The power of artichokes is found in the hearts, which are nearly one third inulin. Inulin is a unique carbohydrate, which mimics the action of insulin. Artichoke hearts are so effective in improving blood sugar control that the requirement for insulin may be reduced significantly. Thus, if you are taking insulin and if you are altering your diet radically, be sure to measure your blood sugar level regularly and/or have it monitored by a doctor. Artificially administered insulin can cause hypoglycemic shock, which may be fatal.

3. Artichokes aid intestinal function. They contain a special type of fiber which gently improves bowel function by increasing the bulk of the stool. Artichokes also contain substances which enhance the growth of the good bacteria. Furthermore, they contain a yet to be discovered substance which promotes the flow of digestive juices, and anything which aids in digestion also improves elimination.

4. Sour mood may be a warning of chemical imbalances in the brain. The most common type of imbalance is disturbed blood sugar regulation. Common symptoms usually deemed "psychological," such as mood swings, irritability, anxiety, and depression, are actually warning signs of poor blood sugar control. In order to function normally, the brain must receive a continuous supply of glucose. If the blood sugar level falls precipitously, mental symptoms usually result. These symptoms include irritability, agitation, moodiness, anxiety, depression, memory loss, confusion, dizziness, bouts of fatigue, sleepiness during the day, temper tantrums, headaches, crying spells, and insomnia. Artichokes are one of Nature's most powerful foods for normalizing blood sugar levels, and this is largely due to their rich content of inulin, thiamine, cynarin, and folic acid as well as blood sugar enhancing trace minerals.

5. If you can't seem to get full when eating, try eating artichokes with meals. Add them to vegetable trays, salads, soups, and stir fry. The inulin and cynarin help balance blood sugar levels and, as a result, create a sensation of satiety. By regulating appetite and blood sugar, artichokes aid in weight loss.

6. If you have a problem with plaque on the teeth, eat artichokes regularly. They contain a chemical which inhibits bacterial growth in the mouth, and this leads to a reduction in plaque. This is readily apparent, because, when artichokes are eaten they create a sort of squeaky or slippery sensation on the teeth.

7. Artichokes are an ideal food for the individual with a sensitive stomach. This is because artichokes are one of the most readily digested of all foods. They are gentle upon the digestive tract and rarely cause allergic reactions. This means they are also excellent for those suffering from chemical or food sensitivities. Artichoke hearts are an excellent source of a type of fiber which is highly digestible, and this aids in bowel function.

8. Inulin is a natural diuretic. If you have a tendency to retain water or if

you have kidney disease, eat artichokes on a daily basis. The water retention will assuredly improve as a result of eating eight ounces of artichokes per day.

9. Currently, there is major interest in plants of the thistle family, because they contain compounds which are useful in the treatment of liver disorders. Certain thistles contain a substance called *silymarin*, which helps protect the liver from toxic chemical damage. Artichokes contain a similar substance, cynarin, and, indeed, may be relied upon as a dietary cure for liver disease. With artichokes regularly on the menu you can eat your way to a healthier liver. The inulin helps prevent the accumulation of fat in the liver, and the cynarin improves the flow of bile. Eat artichokes with every meal if you suffer from liver disease.

Avocados

This precious fruit originated in the forests of Central and South America. The Western world got its introduction when Spanish explorers found it thriving in the forests of Columbia in 1509. The word itself is derived from the Aztec term *ahvactl*. However, it was not until the 19th century, some 400 years after its discovery, that avocados were grown commercially in the United States. Today, America produces more avocados than any other region in the world.

The avocado has been unfairly maligned. This is largely due to its fat content. However, the fat content is no reason to avoid it. Rather, avocados are an exceptionally valuable food. In fact, they are one of the most nutritious of all known foods, containing a greater density of nutrients than more commonly eaten foods, including corn, wheat, oats, dark green leafy vegetables, and even milk. It is possible to live, if not thrive, on nothing but avocados and water, and that can be said for only a minute number of foods.

Avocados are primarily rich in fat, which constitutes some 70 to 80% of the calories, depending upon the variety. This fat occurs mostly in the form of monounsaturated fatty acids, the same type which occurs in olive oil. Monounsaturates are exceptionally valuable as a source of fuel for energy production within the cells, particularly the cells of the heart and arteries.

It is commonly believed that avocados should be avoided by people with high cholesterol. The irony is that avocados, like all fruits and vegetables, are devoid of cholesterol. Yet, dieticians and health practitioners continue to vociferously prohibit avocado consumption in the event of heart disease or high blood lipids. This view is erroneous. In fact, research conducted in Queensland, Australia reveals the gravity of the error. Australian cardiologists tested the effects of eating avocados on their patients' blood cholesterol levels. They immediately recognized that eating avocados cut levels of bad cholesterol significantly. Furthermore, it was discovered that avocados were twice as effective in lowering cholesterol as the low fat diet. The real shocker was the fact that the low fat diet exerted a harmful effect on the good cholesterol (HDL cholesterol), while avocados were beneficial.

It must also be remembered that avocados have been a staple food for the natives of Central and South America for centuries. Yet, despite the fact that they consume a food which is essentially entirely fat, the natives suffer no heart disease.

Avocados are exceptionally rich in a number of vitamins, including biotin, thiamine, niacin, vitamin A, folic acid, vitamin B_6, and vitamin E. They are one of the top food sources of natural vitamin E. Two avocados supply approximately 5 I.U., which makes them richer in this nutrient than any other fruit or vegetable. They contain vitamin E in a pure, complete, natural form. Recent research indicates that vitamin E in food is more active in preventing disease than the vitamin E in supplements. In nature, there are dozens of vitamin E molecules; pills and capsules only contain a few of these, so it is best to get as much vitamin E in the diet as possible. Ensminger lists avocados as a top vegetable/fruit source of vitamin B_6, second only to bananas. Avocados contain a fair amount of phosphorus, as well as magnesium, and are rich in potassium. They are also one of the few fruits rich in carnitine, an amino acid necessary for the transport of fatty acids into the cells.

Carnitine is an invaluable substance. This nutrient is vital for fat metabolism. Carnitine is required for transporting the various fatty acids, such as essential fatty acids, monounsaturates, and saturated fats, into the cells so they can be burned as fuel. Avocados are the only considerable plant source of this essential nutrient, the primary dietary sources being the juices of fresh red meat, poultry, milk, and eggs.

65

Top Avocado Tips

1. Never refrigerate avocados; the cold damages the flesh and disturbs the flavor.
2. After peeling, remove any discolored regions, since the discoloration is a sign of spoilage.
3. Check the avocados carefully for firmness before buying. If they are spongy or if they have soggy pockets, do not buy them.
4. Once avocados are peeled and served, leftovers must be drizzled with vinegar or fresh lemon juice. Both of these liquids prevent spoiling and reduce discoloration.
5. Avocados are one of the finest of all types of baby foods. They are infinitely superior to the typical preformed baby foods. Mash the ripe avocado with pureed carrots or peas for a superbly nutritious infant entree.
6. While the fat in avocados is readily absorbed, digestion is enhanced when they are eaten with lemon juice, vinegar, garlic, and onion. In particular, garlic and onion lend themselves well with avocados, both for flavor and enhanced digestibility. Garlic and onions accelerate the digestion and absorption of fat, plus they help cleanse the blood of any residues of fat.
7. Avocados make a tasty and filling snack. Slice a peeled avocado in half and fill the center with salsa; this is a nutrient packed and delicious snack.
8. Fat lends itself with fat. This means that avocados taste great with other fatty foods. Top salad greens with diced avocados and feta cheese, and drizzle with extra virgin olive oil and tarragon or balsamic vinegar. Add olives and avocados together in salads or on vegetable plates.

Top Avocado Cures

1. Avocados are perhaps the finest food to serve the malnourished individual. In other words, if the individual has difficulty maintaining weight or is suffering from malabsorption, avocados are the perfect cure. To increase weight or muscle mass, eat two or three avocados every day. Avocados are also excellent for malnutrition of the red cells, i.e. anemia. In this case, squeeze lemon juice over the avocado, since lemon juice aids in the absorption of iron.

2. If the individual is suffering from poor complexion or chronic skin disease, avocados should be consumed on a daily basis. Avocados provide special curative oils, which help regenerate the skin and protect it from disease. Pure cold pressed avocado oil makes an excellent emollient for skin and reportedly helps accelerate the growth of new skin cells as well as hair cells. Avocados also help to eliminate fingernail disorders, especially weak or brittle nails. This is due to the fact that the natural oils in avocado make the nail more pliable, and this increases their strength. Eat an avocado daily until the nails are super strong and beautiful.

3. If the appetite is uncontrollable and you can never seem to get full, eat avocados, especially for lunch and breakfast. Avocados are so filling that they will obliterate even the most voracious of appetites. This is because the natural fats in avocados balance the fuel needs of the body and slow emptying of the stomach, so you stay full for longer periods. Furthermore, blood sugar is stabilized for a longer time period.

4. If you are suffering from hair loss, eat avocados daily. For severe hair loss, especially in women, eat up to three avocados per day. Avocados contain special oils which aid in the regeneration of hair follicles, stimulating the growth of new hair.

5. If you can't seem to muster an appetite for breakfast or if you don't feel you have the time to prepare it, try eating avocados. Eat a half or two halves of an avocado filled with salsa, chopped vegetables, or diced onions. This will stimulate digestion as well as create energy.

6. If you have dry, flaky skin, avocados are the food of choice. Eat an avocado per day for two weeks, and the condition will usually improve noticeably. Continue this for a month, and the dry skin will almost certainly be cured. This treatment is most effective if the diet is rich in beta carotene, riboflavin, vitamin D, and vitamin E. For extra beta carotene, include dark green leafy vegetables, for riboflavin, eat eggs or liver, for vitamin D, eat herring or salmon, and for vitamin E eat hazelnuts, almonds, or salmon. Eating avocados with salmon offers a synergistic effect against dry skin: the monounsaturated fatty acids from the avocado and the fish oils from the salmon have both been shown in scientific studies to reverse dry skin and help prevent a variety of skin diseases.

7. If you are plagued with debilitating cardiovascular disease—high

blood pressure, stroke, heart failure, cardiac arrhythmia, or any other type of heart disease—eat avocados. Yes, avocados are a top food for the heart. They are rich in fuel fats needed by the heart for its normal energy production. Remember, avocados are primarily monounsaturated fats, the same type found in olive oil. The types of fats in avocados help cardiac function and can in no way hurt the heart. The point is that eating avocados is not a cause of heart attacks. For instance, in rural Mexico and Central America, where avocados are a staple, there is no heart disease.

The potential value of fat in the diet cannot be underestimated. Obviously, fat serves as a source of calories or fuel. This fuel is critical for good health. In fact, normal function of the body cannot proceed without it. Forget about the common concept of the calorie for a moment. Think instead of the concept of fat as a form of fuel, similar to gasoline in a car. For the car to run optimally it must be provided with the most efficient type of fuel possible with the highest octane—in other words, premium. For the human body the premium fuel is fat. This is because fat contains more than 9 kilocalories of fuel per gram, over twice that provided by carbohydrates. This means that it is the most efficient, that is most biologically useful, form of fuel. It means the individual receives a greater value biologically in terms of enhanced organ function, synthetic activity, and energy when consuming fat versus carbohydrates or protein.

The heart is the only organ in the body which never rests; it must ceaselessly pump blood at essentially the same rate day and night for the duration of our lives. It must utilize the most efficient fuel possible, and that is why hearts love fats. That is right, the heart muscle prefers naturally occurring fatty acids over all other fuel sources. Numerous textbooks of human physiology, including the world renowned Guyton's textbook of physiology, state categorically that only fatty acids are the preferential fuel for optimal cardiac function. Think about it: dozens of civilizations eat large amounts of fat, and they have a lower incidence of heart disease than Americans. For instance, the Eskimos, despite a diet consisting of nearly 80% fat, have no heart disease, that is not until they adopt a Western diet. With the advent of modern civilization Eskimos now have a high rate of heart disease. However, it is the potato chips, candy, soda pop, margarine, cookies, sugary cereals, bread, ice cream, canned foods, and pasta that is killing them, not the natural fats in their native diet.

Basil

Not just a flavoring for tomato sauce, basil has been highly respected for untold centuries because of its curative powers. A member of the mint family, basil originated in India and Persia. Grecian physicians used it to ameliorate nervous disorders. The French esteem it as the supreme of all herbs, calling it *herb royale*, while the Italians deem it a cure for the soul. The Eastern Indians exalt it to such a degree that they grow it around their shrines.

Basil is perhaps best known for its antiseptic powers, which are a consequence of its essential oil content. One of its essential oils is similar to the well known antiseptic eucalyptus. Historically, it has been used to kill parasites and fight bacterial infections. Basil has been known to cure infections of the skin, lungs, liver, spleen, and blood. It is also reported effective for combating diarrhea. In the 1600s it was prescribed by English herbalists for treating venomous bites and stings. Basil is also an excellent remedy for lung conditions of all types, including asthma, a disease for which modern medicine offers no cure. This positive effect upon the lungs may largely be a result of its rich essential oil content, since these oils help soothe irritated bronchial passages and enhance blood flow. According to Ben Charles Harris, author of *Kitchen Remedies*, in Japan fresh basil leaves, steeped in water, are used for alleviating arthritic pain. This makes sense, since the volatile oils in basil are antiinflammatory.

Basil is an excellent source of trace minerals. It is extremely high in calcium, containing a greater amount than dark green leafy vegetables. Incredibly, basil contains over 2100 mg of calcium per 100 gms, over twice as much as cheese. Ensminger lists it as the eighth richest source of magnesium. As a source of potassium it rates third behind coriander and parsley.

Some individuals may be sensitive, that is allergic, to basil. This is largely a result of the fact that basil is a relative of mint, and the entire mint family is fraught with the propensity of inducing allergic toxicity. However, allergy to the more common members of this family, notably spearmint and peppermint, is exceedingly more common than is allergy to basil.

Fresh basil is the best type to use, since its volatile oils are rapidly lost when it is dried. Ensminger notes in *Food and Nutrition Encyclopedia* that the commercial dried variety "can never replace" the fresh. Always use fresh basil instead of the dried spice in recipes that call for it.

Top Basil Tips

1. Avoid using the standard type of commercially available dried basil. It is essentially herbally dead, since virtually all of the active ingredient, the pungent volatile oil, has evaporated by the time you buy it. Use fresh basil instead to obtain the best flavor and to derive the curative properties.

2. Basil should be consumed as soon as possible after purchasing. This is because the active ingredient is a volatile oil, which evaporates with time. This is the oil which is responsible for its antibiotic action. If you cannot use it right away, clean it and immerse it in extra virgin olive oil. The olive oil will retain basil's delicate and vulnerable volatile oils in the form of a natural oil suspension. This "basil oil" may be used later as an incredibly flavorful cooking oil or, preferably, as a salad oil.

3. Use basil in sauces, soups, and entrees, but make sure the recipe contains natural fats. The natural fats help extract the active ingredients, which include vitamins, minerals, and other constituents, such as linalool, methyl chavicol, and eugenol, from the basil leaves, while aiding absorption of these active ingredients into the body. So, if you are adding basil to tomato sauce, be sure to also add ground beef or extra virgin olive oil. Don't prepare low fat tomato or marinara sauce and expect to garnish any of basil's curative powers. This oil/basil combination has been known since ancient times. For instance, pesto sauce, an old Italian recipe, contains basil plus extra virgin olive oil and walnuts. The oil and walnuts retain the volatile basil oil, which is readily dissipated unless it is held in fat. Thus, by making this traditional recipe the active ingredients are preserved indefinitely. Here again, there is sound wisdom to ancient eating habits, and eating basil "vegetarian" or in low fat dishes is poor advice.

4. If you love vinegar and oil, you'll enjoy it even more with basil. Add one or two tablespoons of minced basil leaves to a vinegar and oil mixture. After a few days the mixture will exude the rich aroma and taste of fresh basil, and you will be armed with a salad dressing that tastes fantastic, plus it is a valuable natural medicine.

5. Basil is one of the most readily digested of all foods and is, in fact, a digestive stimulant. Thus, it is ideal for individuals who have sensitive stomachs. If you have difficulty with digestion or if your body reacts negatively to certain foods, it is a good idea to eat basil with each meal.

Virtually anyone, even those with sensitive stomachs, will benefit from eating this gentle spice, the exception being individuals who are allergic to it.

6. Whenever cooking tomatoes or tomato sauce, add basil. Be sure to add a tablespoon or two of extra virgin olive oil to the tomato sauce, since the oil will help extract the active ingredients from the basil and will also protect the active ingredients from being destroyed by cooking. Add freshly chopped basil to your favorite salsa or tomato salad and drizzle with extra virgin olive oil.

7. Make fresh pesto sauce for a dip. It is far healthier than commercial cheese dips. Use pesto as an accompaniment for vegetables or meats or as a spread for whole grain bread or rolls. The recipe can be readily prepared with a food processor or blender. Simply add basil leaves and walnuts to a food processor and chop finely. As an alternative use pine nuts instead of walnuts or perhaps both. Feta cheese may also be added. Immerse all ingredients in a liberal amount of extra virgin olive oil.

8. If you tolerate cheese and love soft cheese, try grinding fresh basil leaves in the cheese. The oils of basil will be preserved by the fat in the cheese. Plus, this herb adds immense flavor to all types of cheese, especially full fat soft cheese and feta cheese.

Top Basil Cures

1. If you have a stomach ache or sensitive stomach, eat fresh basil before or with meals. Thoroughly chew several basil leaves. Hold the macerated leaves in the mouth for a few minutes and then swallow. Usually, this alone will eliminate the stomach ache.

2. If you have a headache, try chewing on several leaves of fresh basil. Hold the basil in the mouth as long as possible. This will permit the volatile oils in basil to be absorbed directly into the blood. The mouth is one of the best sites for the absorption of volatile oils. In fact, while many of these oils cannot be absorbed from the stomach, they are directly and immediately absorbed into the blood through the mucous membranes of the mouth. This allows the individual to derive immediate benefits from its medicinal actions.

3. If you're tired constantly, try eating basil on a daily basis. It stimulates metabolism and provides energy for even the most sluggish of individuals.

4. When intestinal gas is unrelenting, use basil to calm the distress. Eat it several times daily; use it on salads and add it to soups. The natural oils in basil soothe the intestinal tract, thus reducing irritation, cramping, and gas formation.

5. If your life lacks stimulation and if you feel apathetic about everything, try eating fresh basil regularly. Basil rejuvenates even the most forlorn, defeated, and depressed individual, providing mental and physical vigor beyond any conceivable expectations.

6. Nausea is an uncomfortable symptom that meets its match with basil. This herb is effective and safe for combating nausea of pregnancy. Chew basil leaves continuously until the nausea dissipates.

7. If you are suffering from grief or melancholy or if your nerves are on edge, basil may come to the rescue. It is an effective stimulant for a defeated nervous system. Simply add basil to soups, salads, casseroles, and stir fry; expect the mental and nerve-related symptoms to disappear within days.

8. For joint pain or arthritis try the old Japanese remedy of infusing basil leaves in steaming water. Bring 2 cups of water to a boil and turn off heat. Immediately immerse 12 fresh basil leaves in the water. Let steep for 30 minutes and drink immediately. Drink this tea several times daily, if necessary.

9. Spasticity or cramps of the bowel may respond to a basil prescription. Chew several leaves of basil thoroughly to properly release the active ingredient from the fibers; hold mixture in mouth for a minute and then swallow. Repeat this dosage until the pain/cramps dissipate.

10. Since ancient times, basil has been utilized as an effective treatment for headaches. Fresh basil contains a variety of volatile oils, which possess antiinflammatory as well as anesthetic properties. For the treatment of headache combine fresh sprigs of basil and freshly sliced ginger in a pot of hot water. Let steep for thirty minutes and drink while hot. Drink several cups daily for relief of any type of headache. Or, for a more convenient basil remedy take *Aganex*, two or three capsules four times daily until the headache is resolved. Aganex is an anti-migraine herbal formula containing organic basil, wild strawberry leaves, coriander, and ginger, all of which possess anti-migraine actions. For ideal results take it in divided doses several times daily (see Appendix A).

Beef

It has become sort of in vogue to vigorously avoid the consumption of red meat. In America tens of millions of individuals now rarely or never eat beef. Yet, this intentional avoidance of red meat is a relatively new phenomenon. Thirty years ago virtually every American regularly ate meat, and beef was the most commonly consumed type. In other words, beef has been regarded as a highly nutritious and primary food on the American menu for hundreds of years.

Beef is one of the most nutrient rich of all types of meat. It contains a greater density of nutrients than poultry and is a superior source of certain vitamins and minerals than either poultry or fish. Beef contains virtually every known nutrient, including all of the primary amino acids, vitamins, and minerals, a feat accomplished by few foods.

Beef is perhaps the richest source of energy nutrients, containing a greater density of long chain fatty acids and potential hydrogen ions than any other food. Hydrogen is needed to provide molecular energy, and it is found in immense quantities primarily in meat, fish, poultry, eggs, and milk products. Beef is a superb source of hydrogen. The old adage that the individual who is weak of body needs to gain strength by having "a good steak under the belt" is certainly substantiated by the content of hydrogen ions and nutrients in red meat. Thus, the saturated fats and amino acids from beef are invaluable, because they provide great fuel value for cellular combustion. In contrast, Harrow and Mazur note in *Textbook of Biochemistry* that fruits and vegetables, while donating valuable amounts of vitamins and minerals, "contribute...little as sources of energy."

The hydrogen ion content of beef largely explains its potential for increasing energy and strength. Remember, the sun, our most powerful celestial ally, is essentially a hydrogen factory. The most powerful of all bombs is the hydrogen bomb. Hydrogen is pure energy, and the human body requires it for creating internal energy.

Beef is rich in a variety of vitamins and minerals, containing a greater array than most foods. The vitamins found in the densest amounts include thiamine, riboflavin, niacin, pantothenic acid, biotin, pyridoxine, folic acid, and vitamin B_{12}. The minerals found in the densest amounts include phosphorus, magnesium, potassium, selenium, chromium, sulfur, copper, iron, and zinc. Depending upon the cut a large serving of beef may provide as much as 100% of the RDA for zinc plus over 100% of the RDA for iron. It is one of the few commonly available foods rich in chromium, a mineral required for the assimilation and metabolism of fat and sugar. There is only a limited list of foods containing such a massive array of nutrients. Comparable foods include milk, eggs, poultry, and fatty fish. Yet, in many aspects these foods are inferior to beef. For instance, milk is high in protein, but it is quite low in zinc and contains no significant iron; beef is rich in these minerals. Eggs have iron but are much lower in B_{12} and magnesium than beef. Thus, beef provides a unique array of nutrients, which make it a necessary component of a nutrient dense diet.

The brain and nervous system require a wide range of nutrients, many of which cannot be supplied by the vegetable kingdom. Without certain of these nutrients, brain and nerve cells degenerate. Impressively, beef contains a wide range of nutrients required by the nervous system, including carnitine, taurine, tyrosine, tryptophan, chromium, selenium, magnesium, thiamine, riboflavin, pantothenic acid, niacin, folic acid, choline, cholesterol, and vitamin B_{12}. Iron, for which meat is the primary source, is required for oxygenation of the brain. In particular, Italian researchers found that a type of carnitine halts memory deterioration and brain cell degeneration in Alzheimer's patients. As described by Linus Pauling the only considerable source of carnitine is the juice of red meat. Taurine, which is needed for the conduction of brain electricity, is only found in animal products. B_{12} is absolutely essential for the proper function of the neurons. Without it, brain cells, as well as the cells of the spinal cord, die. Other researchers have found that selenium, for which meat is a preferred source, efficiently blocks aging of brain cells.

Obviously, beef is extremely dense in nutrients desperately needed for the function of the nervous system. A vegetable and grain based diet alone fails to provide such a balance of nutrients. The fact is a lack of fresh meat in the diet, if the diet is not carefully balanced and if it is too rich in carbohydrate, will likely cause brain dysfunction. This may be signaled by the fact that mental disorders, such as depression, irritability, panic attacks, anxiety, insomnia, agitation, and belligerence, are relatively common in vegetarian populations. Persistent hostility and anger, which are common in vegetarians, are warning signs of nutritional deficiency.

The consequences of a prolonged vegetarian diet, deficient in vitamin B_{12}, are serious. The fact is the brain and spinal cord, as well as all of the nerves throughout the body, rapidly degenerate if the deficiency is not corrected.

Lately, there has been great concern about microbial contamination of meat, and this is a legitimate problem. However, all meat, not just beef, is subject to microbial infection. The fact is, as a rule, beef is less subject to microbial contamination than poultry, and, since it is a strict herbivore, it is a relatively clean animal. While cases of food poisoning from beef do occur, it is largely a consequence of the way beef is handled. Thus, ground beef is the source of virtually all cases. In contrast, poultry is universally contaminated, primarily with the bacteria Salmonella. According to Dr. Rodrigo Villar of the Centers for Disease Control (CDC) up to 4 million Americans contract this infection every year.

Herbivores are relatively free of microbial infection, that is if they are raised in a natural method. The flesh is essentially sterile as long as it is not contaminated during processing. The main risk is with ground beef. There have been significant outbreaks of infection by E. coli, particularly in pre-formed patties, but this is strictly due to contamination with filth. Disease may also be induced in cattle by errant feeding practices. Thus, any health issues related to beef are man-made. The problem is what is administered to the cow, that is what it is fed and what is injected into it. There is nothing inherently noxious about the cow itself when it is allowed to graze on natural forage.

Mad Cow disease, which has led to the decimation of England's beef industry, is a consequence of human meddling with Nature. Instead of being fed their natural forage, which is exclusively plant matter, cows were being fed commercial feed containing animal by products. Although the precise cause has eluded scientists, the disease is probably instigated by microbes found in the animal by-products, which infect the brains and nervous systems of cows, causing them to exhibit bizarre behavior (thus, the term "mad"). These organisms are most likely viruses or virus-like particles, although recent studies implicate bacteria. Ultimately, the viruses destroy the brain and nerve cells, leading to death. No such disease exists in naturally raised cattle, proving that contaminated feed is the direct cause.

Here is how Mad Cow disease began. For decades cows in England were fed commercial feed containing fecally contaminated meat scraps, notably sheep gut, which is utterly foreign to their diets. The fact is any creature would be vulnerable to develop disease when fed such offal. The British government itself was aware of the danger of such a practice, as a royal commission of scientists warned in 1979 that feeding animal by-products to cows could lead to diseases which might be transmitted to humans. Unfortunately, no one listened. I also predicted that the feeding of herbivores, such as cows and sheep, meat by-products or blood meal would lead to wholesale disaster. In fact, blood meal, which is a type of commercial feed made from blood and animal by-products, has been fed to animals in America, particularly pigs, for decades. Obviously, blood, and such animal parts as ground intestine—a formerly routine component of commercial feed in Britain—are hopeless infested with microbes.

The problem with feeding animal residues to cattle is that it errs against the normal physiology of the animals. Cows are strict herbivores, meaning they only eat plant matter. Herbivores have a unique type of digestive tract geared for digesting cellulose, and they are utterly incapable of digesting animal products. In fact, their stomachs lack sufficient stomach acid, that is hydrochloric acid, for digesting meat. Humans, as well as strict carnivores, such as cats, produce large amounts of stomach acid. Hydrochloric acid is the most powerful natural germicide known, and it continuously protects us from microbial infestation. Without stomach acid, microbes, which abound prolifically in meat scraps, cannot be killed. Ultimately, the cattle became infected and the meat, organs, and milk served as reservoirs for the organism.

Several deaths have been attributed to a disorder in humans similar to Mad Cow disease. Known medically as Cruetzfeld-Jakob's disease, evidence seems clear that it is contracted from infected cattle products. However, the majority of cases of Cruetzfeld-Jakob's disease, even in England, fail to be attributed to beef consumption, rather, they are correlated with surgical contamination during brain surgery. In these instances, the culprit is human blood.

This unfortunate disaster for the British was entirely preventable. This is a man-made syndrome, caused by irresponsible individuals in the feed industry, as well as the government, who sought profit before safety. Cows are strict herbivores, and they thrive on their natural diet. If a strict carnivore, such as the mighty lion, was fed nothing but grass, it would become ill. It too would develop diseases unknown to it naturally and would ultimately die from the erroneous diet.

For Americans there is one major concern: British beef has been imported to the United States for decades, although importation was stopped in 1989. However, it takes several years—10 or more—before Mad Cow disease surfaces after the initial exposure. Furthermore, while the feeding of animal byproducts to herbivores has been discouraged in the United States, there is still no ban on such products despite the Mad Cow scare. Thus, it is possible that some feed lots still utilize animal based feeds.

Range fed cattle is the safest, as well as most nutritious, beef. With feedlot beef make sure it is fed grain rather than commercial feed. Insist on buying the kind which is hormone- and antibiotic-free.

Beef is one of the most healthy, least processed foods available in the supermarket. There are a number of foods, like commercial chicken, which should elicit greater concern. Thousands of individuals contract severe Salmonella infection every year from eating commercial chicken: hundreds die. Many of these infections are contracted in restaurants, but it can also happen right in the home. In contrast, there are currently no cases in the United States of Cruetzfeld-Jakob disease linked to beef consumption. Furthermore, the individual is far more likely to develop Cruetzfeld-Jakob disease as a result of brain surgery and/or hospitalization than from eating beef.

In this era virtually everything we eat or drink is potentially contaminated. Furthermore, some things are generally safe but cause harm when consumed in excess. I saved the life of a women, who was killing herself with water. For some unknown reason she envisioned that she needed to "flush all the poisons" out of her body. Thus, she drank two gallons of distilled water daily for several weeks. My first glimpse of her was utterly revealing: she was pasty in color, exhausted, and limp, a sort of "washed out" appearance. Importantly, the examination revealed a rapid, irregular heart rate. In fact, her primary complaint was that her "heart felt funny." She also said that she "thought she was dying." Indeed, she was close to death with severe cardiac arrhythmia, albeit self-induced, which resulted from washing the electrolytes out of the body. I prescribed sodium chloride (as salt) as well as magnesium and potassium, which aborted her "liquid suicide." The point is that water could kill you and so could just about anything else if done to excess.

If you are concerned about the safety of beef, here are some rules to follow for keeping it on the menu:

a) buy only range fed beef. Cattle which roam about eating their natural forage are relatively free of disease, plus their meat is more nutritious than those fed on commercial feed or fodder.

b) buy beef as fresh as possible. Properly aged beef is also acceptable. Cook it at least medium, but don't heat it to oblivion. Excess cooking destroys much of the nutritional value.

c) opt for chemical free beef, that is beef which is raised without synthetic chemicals such as hormones, pesticides, and antibiotics. Ask your grocer to carry such beef, which is available from local growers and/or wholesalers. Furthermore, health food markets which carry chemical free beef are now found in numerous major cities.

d) consider mail order or special order for fresh chemical free beef if it is not carried locally.

e) check local farmers to see if they would be willing to raise chemical free beef. Often, they raise a special cow for slaughter for their families; perhaps they will sell you a quarter or half of a beef from their chemical free "family" cow or will raise a special one for your family.

Keep in mind that beef contains a wide variety of nutrients, which are of immense value in human nutrition. It's nutrient density is overwhelmingly greater than that of any fruit or vegetable, perhaps with the exception of avocado.

Top Beef Tips

1. Antibiotic and synthetic hormones in foods are unfit for human consumption. Don't add to your chemical burden by eating commercially raised meat. Instead, eat naturally raised beef. If it is unavailable, request it from your grocer or health food store. Create a demand. Start a natural food club. Do whatever it takes to make the marketplace meet your needs.

2. Do not be overly concerned about microbial contamination of beef. Virtually any food can be contaminated by microbes. The fact is a greater number of cases of food poisoning are reported every year from eating contaminated vegetables and fruit than beef. For example in 1996 fatal outbreaks of E. coli were traced to contaminated lettuce, alfalfa sprouts,

and apple juice. In 1997 hundreds of individuals were stricken with hepatitis—the source was contaminated strawberries.

3. When making hamburgers, always add herbs and spices. Finely chopped onions and garlic improve the taste and digestibility of hamburger. Add also curry powder, coriander, and wild oregano or a few drops of oil of oregano (see Oregano section). All of these herbs and spices contain volatile oils, which inhibit the growth of noxious microbes.

4. To tenderize tough cuts of meat, slice it into thin slices and marinate in extra virgin olive oil, chopped garlic, chopped onions, ginger, and vinegar. For added tenderizing power add either cubed papaya or kiwi fruit, both of which are rich in protein digesting enzymes.

In Hawaii fish is served with fresh pineapple for a reason: raw pineapple is rich in protein digesting enzymes. Raw pineapple or the juice from fresh pineapple may be used to tenderize beef. Simply add the pineapple or juice to the meat and marinate overnight. Cook separately or slice the meat and use it in a tropical stir fry recipe using fresh vegetables in a base of coconut milk. In the latter case, add the pineapple chunks to the stir fry so they don't go to waste. Tropical fruit goes well with meat dishes.

5. Don't over-cook steaks; the center of the meat need not be totally grey for it to be safe to eat. Just make sure the steak is heated all the way through, and feel free to eat steak medium or medium rare. It is easier to digest if it is cooked gently.

6. Beef makes an excellent addition to vegetable dishes of all types. Add beef to create a more complete amino acid profile of vegetable soup and stir fry recipes. By providing the balance of nutrients found within vegetables and meat, the cells of the body will be more thoroughly nourished.

Top Beef Cures

1. Beef is an ideal food for children. Because it is so nutrient-rich, it is quite filling. Thus, it represses the craving for sweets and junk foods. Children should eat beef several times per week. Let them eat as much as they desire. Be liberal with beef meals, and restrict the inferior meals such as white flour pasta, macaroni, and pizza.

2. Those suffering from an energy deficit must consider eating more beef. This is because beef is rich in a variety of nutrients needed to create energy. These energy supplying nutrients include amino acids, carnitine, B vitamins, trace minerals, and iron. One exception to this is food allergy. If you are allergic to beef, eating it may make you feel tired or sleepy.

3. Beef is an excellent remedy for a ravenous appetite and/or obesity. The fact is beef is so nutrient dense that even modest portions induce a sensation of fullness. Perhaps the individual remembers how full the stomach feels after eating a good sized steak. Curb your cravings for sweets and starches by eating hefty portions of beef.

4. Organic calf liver provides a wealth of nutrients which enhance the immune system, improve vision, accelerate digestion, and calm the nerves. Eat it several times per month if you have health problems of any kind. Calf liver is preferred over beef liver, since it is less likely to be contaminated with harmful chemicals.

5. Beef is the ideal food for reversing anemia. Regardless of the cause, if you have a low blood count, beef should be on the daily menu. This is because it is rich in virtually every nutrient needed to produce healthy red blood cells: iron, copper, manganese, zinc, selenium, riboflavin, folic acid, vitamin B_{12}, and amino acids. Beef will help cure anemia if it is eaten regularly. For extremely low blood counts, as measured by a hemoglobin of under 12.0, eat at least 18 ounces of beef daily. For moderate anemia eat at least 12 ounces daily.

6. Surprisingly, eating beef can help improve the complexion. This is because it supplies a variety of nutrients needed for the creation of skin cells, including riboflavin, niacin, pantothenic acid, folic acid, vitamin B_{12}, copper, zinc, and amino acids. Recently, researchers have discovered that saturated fats, in which beef is rich, help block the toxicity of ultraviolet rays, while unsaturated fats, such as the type found in commercial vegetable oils, increase the risk for sun-induced skin damage. Furthermore, pale skin and/or poor complexion is a symptom of both iron and vitamin B_{12} deficiency, and beef is the top commonly available source of these nutrients.

7. For sugar sensitive individuals beef is an ideal food. It is devoid of carbohydrate, consisting instead of protein and fat. For Americans toxic reactions to sugar are common. This is because the excessive consumption of refined sugar damages the body's capacity to handle

sugar. Initially, this sugar sensitivity is manifested by hypoglycemia and in the later stages diabetes. Eventually, the individual becomes so sensitive to sugar that even a tiny amount, like the amount found in a piece of chewing gum, creates symptoms or reactions. The best way to recover from sugar sensitivity is to eat a diet free of refined sugar and consume the majority of the calories in the form of protein and fat rich foods. This carbohydrate fasting will eventually improve the body's ability to process sugar, and, thus, the heightened reactivity to sugar will be diminished. The following is a list of foods which are ultra low in carbohydrates and/or sugar:

beef	chicken
turkey	lamb
liver	fish
shrimp	crab
lobster	avocado
butter	cheese
yogurt	olives

8. If you have trouble digesting food, eat beef. This grand meat is one of the most readily digested of all foods. According to Proudfit and Robinson beef is "almost completely digested and absorbed" with "little if any residue in the intestinal tract." This is in contrast to the common but unsubstantiated perception that if you eat beef, it will fail to digest and will "putrefy" in the bowel. The fact is beef protein is infinitely more digestible than the commonly touted alternatives such as bean, soy, and grain protein.

Beets

Known for their valuable effects upon liver function and blood cleansing, beets are one of the most internationally renown of all medicinal foods. They have been used as medicine since ancient Egyptian times and perhaps prior.

Beets are root vegetables. In fact, in Britain, where beets are a staple food, they are called beetroot. Because of their immense popularity in

Britain, France, Germany, Russia, and Poland (borscht, pickled beets, etc), it would seem that beets are originally European. Actually, they are Mediterranean in origin and once grew wild in North Africa as well as throughout the Fertile Crescent. The wild version was entirely different than the type available today. With the ancient plant the roots were small and were used strictly as medicine. Only the beet greens were consumed as food. Although it took many centuries of careful cultivation, the wild medicinal beet was eventually converted into the current variety. Unfortunately, as a result much of the medicinal value has been lost.

Beets derive their color from a flavonoid called *betanin*. The more commonly known active ingredient is betaine, which is similar to choline in structure. This substance has been found in scientific studies to aid in the regeneration of cells throughout the body, particularly blood and liver cells. Beets contain a fair amount of sugar, and this explains their pleasant taste. It is an oddity that commercial beets often contain added sugar, usually in the form of corn syrup. This is nutritional travesty, since there is an abundance of natural sweetness in beets without the adulteration.

Beets are a significant source of minerals and are particularly rich in phosphorus, which they aggressively concentrate from the soil. They are also high in iron and contain a fair amount of copper. Potassium is their most significant mineral, and one source indicates that it accounts for some 20% of dry weight. A cup of raw beets contains the potassium equivalent of two small bananas. Fresh beets also contain valuable amounts of vitamin C and folic acid. Since all of these nutrients are readily lost in cooking, save the beet juice and add it to soups and sauces or, better yet, drink it.

Beets and beet tops have been a favorite remedy of herbalists and physicians, as well as common folk, since the earliest times. The Romans and Greeks dispensed beets for dozens of illnesses. Records from the 16th century indicate that beet juice was dripped into the ear to cure ear aches. Beets and beet juice have also been used to eradicate gallstones, kidney stones, bladder disorders, and kidney disease. In early America colonial physicians recommended fresh beet juice for combating headaches and toothaches. Recently, researchers have determined that beet concentrates are useful in reversing the toxicity of x-irradiation and chemical poisoning.

Top Beet Tips

1. If possible, always serve beets with beet tops. This increases their nutritional value ten-fold. Clean the tops and roots thoroughly. Cook the root portion in a minimum of water just until tender, cool with cold water, and peel the stem and skin. Gently steam the tops. Remove from heat and serve with sliced or chopped beet root while the greens are still brightly colored and crisp. Add vinegar and chopped onions for additional flavor.

2. Use fresh beets whenever possible. Some brands of canned beets are acceptable, but most commercial beet products, such as pickled or diced beets, contain added sugar in the form of cane sugar, beet sugar, or corn syrup. Pickle your own beets in vinegar and spices. Beets are naturally sweet, so why add sugar?

3. Add beet tops to salads. There is a greater amount of nutrients in the tops than all of the other ingredients of a typical dinner salad combined. Shredded beets also make an excellent addition to salads and offer natural sweetness. Remember, commercial salad dressings contain sugar. So, instead of using these drizzle vinegar and extra virgin olive oil; add shredded or sliced beets for sweetness.

4. If beets are boiled, do not discard the juice. Either drink it right away, or decant it and use it later in soups or salads. The majority of the nutrients are found in the juice.

5. For a quick, refreshing, and nutritious "salad," try adding diced pickled beets in whole fat cottage cheese. The fat in cottage cheese extracts the pigments in the beets and helps accelerate their absorption into the blood. Beets provide that sweetness of the typical cottage cheese and fruit salad but with much less sugar than fruit.

6. Soup is perhaps the most ideal way to serve beets. By retaining the cooking fluids, all of the nutrients and pigments within beets are preserved. The pigments are the primary source of the curative power, and they are readily lost in cooking and processing. This is apparent simply by placing beets on the plate; the pigment leaches from the beets onto the dish. Beets may be added to any soup, but they lend themselves particularly well to cabbage soup, known in Europe as borscht.

7. Beets are the perfect side dish when serving fish. This combination is an old European tradition. Remember the previous discussion about choline? Fish is one of the richest dietary sources of this nutrient. The betaine in beets and the choline in fish work synergistically for aiding

protein synthesis and liver function. For Europeans, who love fish and beets, it wasn't research but was instead common sense and instinct which determined a simple fact: that beets and fish are good for overall health.

8. To retain the beautiful color of the beet root, add some form of acid such as vinegar or lemon juice. It also helps diminish the earthy flavor of fresh beets.

Top Beet Cures

1. If you have liver disease, eat beets as often as possible. The health benefits will be accelerated if the beets are cooked with the tops. Beets contain a chemical called betaine, which exerts special protective actions on liver cells. Betaine greatly aids in the regeneration of this organ. This choline-like molecule functions in part by assisting protein synthesis and fat metabolism. Since betaine is similar in structure to choline, the regenerative effects are potentiated by eating choline rich foods. Such foods include eggs, organic liver, soy beans, wheat germ, rice bran, and fresh meat. Lecithin is an ideal choline supplement. Yet, not all lecithin is the same. Much of the lecithin available in the market contains oil residues, or oil is added during manufacture or encapsulation. Refined vegetable oils may induce spoilage, causing the lecithin molecules to become rancid. Granular or dry lecithin is the obvious answer to this dilemma. *Nutri-Sense* is an excellent supplement offering a high concentration of natural lecithin in a pure granular form, plus it contains the naturally occurring lecithin found in rice germ and bran. With Nutri-Sense you receive a double dose of natural lecithin from two unique sources. Take three tablespoons per day in milk, juice, soup, hot cereal, or water to gain a power-packed natural choline boost.

Choline, as found in lecithin, is invaluable for brain function. Scientists at Massachusetts Institute of Technology found that the consumption of lecithin dramatically improves nerve transmission in the brain by increasing the synthesis of the critical brain chemical acetylcholine. The synthesis of this critical substance is also highly dependent upon thiamine and pantothenic acid. This means that Nutri-Sense, rich in B vitamins and lecithin, is pure brain nourishment.

It must be remembered that our livers are under siege. Every day they are being bombarded with all manner of poisons. America is one of the most toxic regions in the world, and this means that the livers of virtually all Americans are toxic. While the liver possesses great regenerative powers, eventually the toxic burden overwhelms it, and dysfunction or disease results. Beets, betaine, lecithin, and choline, taken on a daily basis, will help the liver reverse much of the toxic damage.

2. Beets work best in ameliorating liver disease if combined with fat. Eat beets with full fat cottage cheese. This fat/beet combination aids in the delivery of the active ingredients of beets to the liver. If adding beets to salad, be sure to also add extra virgin olive oil.

3. Be aware that when eating large quantities of beets, the pigment may reappear in the urine or stool. In particular, if the stools turn dark or have a reddish color after eating beets, don't become alarmed and think it is blood. The pigment is never totally digested, and it is normal for it to appear in the stool.

4. If you are anemic, eat beets. They contain chemicals which stimulate the formation of red blood cells. To be effective a considerable amount must be consumed: at least one bunch of fresh beets or three cans of beets daily—no sugar added.

5. Beets are an ideal vegetable for combating cancer or for preventing cancer. According to the herbal researcher Joseph Kadans, PhD, fresh mashed beets are effective in the treatment of solid tumors as well as leukemia. The trick is to eat enough of them: those who overcame cancer ate 2 pounds of mashed beets daily. A superior formula would be to include the tops with the beets. The tops would obviously taste better steamed with a bit of butter or olive oil along with your choice of spices.

6. If your nerves are on edge or if you are irritable, moody, depressed, or anxious, try eating beets on a daily basis. Eat a meal of beets plus fish every day. The betaine in beets fights nervous disorders, as does the choline in fish. Both betaine and choline are necessary for the production of neurotransmitters, the chemicals responsible for maintaining the channels of communication within the nervous system. Choline is a component of naturally occurring fats, and, thus, it is found in the richest amounts in fatty fish. Salmon, albacore tuna, sardines, bluefish, herring, mackerel, and anchovies are richest in choline. Another way to receive the betaine/choline combination is to add beets to omelets or to serve them as a side dish with eggs. Eggs are the richest dietary source of choline. Eaten together, they give the nervous system an immense boost.

85

Blueberry

These tasty and nutritious berries grow on shrubs native to North America. They may be found growing wild in the Northern reaches of the United States, as well as Canada, and are raised commercially primarily in Michigan, Maine, and New Jersey. Interestingly, blueberries are one of the few fruits which are exclusively North America in origin, although a close relative, the bilberry, grows wild in Europe.

Blueberries were a favorite food of Native Americans, who used them to make pemmican, which is a combination of dried meat, meat fat, and berries. Native Americans sun dried the meat and berries, ground them together, and mixed them with fat. The animal fat acted as a natural preservative, extending the shelf life of the mixture indefinitely.

Commercial blueberries are less nutritious than the wild type. Only commercial berries are readily available. However, few people realize that much of the modern blueberry crop comes from "wild" commercial blueberry plants not found in plantations, in other words, plants which have grown voluntarily as a result of the dissemination of the seeds by animals, birds, wind, and weather. As a result, it may not be necessary to forage in order to eat wild berries.

Blueberries are one of Nature's finest fruits in terms of curative powers. According to herbalist Dr. Joseph Kadans blueberries are notable for their ability to purify the blood as well as their antiseptic powers. C.B. Harris mentions in *Kitchen Remedies* that they have been utilized historically as a tonic for the kidneys, because they promote the healthy flow of urine. Blueberries also help block the formation of kidney stones. They have also been found invaluable in the treatment of diabetes. A book on herbal pharmacy from the 1940s describes how blueberries successfully cured a number of cases of diabetes. The cure was even more effective when an extract of the fresh leaves was dispensed. There is one problem with the blueberry remedy: being fruit, blueberries, contain a fair amount of sugar, and this restricts their use in diabetes. The exception might be wild blueberries, which are lower in sugar or, preferably, herbal tea made from blueberry leaves.

Perhaps the reason blueberries are so valuable for diabetics is that they are rich in manganese, a mineral needed for carbohydrate metabolism. Horatio Wood, author of a 1940s natural medicine textbook, attributes the anti-diabetic action to an unknown substance called *myritillin*, named after blueberry's botanical name *Vaccinium myrtillus*. Researchers have yet to discover just what this substance is, but one fact is certain: it does help normalize blood sugar levels.

Contrary to popular belief blueberries are relatively low in calories. In fact, they are lower in sugar than many fruits, being less than 15% sugar. They contain a fair amount of niacin, vitamin C, and iron. Furthermore, they are one of the few fruits rich in manganese. Incredibly, a heaping cup of blueberries contains as much as one half milligram, which is about 30% of the daily need. While wild blueberries are relatively rich in vitamin C, commercial blueberries are not a dependable source, unless they are eaten freshly picked.

Blueberries' greatest nutritional strength comes from substances other than vitamins and minerals: they are rich in pigments called *anthocyanosides*, a category of bioflavonoids. This is where the greatest curative powers of blueberries arise. All berries contain anthocyanosides, but the greatest concentrations are found in wild berries. However, commercial berries also contain valuable amounts. The type found in blueberries has a particularly critical effect upon the eyes. Perhaps this is why wild creatures that depend upon these berries, such as birds, bear, and deer, have such stupendous vision. The anthocyanosides are particularly important for enhancing night vision. It has long been known that the eye contains a substance called *visual purple*. This substance is found within the retina, primarily in tiny organelles called rods. When light passes into the eye, it strikes the retina and enters the rods. These rods act to decode the light message and help the brain interpret it. In essence, the rods act as an absorptive surface, capturing the light long enough so that the nervous system can interpret the message. The rods are ultra sensitive to light and are able to absorb it to such a degree that they give humans the power to see even in the most dim light. Without them, night vision is dramatically diminished. Here is the point; when light strikes the rods, visual purple, which is a purple colored chemical found within them, is activated. It then sends chemical messages to the brain, describing what the eye is seeing. Ultimately, as a result of repeated exposure to light, the visual purple is depleted, and it must be replaced for night vision to remain normal. The warning signs of visual purple deficiency include night blindness, sensitivity of the eyes to bright light (especially at night), tired feeling or heaviness of the eyes, spots before the eyes, nearsightedness, and farsightedness.

Other organs besides the eyes benefit from blueberry antioxidants. A recent U.S. government study found that of some forty fruits and vegetables tested blueberries were the most potent in antioxidant action. Incredibly, about one-half cup of blueberries showed more antioxidant strength than the RDA of vitamin E or C.

People who work with bright lights, such as photographers, computer operators, and TV crews, are highly vulnerable to developing visual purple deficiency. Fluorescent lighting also accelerates its destruction. The primary nutrients needed for the synthesis of visual purple are vitamin A, zinc, riboflavin, and anthocyanosides. Regarding the latter, blueberries are the top dietary source, because they contain a special type of anthocyanoside which is utilized directly in the formation of visual purple. It should be no surprise that purple colored berries, particularly blueberries, blackberries, mulberries, boysenberries, and bilberries, are richest in the substances which feed visual purple. Thus, it is a simple rule that if you eat purple pigments of any sort, it will aid in visual purple formation. The darker berries are in color the more helpful they will be in enhancing vision. Blueberries are among the darkest.

It makes sense that if an individual has a "pigment" deficiency, the best way to correct it would be to eat pigment. This is why the anthocyanosides are so valuable. These fruit pigments rapidly regenerate visual purple, resulting in virtually an immediate improvement in vision. The rate of improvement is dependent upon the severity of deficiency. In some individuals it may take weeks or months to fully restore the levels of visual purple to normal.

An additional benefit is due to the role played by anthocyanosides in strengthening the walls of blood vessels, especially the tiny ones that supply the eyeball. Known as capillaries, these are the tiniest blood vessels of the body, and they serve it by coursing tortuously over untold billions of miles. They are found in a high density in regions requiring large amounts of oxygen such as the eyes and brain.

Anthocyanosides found in commercial and wild berries are useful for virtually any visual disturbance ranging from night blindness to macular degeneration because of their immense role in improving capillary circulation. If vitamin A and riboflavin are added to the protocol, the beneficial effects upon both circulation and visual purple formation will be greatly accelerated. It is reasonable to presume that almost any visual disturbance will improve if fresh wild or commercial berries are regularly consumed.

Top Blueberry Tips

1. When buying blueberries be sure to look for bruising or mold. Blueberries are "out of season" for the vast majority of the year. Hence, in order to make them available all year they are stored for prolonged periods. Do not buy blueberries that appear wilted, and return them if they are moldy. Be sure to eat them soon after purchasing, because they spoil readily.

It is interesting to note that wild blueberries are highly resistant to spoiling. Once I kept a bowl of wild blueberries refrigerated for over three months, and they were still unspoiled and edible.

2. Add blueberries to hot cereal; use them in place of sweeteners. They not only taste luscious but enliven the appearance of the cereal. Oat bran, Red River, and Triple Bran are three excellent high fiber-low starch cereals which taste wonderful with blueberries. Add Nutri-Sense to the cereal to enhance the B vitamin content (see the section on rice bran).

3. When making the batter for muffins, pancakes, or waffles, always add blueberries. Baking enhances the digestibility of blueberries, liberating the anthocyanosides. Furthermore, it is healthier to rely on the natural sweetness of blueberries and reduce the amount of sweetener used in baking.

4. The traditional recipe of blueberries and cream is a nutritionally sound dessert. This is because the fat in cream helps liberate certain nutrients in the blueberries that are fat loving. These nutrients include beta carotene, anthocyanosides, and bioflavonoids. Have you ever noticed how cream turns blue when it is added to the berries, whereas if you add only water, the water won't be deeply colored? This is evidence of the fat in cream liberating the fat-soluble nutrients from the berries.

5. Don't overdo it with blueberries. Have them as an occasional treat, and use them in baked goods, while reducing the amount of added sweetener. Blueberries contain a fair amount of natural sugar, and cooking increases

the sugar content. It is possible to overdo it on sweet fruits, especially if you are sensitive to sugar; and who isn't? However, with wild blueberries picked right off the bush you can eat as much as you desire.

6. If you are eating blueberries to improve vision, be sure to add vitamin A, riboflavin, and zinc. This nutritional foursome aids in reversing practically every conceivable eye condition, including night blindness, nearsightedness, farsightedness, uveitis, iritis, and macular degeneration. Nutritional supplements may be of value; for vitamin A, use cod liver or halibut liver oil, and for zinc, use chelated zinc. Foods rich in vitamin A include organic liver, butter, eggs, and fatty fish. Foods rich in zinc include fresh meats, organ meats, eggs, crab, oysters, peanut butter, and tahini.

It is important to realize that the absorption and utilization of synthetic riboflavin is questionable. Food sources are organ meats, eggs, cheese, and fresh whole milk. Remember that riboflavin is easily destroyed by light, making it perhaps one of the most difficult of all vitamins to sufficiently ingest.

7. Blueberries are a preferred fruit for individuals suffering from diabetes or individuals blood sugar disturbances. This is because they are lower in sugar than the more commonly consumed fruits such as apples, oranges, cherries, pineapple, and grapes. However, if the blood sugar is completely out of control, as occurs in severe diabetes, don't eat blueberries or any other type of fruit. Eat instead sweet tasting vegetables such as red bell peppers, yellow bell peppers, fennel, tomatoes, and romaine lettuce or low sugar fruit such as grapefruit and melons. Despite their sweet taste these fruits and vegetables are relatively low in sugar and may be well tolerated by diabetics and hypoglycemics. Yet, raw wild blueberries are assuredly the best type for diabetics. Wild blueberries contain substances which are beneficial in the treatment of diabetes, and they are lower in sugar and richer in trace minerals than cultivated berries. They are particularly curative for hypoglycemia.

Broccoli

The name broccoli is derived from a Latin term, meaning "branch or arm." The Romans named it after observing that broccoli spears resembled the branches of trees. Most reports place broccoli's origin in Europe, probably Italy, where it was apparently developed from wild cabbage, although some believe it to be originally a Middle Eastern or North African plant.

Broccoli is a newcomer to America and has been grown commercially only since the 1920s. It became popular during the 1960s and 70s but reached its height in the 1980s, when consumption increased by some 800%. Contrary to popular belief, broccoli is not a vegetable, but it is a flower. Botanically, it consists of "aborted flowers," that is little buds of sterile flowers.

Lindelaur, one the modern world's first nutritionists, called broccoli the "perfect...food." He correctly observed that it is extremely rich in vitamins and minerals, especially vitamin C, vitamin A, folic acid, pyridoxine, calcium, magnesium, potassium, and sulphur. Broccoli is unusually rich in vitamin C; one cup contains more vitamin C than two oranges. Like all heavily colored vegetables, it is rich in bioflavonoids. Broccoli is one of the few vegetables high in protein, containing more per serving than corn, the latter being traditionally regarded as a good vegetable source. Yet, broccoli contains additional compounds which may prove of greater value than even its vitamin, mineral, or protein content. These compounds are known as *indoles*. The indoles are specialized chemicals which are highly effective in protecting human cells against cancer. Yet another compound, *sulforaphane*, blocks cancer by stimulating the liver to produce protective enzymes such as glutathione. These actions may explain why in societies where broccoli is a regular part of the menu the cancer incidence is low.

Broccoli is an excellent source of minerals. It is particularly rich in calcium. A large serving (1½ cups) contains about 200 mg of this mineral. Broccoli also contains significant quantities of potassium and magnesium. It is one of the rare vegetables which supplies a worthy amount of zinc and copper, and, with the exception of turnip greens, it is the richest vegetable source of these minerals.

To achieve the top benefits of broccoli's calcium content, be sure to eat only fresh broccoli, because up to 60% of the calcium is lost when broccoli is frozen. Furthermore, calcium is water soluble, and much of it is leached into cooking water. Reserve the cooking water, and use it in soups or sauces to gain the greatest benefits of broccoli's intense nutritional powers.

On the negative side broccoli is high in goitrogens, which interfere with thyroid function. Goitrogens impede the absorption and utilization of iodine, which is essential for normal thyroid function. Fortunately, the majority of goitrogens are inactivated by cooking.

Top Broccoli Tips

1. Never eat raw broccoli. It is indigestible unless cooked. Raw broccoli is not only difficult to digest, but it also contains tiny microscopic spicules which may irritate or damage the digestive tract. Furthermore, · the vitamins and other therapeutic substances in raw broccoli, especially the indoles, vitamin E, vitamin K, and beta carotene, are poorly absorbed, since they are bound firmly to its fibrous elements. These substances are liberated through cooking. As mentioned previously raw broccoli also contains the anti-thyroid goitrogens, which are readily destroyed by cooking.

2. Be sure to cook broccoli in a small amount of water. There is no reason to boil it for prolonged periods in a large amount of water, that is cooking it until it turns to mush. This leads to losses of up to 90% of its nutrients. Rather, to cook it properly, heat for just a few minutes. Steam it or boil it gently in a small amount of water. Cook it only until it turns bright green. When the color change occurs, turn the heat off immediately. At this point it should be firm or crisp. The small amount of water that remains should either be drunk or reserved for soups or sauces.

3. Try the scalding method for cooking broccoli. Simply heat a small amount of water, $1/2$ cup or less, in a one or two quart pot until boiling. Immerse broccoli and continue heating until the color changes to bright green. This type of cooking minimizes nutrient loss. Serve hot with butter and salt. Be sure to drink the mineral/vitamin rich water which remains after it cools.

4. Don't just eat the sweet tips of broccoli. Cook and eat also the stems. While lower in vitamins and minerals, the stems provide valuable fiber and are, in fact, a superior source of fiber than bran. This is because vegetable fibers are less harsh on the digestive tract and are partially digestible, which makes them a more valuable source of nutrients than indigestible fiber sources such as psyllium and wheat bran.

5. Feel free to serve broccoli with fats that are traditionally served with it. Yes, it is perfectly fine to melt a pat or two of butter on broccoli spears. Fat aids in the absorption of the vitamin A (in the form of beta carotene). Alternative fats in the event of butter or cow's milk allergy include extra virgin olive oil, hazelnut oil, avocado oil, and coconut fat. The latter tastes similar to butter when melted over broccoli. Another method is to cook broccoli directly in the fat by adding a few pats of butter, a tablespoon of coconut fat, or a few tablespoons of extra virgin olive oil. Simply cook the broccoli in the oil until the color changes to bright green.

6. If cooking broccoli on the grill (it tastes wonderful when prepared in this manner), be sure to brush it with extra virgin olive oil, coconut fat, or pure butter. These oils enhance the richness of taste, and the oil also protects the vitamins from being destroyed by heat.

7. When preparing stir fry don't forget to add broccoli. Broccoli tips enhance the taste of any stir fry dish and provide valuable vitamins and minerals that are retained within the stir fry sauce.

8. Don't buy broccoli that is discolored. It should be green throughout with no brown or yellow spots. Blemished broccoli could carry disease, but usually it is an indication of a lack of freshness and, therefore, a loss in nutrient content, especially vitamin C. Untarnished fully green broccoli contains a better complement of antioxidants, because a reduction in the intensity of green means the antioxidants are depleted.

9. If cooking broccoli in a pot, be sure to place it stems down. In other words, allow the florets to stand out of water. The reason is that the stems take longer to cook than the florets, and the latter usually get soggy by the time the stems are done. In this manner the florets will remain crisp.

10. To achieve the daily allowance for vitamin C, don't just rely on fruit. By weight, broccoli is richer in vitamin C than most fruit. A single spear contains over twice the RDA for the vitamin. To garnish the greatest amount be sure to use the cooking juice—that is where the majority of the vitamin C will be found.

Top Broccoli Cures

1. If you have difficulty relaxing at night, eat broccoli for supper. The high content of calcium will help relax the nervous system. Calcium is a natural sedative.

2. If you suffer from constipation, eat broccoli twice daily and include the stems. To gain the greatest benefits from the fiber, be sure to cook it gently. If broccoli is served firm or slightly crunchy, the cooking process was correct. Here is the rule of thumb: if the broccoli is cooked properly, it should stand on end without buckling. If the stem buckles under its weight, it is overcooked.

3. Those who are stricken with cancer or who have a significant family history of cancer should eat broccoli every day or at a minimum three times weekly. Broccoli contains a plethora of anti-cancer substances, including vitamin C, bioflavonoids, beta carotene, calcium, vitamin E, and indoles, as well as specialized sulfur compounds known as sulforaphanes.

4. If your immune system is incapacitated, be sure to eat broccoli at least three times weekly. Add it to soups and stir-fry. The rich content of vitamins and minerals provides much needed nourishment to the immune organs, increasing their anti-infection and anti-cancer powers. The immune boosting power of broccoli should not be underestimated. In addition to its rich nutrient supply, which includes significant quantities of vitamin C, beta carotene, magnesium, potassium, and folic acid, it contains a plethora of anti-tumor substances, including chlorophyll, indoles, and sulfones.

5. If you have a sensitive stomach or an irritable colon, you will probably tolerate broccoli better than most other vegetables. This is partly due to the fact that broccoli is a flower rather than a vegetable, and it is quite gentle upon the gut. There is a word of caution: be sure to cook the broccoli (steaming is best). Raw broccoli may irritate the digestive tract in some individuals.

6. If you have a thyroid problem, never eat raw broccoli. Like all cruciferous plants, broccoli contains thiouracil derivatives, known commonly as goitrogens, which interfere with the synthesis of thyroid hormones. Cook the broccoli well (but don't murder it), since cooking destroys the goitrogens. Goitrogens are also neutralized by iodine, lending credence to cooking/serving broccoli with shrimp or fish. Remember, only salt water fish contain iodine.

94

7. For those suffering from bleeding disorders, such as bleeding gums, easy bruising, nose bleeds, or weak blood vessels, broccoli may provide relief. This is because it is inordinately rich in four key anti-bleeding nutrients: vitamin C, calcium, bioflavonoids, and vitamin K. Because of this, broccoli boosts the body's ability to reverse disordered blood clotting. Furthermore, it aids in the prevention of vascular diseases such as hardening of the arteries, vasculitis, edema, hemorrhoids, and varicose veins. The vitamin C and vitamin K in broccoli also protect against life threatening diseases such as heart attacks, internal hemorrhaging, bleeding ulcers, hardening of the arteries, blood clots, ulcerative colitis, and strokes. Eat broccoli on a daily basis if you suffer from any of these conditions.

Cabbage

Cabbage is an important food world-wide. A versatile plant, it grows in virtually all climates and is a staple of dozens of cultures, particularly European. It is believed that cabbage was first cultivated in the Mediterranean, where it was a favorite food of the Greeks and Romans. However, the type they consumed is entirely different than the kind we eat today; it was more leafy and herbal. For the Romans cabbage was the number one vegetable cure. The fact is cabbage has been consumed since time immemorial as a health food and medicine.

In Europe, as well as many other parts of the world, cabbage is perhaps the most popular vegetable. Eaten raw it is tangy, while when cooked, it becomes slightly but pleasantly sweet. When fermented it becomes incredibly sour.

Cabbage belongs to the cruciferous vegetables along with Brussels sprouts, cauliflower, kale, kohlrabi, and broccoli. While mostly fiber and water, it is relatively rich in vitamin C, containing over 50 milligrams in a four ounce serving. Red cabbage contains an even greater amount than the green type, offering over 100% of the RDA for vitamin C per four ounce serving. During the colonial era cabbage was used as a scurvy cure. Yet, it possesses chemicals of far greater import than the vitamin C content: the indoles. These nitrogenous compounds are regarded as among the most potent anti-cancer substances known.

Few people realize that cabbage is a good source of calcium; a large serving contains about 100 mg of the mineral. It is also relatively high in phosphorus and contains calcium and phosphorus in the perfect ratio: 2 to 1. Its potassium content is valuable. A large head of cabbage contains several thousand milligrams. Cabbage could be an excellent source of selenium, the anti-cancer mineral, depending upon where it is grown. The selenium content of food is directly correlated with soil concentrations. If the selenium content of the soil is high, cabbage aggressively concentrates it. For instance, cabbage grown in the selenium rich soils of Wyoming and the Dakotas in essence becomes a selenium supplement. Summer cabbage probably comes from California, but, unfortunately, selenium rich soil is found only in certain regions of California. Furthermore, agricultural practices have destroyed much of the soil selenium. During the winter the majority of the cabbage comes from California, Florida, and Texas. Cabbage grown in Texas is most likely rich in selenium, since the soil is abundant in this mineral.

Cabbage is unusually high in a number of other trace minerals, including iodine, chlorine, and sulfur. Regarding minerals perhaps its greatest nutritional claim is related to its sulfur content in which it is inordinately rich. The sulfur acts as an antiseptic, plus it is used by the body for the synthesis of valuable proteins needed for structure and immunity. Sulfur is also responsible for the disconcerting intestinal gas that cabbage often produces. Cabbage rich in selenium is a super-nutrition food; the selenium and sulfur work in unison in the formation of tissue proteins and in the prevention of degenerative disease.

Top Cabbage Tips

1. Follow the old European adage and add cabbage to soups. Instinctively, Europeans realized that the rich nutrition of cabbage would be compromised by cooking it in water and discarding the fluid. They conserved the nutrients by adding cabbage to soups. Thus, the vitamin content is retained where it is best served: within the human body, not down the sink.
2. Don't throw away the outer dark green leaves of cabbage. Remove and discard any discolored portions; wash thoroughly and then eat them,

either raw or cooked. The outer leaves contain the richest supply of vitamins, particularly vitamin K and vitamin C. In fact, their vitamin K and C content may be as much as twelve times greater than that of the inner leaves. That dark color is providing an important clue.

3. When making cole slaw be sure to add plenty of lemon juice or vinegar. Both help prevent the cabbage from oxidizing (or discoloring) by blocking the loss of valuable vitamins.

4. Sauerkraut is an excellent way to consume cabbage. Because it is fermented, it is easier to digest than raw cabbage. Furthermore, sauerkraut contains the additional benefit not found in plain cabbage: Lactobacillus acidophilus bacteria. In fact, sauerkraut is one of the top dietary sources of natural acidophilus. These bacteria are useful to us, because they help maintain ideal health in the intestinal tract by inhibiting the growth of harmful microbes. Researchers have determined that the regular intake of acidophilus bacteria greatly strengthens immunity. Furthermore, the consumption of acidophilus blocks the development of a variety of diseases of the digestive tract, notably, irritable bowel syndrome, gastritis, esophagitis, diverticulitis, constipation, pancreatitis, and hepatitis. Even seemingly unrelated disorders, such as acne, eczema, psoriasis, and staph infection, improve with the acidophilus dispensation. Acidophilus also exerts significant protection against intestinal cancer as well as stomach cancer. Thus, with sauerkraut the individual gains a double effect: the anti-cancer powers of the cabbage plus the cancer fighting capacities of the acidophilus. However, after serving sauerkraut be sure to drink the leftover juice: it is rich in nutrients as well as acidophilus.

5. Fresh cabbage juice should be consumed immediately; don't refrigerate it for later use. The active ingredients in the juice are rapidly destroyed by exposure to the elements; the vitamin C and vitamin K are particularly vulnerable. If you make more than you can drink, add lemon juice or vinegar. They act as a preservatives and help prevent the loss of nutrients.

6. Certain individuals with sensitive stomachs or irritable intestines are unable to tolerate cabbage and sauerkraut. The intolerance, which may be manifested by bloating or gas, can be minimized by taking digestive enzymes with meals. Try a high quality plant-based digestive enzyme, two or three capsules with each cabbage-containing meal.

7. Use red cabbage as a frequent addition to vegetable dishes. This type of cabbage contains a higher content of vitamin C and bioflavonoids than the

green variety. Shred the cabbage and add it to stir fry and soup. Top salads with a generous portion of shredded red cabbage. This will provide much needed natural vitamin C plus valuable anti-aging and anti-cancer bioflavonoids.

Top Cabbage Cures

1. For stomach ulcers cabbage is the ideal remedy. More importantly, drink cabbage juice. Cheney's monumental research, performed at Stanford University in the 1950s, thoroughly documented that cabbage juice healed stomach ulcers. Cheney studied a number of humans with stomach ulcers, proven on x-rays, and attempted a cabbage cure. After the administration of several cups of fresh cabbage juice made from green cabbage, he repeated the x-rays. Amazingly, he found that the x-rays were negative: the cabbage juice induced complete healing of the stomach ulcers. Dr. Cheney recorded cases where ulcers healed completely in as little as 7 days.

No one knows for sure why cabbage juice heals ulcers. There may be a yet to be discovered protein, perhaps a growth factor, which induces the healing. Possibly, the rich mineral content of cabbage heals the gut wall and helps normalize digestion. Cheney coined the term "vitamin U" for the substance. Perhaps it is the vitamin C, bioflavonoids, folic acid, sulfated amino acids, or vitamin K that is responsible, or perhaps it is a joint effort of all of these compounds. Some researchers claim that vitamin U is actually a compound known as *S-adenosylmethionine*, which is, in fact, an amino acid. What matters is that it works and is non-toxic.

The treatment must be administered as follows: take several heads of cabbage (organically raised is preferable) and wash thoroughly. Chop the cabbage into thick slices and run through the juicer. Make one liter of cabbage juice daily and be sure to drink it that day. Continue this treatment for 2 weeks. The ulcer should heal completely.

Only raw cabbage is capable of inducing ulcer healing. No matter how much cooked cabbage or sauerkraut you eat, it will fail to produce this effect. Eating raw cabbage might help somewhat, but you have to eat a great deal of it, like a head of cabbage a day. Eating that amount might create discomfort, gas, or bloating. When the fiber is removed, as in juicing, the digestive side effects are essentially eliminated.

2. If you have a cold or flu and lack an appetite, try munching on raw cabbage, especially the purple variety. Raw cabbage is inordinately rich in vitamin C, and it also contains substances which soothe the stomach, normalize appetite, and rejuvenate energy reserves.

3. If you are constipated, drink sauerkraut juice. Drink one can every morning until the constipation is resolved. This beverage provides natural laxative action plus much needed acidophilus bacteria, which increase the natural bulk of the stool. The laxative action of sauerkraut juice is likely due to its high content of acetylcholine, an important nutrient which is a tonic for the nerves. Acetylcholine acts directly upon the nerves of the digestive tract, increasing the secretion of digestive juices and stimulating the movement of the colon.

4. If you have cancer or if there is a significant family history of cancer, you must eat cabbage regularly. This is because cabbage possesses a plethora of anti-cancer chemicals, the most powerful of which are known as indoles. The fact is cabbage contains a higher percentage of indoles per weight than virtually any other food. It also contains a variety of sulfated amino acids, all of which exhibit anti-cancer action.

5. If you have a poor appetite and can't stand the thought of eating breakfast, try eating a wedge of raw cabbage upon arising. Cabbage contains chemicals which stimulate stomach and digestive function, and this leads to the creation of a vigorous appetite. Eat a wedge of cabbage a day for one or two weeks, and you'll relish the thought of eating and find that you cannot live without it.

6. Cabbage effectively fights pancreatic disease. A liter of fresh cabbage juice per day is an effective remedy for pancreatitis. Usually, when individuals with pancreatitis are hospitalized they are placed on an "n.p.o." diet, meaning they are given nothing by mouth. This is a judicious prescription. However, when no other food or beverage can be tolerated, green cabbage juice is usually readily digested. Cabbage juice may also be helpful in early pancreatic cancer. Furthermore, cabbage and cabbage juice are ideal remedies for fighting cancer-induced loss of weight, strength, and appetite, a condition known as *cachexia*. The juice is superior versus the plain vegetable as an anti-cancer remedy, since juicing concentrates large amounts of the active ingredients. Regular consumption of prodigious amounts of cabbage and cabbage juice is perhaps the most effective remedy for preventing pancreatic cancer.

There is one precaution with consuming large amounts of raw cabbage. Like all cruciferous vegetables, raw cabbage contains chemicals which block the function of the thyroid gland (i.e. goitrogens). Individuals with a history of low thyroid function may be unable to tolerate large amounts of it. If you have a thyroid condition and wish to eat/drink large quantities of cabbage, iodine must be consumed contiguously. Iodine neutralizes much of the goitrogenic effects of raw cabbage. Be sure to salt the cabbage or cabbage juice with iodized or sea salt, and take at least .5 mg of natural iodine per day if you are a regular consumer of cabbage. Another means of neutralizing goitrogens is to eat iodine rich foods such as herring, ocean (versus farm raised) shrimp, halibut, and crab. Add seaweed to soups, or eat the oriental Miso soup. Ideally, the cabbage remedy should be utilized short term, for instance, a glass of cabbage juice per day for one or two weeks. This prescription may be repeated occasionally.

8. Cabbage should be a regular part of the diet for anyone with a family history of breast cancer. Cabbage contains compounds which help normalize estrogen synthesis. In other words, eating cabbage may help prevent the buildup of excessive amounts of estrogen, and this significantly diminishes the risk for developing breast cancer.

Cantaloupe

Cantaloupe is an immensely valuable food and is one of the most nutritious of all fruits. While it is becoming increasingly popular, few people appreciate the enormity of its nutritional content.

Despite its rich, sweet taste cantaloupe is low in calories, containing a mere 190 calories for an entire melon. It is mostly water and is excellent for hydration. A half cantaloupe gives the entire RDA for beta carotene and a greater amount of potassium than three bananas. Cantaloupe provides significant quantities of pyridoxine, with a half cantaloupe providing over 30% of the RDA. It is one of the few fruits containing good amounts of biotin; a half cantaloupe is 300% richer in this nutrient than an orange. It is also an excellent source of folic acid; a large cantaloupe contains over 100 mcg, which is one-third the RDA. The vitamin C content is tremendous; 8 ounces (about 1/2 cantaloupe) provides 90 mg, the equivalent of a large sun-ripened orange. Cantaloupe contains such a unique array of nutrients that it should be regularly included in the menu perhaps more so than any other fruit. Indeed, cantaloupe is the most nutrient dense of all melons.

Cantaloupe makes a refreshing addition to virtually any meal. It is easy to digest and is usually well tolerated even by those with sensitive stomachs. It is an ideal fruit for infants and children, because, while it is sweet in taste, it is lower in sugar than the usual fruits children eat. Plus, it is higher in nutrients than apples, oranges, bananas, peaches, and pears. This is certainly one of the most nutritious and readily digested of all fruit.

Top Cantaloupe Tips

1. The taste of cantaloupe depends upon ripeness as well as the way it is grown and the type of soil it is grown upon. To detect a ripe cantaloupe first smell it. If it smells sweet, then it is ripe. If there is no or a slightly sweet odor, then it is green and the taste will be compromised. If it smells musty, then it may be overripe and moldy. The best place to smell is the bare end where the vine attaches. Another hint is to look for cantaloupe with orange color on the skin. Firmness is another guide. If the cantaloupe is rock hard, it is unripe. If it gives a bit, it is ripe. If it is soggy, it is too ripe.
2. Cantaloupe is available in most supermarkets all year, but the winter varieties are less tasty and often moldy. This is because growers store summer cantaloupe for the winter market.
3. The nutrients in cantaloupe, particularly the vitamin C, potassium, and beta carotene, may be rapidly lost once it is cut open. One way you can keep the remainder fresh is to add a wedge of lemon or lime. The antioxidants in the lemon and lime prevent spoilage by minimizing the loss of valuable vitamins and minerals.
4. Make sure the cantaloupe is washed thoroughly before slicing. Cantaloupe is the fruit of a vine, and, thus, it lies on the ground. As a result, it is often contaminated by microbes. In fact, thousands of instances of food poisoning have been traced to unclean cantaloupe. If there is obvious dirt or sand, scrub it with a brush. Even if it appears clean it should be well rinsed. One way to ensure sterility is to dip the cantaloupe in a solution of water and oil of oregano. Simply add a few

drops of oil of oregano to a half gallon of water. Dip and scrub the cantaloupe with the water. This method may be used to sterilize any fruit or vegetable. Oil of oregano is non-toxic. Do not use bleach. It is toxic: when used on vegetation, it destroys, that is oxidizes, the vitamins, minerals, and proteins.

5. Use cantaloupe as a main ingredient in fruit salad. Dice a half or whole cantaloupe and add to any fruit salad recipe. Top with ground nuts and/or whipping cream, if desired. The fat aids in beta carotene absorption. Make melon salad from equal parts of cantaloupe, watermelon, and honeydew melon.

6. Children tolerate cantaloupe exceedingly well, and it is a healthy alternative to citrus fruit or apples. The latter is more likely to cause allergic reactions, and allergy to cantaloupe is relatively rare. Plus, although cantaloupe is sweet tasting, it is much lower in sugar than the typical fruit children eat. So, if your child is sensitive to sugar, feed him/her cantaloupe and other low sugar fruit such as honeydew melon, watermelon, papaya, and grapefruit.

7. For a fruit treat filled with pyridoxine eat cantaloupe and avocado, both of which are rich in this nutrient. Simply cut a cantaloupe in half, seed, and fill the center with diced avocado. Or, dice both and eat as a fruit salad topped generously with filberts (which are also rich in B_6). This Pyridoxine Fruit Salad provides fully half the RDA for this nutrient.

Top Cantaloupe Cures

1. If you have a heart problem or high blood pressure, cantaloupe is perhaps the number one fruit to eat. This is because heart ailments are associated with potassium deficiency, and cantaloupe is exceedingly rich in this mineral. One whole cantaloupe contains as much potassium as several small bananas. Plus, it is rich in beta carotene and folic acid, which researchers have proven help prevent heart disease. If you are taking heart or high blood pressure medications, it is especially important to eat cantaloupe on a regular basis. A cantaloupe per day is an appropriate dispensation. What a wonderful prescription this is; something healthy that the individual can actually look forward to. Heart patients need the extra potassium which cantaloupe supplies, because

virtually all cardiac medications deplete potassium, and the loss of this mineral further weakens cardiac function. Cantaloupe builds strong hearts by providing several nutrients known to aid cardiac function, including potassium, folic acid, beta carotene, and vitamin C.

2. Individuals with allergies benefit from cantaloupe. This is because it is one of the least likely fruits to cause allergic reactions. Plus, it contains an abundant supply of potassium, beta carotene, folic acid, bioflavonoids, and vitamin C. These nutrients strengthen immunity and boost adrenal function, and the result is enhancement of the body's ability to combat allergic reactions. While allergy to cantaloupe is uncommon, it does occur. If you tolerate it poorly, this may be a sign of mold sensitivity, since this fruit may grow mold especially if it is too ripe.

3. If you abhor eating breakfast and/or if your appetite in the morning is poor, try a half cantaloupe first thing. This is one of the easiest of all foods to digest, plus it is nutrient dense. Furthermore, it is mostly water, and, thus, it aids in hydration. As a result, it is highly refreshing and invigorating as a morning food. Potassium and folic acid, in which cantaloupe is rich, are digestive and energy stimulants.

4. Poor complexion is a sign of nutritional deficiency and, often, it signifies impaired circulation. Potassium deficiency is a likely cause of sluggish circulation, and, once the potassium level becomes normal, circulation is improved. The result is a vibrant complexion. In many respects, cantaloupe is essentially a tasty potassium supplement. To gain normal potassium levels, eat a cantaloupe per day for a month. Thereafter, be sure to eat at least one or two cantaloupe per week.

5. Cantaloupe is the fruit of choice for children who suffer from chronic respiratory infections such as ear aches, bronchitis, pneumonia, colds, or sore throat. While citrus fruit may aggravate these problems, cantaloupe eases them and enhances immunity. It is an ideal food and can be consumed in large amounts during respiratory infections or for any other childhood debilitation. For children a quarter or half of a cantaloupe per day will do more to help keep children free of medical need perhaps more than any other fruit.

Chicken and Chicken Soup

Grandma was correct when she made chicken soup to defeat disease. Yet, it is not just the chicken, but it is also what is put in the soup that makes the difference.

Chicken provides the body with much needed protein, as well as fatty acids, which are needed for fuel. Furthermore, chicken fat and skin are rich in an essential fatty acid known as linoleic acid. This fatty acid is needed for the formation of normal skin, hair, and nails. Plus, linoleic acid is a major building block needed for the synthesis of hormones as well as prostaglandins.

Cooking chicken as soup is the perfect medium for liberating its nutrients. Soup mobilizes the fuel fats and the linoleic acid. It renders the calcium, phosphorus, and magnesium readily available for digestion, because these minerals are extracted from the bones. Therefore, the broth is nutrient dense. To increase the nutrient density the chef adds all manner of vegetables, which disseminate their nutrients into the broth. The broth becomes veritably a nutritional power plant, rich in vitamins, minerals, proteins, and fatty acids. No wonder people have used chicken soup over the ages to ease the common cold or cure whatever might ail humanity.

Chicken is an excellent source of minerals, notably phosphorus, iron, copper, silicon, magnesium, and zinc. It is also a top source of vitamins B_6 and B_{12}, and it supplies high amounts of biotin, niacin, pantothenic acid, riboflavin, choline, and thiamine. In essence, chicken serves as a tasty B complex supplement. Furthermore, it is one of the few foods containing vitamin A, which is found in both the flesh and chicken fat.

After removing the fat, chicken is essentially pure protein. It has a higher protein content than virtually any other meat, and its protein is easily digested. According to K. Platt, M.D., author of *Food: Its Use and Abuse*, the digestibility of protein is a function of how long or short are the protein fibers within the meat. Chicken has short fibers, and white meat is shorter than dark meat. This becomes evident when the meat of chicken breast is lifted with a fork from the bone; the short fibers are readily seen when the meat is peeled off. What this means is that chicken protein is rapidly and efficiently digested, and this may be why it is so useful for sluggish immunity. The protein is needed for rebuilding immune cells, as well as antibodies, so that the invaders can be destroyed.

Top Chicken Tips

1. Make sure that the chicken carcass is thoroughly scrubbed and rinsed before cooking. This ensures removal of bacteria and parasites through the mechanical action of the scrubbing and rinsing. Then rub with oil of oregano for ultimate germ protection. Commercial poultry is commonly contaminated by microbes, and the risk of contracting infections can be dramatically reduced by carefully cleaning the carcass. Always clean hands thoroughly after dressing poultry. Also be sure to clean all work surfaces, since bacteria contamination can spread to other foods which are being prepared in the same work area.

2. Urge the supermarket to carry guaranteed chemical free or range fed chicken. This type of chicken is less likely to carry disease or microbial infection. Range fed/organic chickens roam free and eat their natural forage. They are not fed food laced with chemicals and antibiotics. The difference in taste alone is incredible. Remember that consumer demand dictates what is supplied in the market place. Your request does count, and good food is mandatory for good health.

3. Be sure to always cook chicken thoroughly. Never cook it in a microwave. The latter cannot dependably sterilize the meat as does normal cooking.

4. Cook chicken in soups as often as possible. Use the entire bird; there are valuable nutrients in the skin, flesh, and bones. Recent research documents how soup made with animal bones is super-rich in calcium. The calcium is readily leached from the bones into the broth, especially if acid is added to the soup such as tomato sauce or lemon juice.

5. Always cook poultry completely. Never cook it partially with the intention of finishing the job latter. Such a process encourages the growth of potentially toxic bacteria even if it is refrigerated.

6. When making dressing the safest method is to cook it separately, and add it to the bird when serving. The stuffing may interfere with the achievement of top core temperature for cooking the bird thoroughly, plus, the stuffing itself may not be thoroughly cooked.

7. Avoid commercial chicken livers. They often contain residues of antibiotics and steroids, which are added to the feed and are, therefore, concentrated in the liver. They are also heavily contaminated by microbes, some of which may cause cancer.

Top Chicken Cures

1. Make chicken soup whenever you have a cold or flu. In my first book, *How to Eat Right and Live Longer,* you will find a recipe called *Cure a Cold Chicken Soup.* About a year after this book was published I received a call from a colleague, a dentist in my locale. The dentist had contracted a cold and was suffering in utter misery. As she had a copy of the book, she decided to avail herself of the soup. She ecstatically reported, "I can't believe it, but in 24 hours I whipped this cold thanks to your soup." You too can defeat a cold, as well as the flu, with this soup. Since it is necessary to drink several cups of broth a day, be sure to make an extra large batch.

2. If you have blood sugar disturbances or if you are suffering from diabetes, eat chicken often as a snack. Since it is essentially devoid of carbohydrate, chicken is an ideal blood sugar controlling food and is particularly valuable for diabetics. Chicken is rich in protein and B vitamins, which makes it the ideal blood sugar balancing snack. Bake a tray of favorite chicken parts. Spice them with paprika, garlic, and onion powder. For additional taste and curative power, spice the chicken with HerbSorb. This nutritional supplement contains several herbs which combat both low and high blood sugar. *HerbSorb* consists of the edible herbs, fenugreek, coriander, cumin, black caraway, and cardamom, which make a luscious addition to virtually any menu, especially meat or starchy dishes. These herbs exert the added benefit of improving blood sugar control. Add HerbSorb to chicken recipes containing starchy foods such as rice, potatoes, whole grain pasta, and squash. Simply open the capsules and sprinkle the contents over the chicken parts or starchy dishes before cooking. Sprinkle it directly on chicken parts before baking. To help the spices hold better on the chicken, brush the chicken with extra virgin olive oil before sprinkling (See Appendix A).

3. If you can't sleep at night, eat your fill of chicken thighs or legs. Dark meat is high in niacin, thiamine, and amino acids, which relax the nervous system as well as improve blood sugar control. Be sure to salt the chicken, since sodium normalizes adrenal function, and this will help you to relax.

4. If your appetite is sluggish in the morning, try eating ground chicken patties. They are healthier than sausage and are essentially pure protein, which helps stimulate the flow of digestive juices. Eat one or two ground

106

chicken patties with a side order of eggs. This breakfast provides a tremendous boost in energy, as it is loaded with protein, minerals, and B vitamins. Plus, it helps curb the appetite, preventing uncontrollable snacking binges. As a result, the egg and chicken patty breakfast is an ideal one for those suffering from obesity and bulimia, and it is also valuable for sugar addicts.

5. Constant fatigue is often a sign of protein deficiency. Chicken is essentially pure protein and is one of the most readily digested types of protein. It is a complete protein, containing all eight essential amino acids.

The diet of the majority of Americans is excessively high in sugar and starch. The problem is that starchy foods displace more nutritious protein-rich foods. This is why the diet of the average American is relatively low in protein. Another reason it is low in protein is because of the current low fat craze. Foods that are high in fat, such as eggs, meat, cheese, and nuts, are the primary sources of protein. If high fat foods are avoided, so are high protein foods. Yet another factor is reticence to eat meat or other animal proteins. Tens of millions of Americans are either full fledged vegetarians or pseudo-vegetarians, the latter being those who occasionally eat meat such as chicken and fish. Because of these factors, low protein intake is exceedingly common. In some individuals the amount of protein consumed on a daily basis fails to meet even the minimum requirement. This reduced protein intake, if occurring continuously, will lead to ill health and may even cause permanent organ damage. Ironically, instead of eating high protein, such as eggs, fresh meat, poultry, fish, and milk products, the diet of the average American is rich in sugar, white flour products, and various junk/processed foods, all of which are low in protein. Since the high starch/sugar diet is a major cause of fatigue, eating chicken as a major portion will certainly provide an energy boost.

6. To increase nutritional stores of protein and vitamins it is important to eat meat, and chicken is one of the most readily digested of all types. An eight ounce serving supplies considerable nutritional density, accounting for virtually 50% of the minimum daily ration for protein, as well as the following minimal needs for vitamins and minerals:

      a) 30% of the phosphorus
      b) 40% of the iron

c) 3% of the vitamin A
d) 50% of the thiamine
e) 20% of the riboflavin
f) 60% of the niacin

The above is an average nutritional analysis for meat, and the percentages may vary slightly depending upon feeding practices and the type of meat. Even so, this is an incredible array of nutrients, which cannot be easily matched. A bowl of pasta or, for that matter, several bowls of pasta, is deficient in comparison to a half roasted chicken in terms of overall nutritional density.

Cilantro/Coriander

Cilantro is the Spanish term for an herb known in English as coriander. The plant originated in the Middle East. From there it was taken to Spain by Islamic conquerors. The Spaniards brought it to Central America, where it became a staple. When Mexicans use this term today they are referring to the leaves of the coriander plant, as this is the part they generally consume.

Coriander has been administered as a medicine since the earliest eras of human history. The early Greeks, Hebrews, and Hindus held it in the highest esteem and relied upon it as more of a medicine than a food. The fact that it was used in ancient Egypt is no surprise, since it is mentioned in the Old Testament and the Biblical prophets knew of it. Muhammad, after ruling out cancer, dispensed it as a cure for virtually all illnesses.

A member of the parsley family cilantro is more correctly described as an herb rather than a vegetable. It is rarely eaten by Americans, but Latinos utilize it regularly in a variety of dishes. The leaves exude a powerful smell and taste, due to the existence of a variety of volatile oils.

When eaten, cilantro/coriander behaves more like a medicine than food. For untold centuries it has been used as a digestive stimulant as well as a mild laxative. It is believed that coriander aids digestion and elimination in part by strengthening the intestinal muscles. Coriander invigorates metabolism and accelerates cellular actions. It nourishes and tones the nervous system. It fights inflammation and strengthens immunity. While these actions are largely a consequence of its essential oil content, a review of this herb's nutritional profile also tells why it is so valuable and curative. Cilantro leaves are one of the top sources of potassium. The fact is the only item which supercedes them is seaweed, which is rarely consumed except in the Orient. This means that cilantro leaves are the top supermarket food source for potassium. Cilantro leaves provide valuable fiber in a form which is gentle on the digestive tract. Yet, the seeds are even higher and are listed by Ensminger as the number one food source of edible fiber. Perhaps this explains why coriander seeds have long been used as a mild laxative.

Top Cilantro/Coriander Tips

1. Add cilantro as often as possible to milk products, particularly cheese, yogurt, and sour cream. The fat in milk helps preserve the delicate essential oils in cilantro. Plus, combing fat with cilantro aids in the absorption of the essential oils into the bloodstream. Chopped cilantro enlivens the taste of yogurt and sour cream, while significantly boosting the nutritional quality and can be used in the latter instead of chives.
2. Use all varieties of cilantro and coriander. Both fresh and dried leaves may be purchased. Powdered coriander seeds is an ideal spice for meat and vegetable dishes.
3. Store cilantro in brown paper bags, cellulose bags, or porous plastic bags. Commercial plastic bags exude hydrocarbon fumes, which deplete nutrients and damage the delicate essential oils. They also encourage microbial growth and cause food to be spoiled more readily. For optimal health the human body requires all of the possible nutrients that the food can supply. Essential oils tend to be delicate and are readily lost from foods. Precautions must be taken to protect these precious nutrients in every way possible. Of course, all foods should be eaten as fresh as possible.
4. Cilantro and coriander help meat digest, largely because it is high in potassium, the latter being a generalized tonic for the digestive tract. Add it to meat dishes. Sprinkle ground coriander over steak, roast, seafood, or poultry. Garnish the plate with several sprigs of fresh cilantro. Add dried or fresh cilantro to stir fry or stew.

5. Coriander and/or cilantro should be added routinely to hamburger. Both contain natural antibiotic-like substances, which prevent the growth of bacteria.

6. Use cilantro leaves on salads as often as possible. Head and leaf lettuce are comparatively low in potassium, so adding cilantro makes the salad potassium rich. A third cup of cilantro leaves not only enhances the taste of any salad but also makes it super rich in potassium.

Top Cilantro/Coriander Cures

1. If the blood potassium level is low, cilantro is the food of choice. It is so rich in this mineral that it may be regarded as sort of a potassium medicine. Use it in all forms. Coriander powder, which is made from the seeds, is even richer than the leaves. Add it to soups, sauces, entrees, and casseroles. The blood potassium level will certainly rise, and the doctor will believe you are a good patient for "taking your medicine."

2. Cilantro and coriander are good for the muscles. Add it regularly to the diet for reversing leg cramps, muscle aches, and muscular fatigue. Make a potassium broth by adding it to soups along with other potassium rich foods such as dill weed, tomatoes, red peppers, spinach, potatoes, Brussels sprouts, beets, broccoli, cabbage, parsley root, and chard.

3. If fatigue is a constant problem, potassium deficiency is likely. Potassium is needed for the creation of cellular energy. It is also needed for the transmission of impulses within the nervous system.

Energy production is controlled to a great extent by the nervous system. Extreme potassium deficiency disables the nervous system's ability to transmit impulses, and this results in a variety of symptoms, including fatigue, muscular weakness, headaches, leg cramps, heart arrhythmia, numbness/tingling, irritability, and sluggish mental function. Usually, a mild or moderate deficiency cannot be detected by blood testing and must be diagnosed via symptoms. A large percentage, perhaps as much as half the body content, may be lost before it shows up in the blood. Thus, a low blood potassium level is a warning of extreme deficiency, and this can be life threatening. Symptoms of extreme potassium deficiency include severe fatigue, digestive disturbances, constipation, joint aches, heart rhythm disturbances, insomnia, depression, irritability, anxiety, confusion, memory loss, apathy, muscular exhaustion, tingling or numbness of the nerves, muscle aches, and cold extremities. If you are plagued with such symptoms, consider a medical evaluation; request a blood test for potassium. Consume fresh cilantro and/or coriander seed in as many recipes as possible. Take a natural source potassium supplement such as HerbSorb. This supplement contains coriander seed, cumin, fenugreek, cardamom, and black caraway seed, all of which are top sources of natural potassium. For a more detailed list of the warning signs of potassium deficiency see the *Self Test Nutrition Guide* (Knowledge House, 1994).

4. Cilantro is an ideal food for diabetics. Not only does it help lower blood sugar levels, but it is also a tonic for circulation, which diabetics desperately need. Because of its rich content of trace minerals and volatile oils, cilantro increases blood flow to all organs, including the skin. Plus, it provides much needed potassium, which is itself a circulatory and cardiac tonic. Remember, the nerves of the heart are dependent upon potassium to operate properly. If potassium deficiency occurs, the heart will misfire. In the extreme it may even stop beating, leading to death. To procure these potassium-induced benefits you must eat a considerable amount of it, like one half or a whole bunch per day.

5. Disorders of the nervous system respond rapidly to the cilantro and/or coriander prescription. Numbness, tingling, and weak muscles may be associated with potassium deficiency. Regular consumption of cilantro/coriander helps rebuild the levels of potassium in the nervous system. This is why the herb may help relieve the symptoms of diseases such as carpal tunnel syndrome, sciatica, atrophy, and neuropathy, if they are due to potassium deficiency. However, numbness and tingling may be caused by mild potassium deficiency and may not be the result of outright disease. In order to reverse the deficiency a considerable amount must be consumed: at least a bunch per day.

6. If the mind is in disarray and the memory is dubious, it is important to consume cilantro. Its volatile oils help activate energy metabolism in the nervous system, and its rich content of potassium accelerates the activity of the neurons. The result is an increase in mental acuity and improved memory. In other words, cilantro can help calm an upset mind or activate an apathetic one.

Cilantro can spark a degree of happiness in the saddest of faces. Do a test on yourself. If you are feeling depressed or if you are mentally sluggish, snack on a bunch of cilantro. Certainly, an improvement will be noted almost immediately. To potentiate the effect dip the cilantro sprigs in a mixture of extra virgin olive oil and vinegar. As a result you should feel significantly better, mentally and physically.

7. Cilantro is a boost for fatigue regardless of the cause. The improvement in energy is virtually immediate, especially if fresh cilantro leaves are consumed.

Cumin

A strong smelling spice, cumin is derived from the seed of a delicate plant belonging to the parsley/celery family. Seeds may be purchased in whole or ground form. Cumin seeds are rich in oil and may be processed to produce an edible essential oil.

Cumin is an impressive and invaluable supermarket cure, because it is both medicine and food. In ancient times it was used mainly as a medicine. As described by Mathias in *Economic Botany* plants of the cumin family have been used since humanity's "earliest written records." Cumin was a favorite spice of the Babylonians, and the ancient Egyptians adored it. It is mentioned in the Bible in Isaiah (Chapter 28:25,27) and Matthew (Chapter 23:23). Hippocrates, describing medicinal attributes, claimed that it was helpful for heart, digestive, and skin disorders. Today, it is rarely used, largely because of its strong taste and smell. Yet, in the Middle Ages cumin was used in Europe and Asia as a favorite medicinal herb. Grieve, in *A Modern Herbal*, notes that the ancients relied upon cumin for a wide range of illnesses, including heart problems, migraines, poor skin tone, sour stomach, indigestion, and excessive gas. The ancient Greeks were particularly impressed with its value in circulatory disorders. Currently, it is used in the Middle East as a reliable tonic for heart disease. It is also well known as an aphrodisiac as well as a cure for impotence.

Modern research confirms the medicinal powers of cumin. Numerous researchers document how cumin, especially cumin oil, dramatically improves the function of the liver. If liver function improves, all organ systems benefit. Other studies point to its protective effects upon the pancreas. In Pakistan a study determined that cumin (and, therefore, oil of cumin) has insulin-like actions. The conclusion was that cumin "can significantly reduce the blood glucose."

112

As delineated by an article in *Phytotherapy Research*, cumin oil exhibits potent antioxidant actions. Researchers found that the oil boosts glutathione levels within the tissues by as much as 700%. This is an incredibly large increase. Glutathione is the body's front line defense against aging and toxicity. Research published in the *Journal of Food Science* noted that cumin is significantly more effective as an antioxidant than garlic, onion, and similar common spices. Cumin oil also exerts positive actions on liver cell function. Researchers note that it increases the liver's ability to synthesize important compounds, while dramatically improving the flow of bile. Other research points to impressive antiseptic powers. A report in the *International Journal of Food Microbiology* lists cumin as an effective antifungal agent, more effective than most drugs. Cumin oil also blocks the formation of fungal poisons such as aflatoxin.

Top Cumin Tips

1. Add cumin to any meat dish. It enlivens the taste, while aiding digestion. Cumin stimulates the flow of bile, which is needed for the digestion of the fats in the meat.
2. For a more tangy cheese dip add a few cumin seeds. They give a taste much like caraway seeds, although a bit stronger.
3. Oil of cumin is a powerful flavoring agent. Add a maximum of one or two drops in hot or tangy dishes, especially stews, curries, or stir fry.
4. Cumin lends itself well with chicken. Dust baked chicken with cumin powder as well as other spices. Add a small amount of cumin powder or seed to stir fry or soup. For a more balanced taste of exotic spices use HerbSorb. Add the content of two or more capsules to any chicken dish.
5. When making chili try adding fresh cumin seeds. Cumin is a major ingredient of chili mixes; the fresh seeds offer a gourmet taste, plus they are higher in the flavorful essential oil than commercial cumin powder.
6. Cumin oil is strong smelling and tasting. Thus, it may be necessary to use gelatin capsules to administer it. If you wish to avoid the taste, put the oil into an empty gelatin capsule and take it with meals. However, the taste is acceptable in tomato or V-8 juice as well as grapefruit juice. To order natural edible oil of cumin or HerbSorb call 800-243-5242.

Top Cumin Cures

1. For liver disorders cumin is ideal. This spice has a dominant action upon the liver, aiding protein and bile synthesis. Cumin, especially the oil, dramatically increases the liver's ability to produce enzymes. Of note, hepatic production of glutathione-S-transferase, the liver's anti-toxic and anti-cancer enzyme, is induced by nearly 700% just by taking cumin oil. This enzyme is highly protective of the liver against toxic damage, plus it greatly speeds healing once damage occurs. Oil of Cumin, by North American Herb & Spice, is the purest possible cumin oil. Assays show it is rich in the active ingredient, *cuminaldehyde*, which is responsible for these effects.

2. Cumin combats sexual weakness, especially impotence. This is because it is rich in phospholipids, which are needed for the production of sperm as well as sex hormones. It is also because it contains substances which improve blood flow. Use cumin seed regularly in food. Take HerbSorb, a cumin-based supplement, 3 capsules twice daily. Take also cumin oil, 10 drops twice daily (in tomato or V-8 juice or in a gelatin capsule).

3. Cumin oil is a powerful tonic for the nerves. Take it to fight depression, anxiety, and irritability. Oil of Cumin by North American Herb & Spice Co. is made from the highest grade cumin possible and contains a high percentage of the active ingredient needed for mood elevation.

4. Oil of cumin is ideal for combating genital infections, particularly yeast infections. Use it vaginally as a rub. As a douche add 10 drops per cup of water. For jock itch apply it to the involved region twice or more daily. There is a word of caution: although it is gentle, it does have a strong, interesting smell.

5. Cumin is good for the brain. It is extremely rich in phospholipids, especially phosphatidylethanolamine, a special substance needed by the brain for the regeneration of its cells. Cumin is also rich in choline and inositol, both of which nourish the brain. For a boost in memory use cumin regularly. Take HerbSorb, two capsules three times daily. Take oil of cumin, 5-10 drops twice daily.

6. If you are aging rapidly, take cumin and cumin oil. Signs of excessive aging include wrinkling of the skin, bone loss, age spots, chronic disease, weak immunity, and visual loss. Researchers in India discovered that

cumin is one of the most powerful antioxidants of all spices tested. Other research points to cumin's ability to block DNA, that is chromosome, damage.

7. For diabetes cumin is a boon. This is because it contains substances which have insulin-like actions. Research points to cumin's ability to lower, even normalize, blood sugar levels. HerbSorb is the ideal cumin supplement, because it also contains fenugreek, another blood sugar normalizing agent. For natural blood sugar control take 2 or 3 HerbSorb with each meal. Take also oil of cumin, 5-10 drops three times daily.

8. Cumin is also invaluable for combating hypoglycemia (low blood sugar). Symptoms of this condition include lightheadedness, irritability, agitation, mood swings, anger spells (temper tantrums), crying spells, anxiety, depression, paranoia, hot flashes, panic attacks, fainting spells, sluggishness, mental confusion, apathy, fatigue, rubbery feeling of legs, insomnia, nightmares, sleep walking, and poor concentration. Furthermore, individuals with low blood sugar usually have ravenous sugar cravings, and they may also crave starchy foods, particularly grains, bread, and potatoes. To treat this take HerbSorb, 2 or 3 capsules with meals. Also, take it between meals to help block sugar/starch cravings. Take oil of cumin, 5-10 drops twice daily.

9. Cumin stimulates the antioxidant and, therefore, anti-aging defenses. Research points to its ability to raise glutathione levels within the tissues by as much as 700%. Gutathione is the key substance produced by the body for combating the chemical reactions that cause aging. Thus, cumin could act as sort of a natural preservative. Interestingly, the ancient Egyptians used cumin for mummification. Furthermore, it was highly regarded by the ancients for its ability to beautify the skin. Perhaps cumin was the secret ingredient accounting for Cleopatra's beautiful skin.

Dill weed

Dill is not just for pickles. It should be used as an herb and spice for daily cooking. This discussion regards dill weed, not the seed, the latter being typically added for pickling. Fortunately, fresh dill is now available in many supermarkets, and, if it is not, it can be ordered by special request.

A relative of the carrot family, dill apparently originated in southern

Russia. From there it became popular in Scandinavia, which may explain its frequent use in fish recipes. Dill is rarely used in American fare, nor is it used in French cooking. This is largely because it lends such a unique and delicate flavor that it must often be used alone; in other words, few other herbs blend readily with it. Furthermore, few people appreciate its immense nutritional content.

The ancients used dill perhaps more as a medicine than a food. Dioscorides dispensed it as a cure for hiccups. Later, Culpeper noted that it was a reliable tonic for the brain and that it enhanced memory. This latter benefit may be explained by dill's abundant content of magnesium and potassium, minerals which are required for the production of brain chemicals known as neurotransmitters.

Dill is one of the richest sources of trace minerals of any food, being exceptionally high in magnesium as well as potassium. Both of these minerals are lacking in the American diet. The potassium content of dried dill weed is particularly massive: a mere heaping teaspoon contains over 50 mg, and a cup of it contains over 3,000 mg.

Top Dill Tips

1. Dill imparts an incredibly rich taste to sour cream, yogurt, and cheese and is commonly added to such foods in Europe. It is the perfect addition to cheese dips. It enlivens the taste of sour cream and may be used in it along with chives for baked potatoes.
2. Lemon and dill is a traditional European marinade or sauce for fresh fish. Marinate fish overnight in fresh lemon juice, extra virgin olive oil, and fresh or dried dill weed. Or, add a mixture of these ingredients to the fish while sautéing or baking. If you are sensitive to citrus, use vinegar instead of lemon. Place a sprig of fresh dill on the fish plate when serving. For a dill sauce simply add fresh cream and dill, as well as a hint of garlic, in a saucepan; heat and pour over fish and garnish with lemon wedges.
3. Chopped dill tastes great on salads. Mix dill, garlic, extra virgin olive oil, and vinegar for a nutritious and invigorating dressing. Let blend overnight and use as a salad dressing. This mixture may also be brushed on baked fish. Add fresh lemon juice, if desired.
4. As they are relatives, dill blends well with carrots. Add fresh or dried dill weed to dishes containing cooked carrots. Sprinkle it on steamed or

boiled carrots; it tastes especially good when carrots are buttered. Dill gives magnificence in taste and color to carrot soup or soufflé.

5. Dill makes a beautiful garnish, but if you use it for this purpose, be sure to wash it thoroughly. This is because you'll want to be certain to eat it and not just look at it.

6. If you pickle or can food, always add fresh dill weed along with the standard pickling spices. Not only will this give wonderful flavor, but dill weed also provides preservative and natural antiseptic powers.

Top Dill Cures

1. Despite consuming a high fat diet numerous European countries have a lower incidence of heart disease than we do in America. In many of these countries dill weed is on the daily menu. Dill is a top source of magnesium and potassium, which are important minerals for the heart. Magnesium deficiency is epidemic in the United States, where the average individual has never tasted fresh dill. Because of its high content of minerals, it should be a staple in the diet of heart disease patients.

2. If you suffer from poor circulation and/or cold extremities, eat dill regularly. Historically, dill weed has been used to improve blood flow. Its positive effects upon circulation may be largely explained by its rich content of magnesium and potassium, both of which enhance the heart's pumping powers.

3. Abnormal menses, particularly severe cramps and pain, should be combated with dill weed. If you are plagued with PMS, ovarian cysts, or other menstrual disorders, use large amounts of fresh or dried dill on salads, in soups, or with entrees. Improvement should be evident by the next menstrual cycle.

4. Dill weed is a folk remedy for high blood pressure. According to the latest research high blood pressure might be regarded as sort of an indication of a *dill weed deficiency*. Actually, it is directly related to magnesium deficiency, of which dill weed is one of the best sources. Ensminger lists it as one of the top ten sources of magnesium, placing it higher than virtually any other herb.

Magnesium is required for muscular relaxation, and this helps prevent hypertension. The arterial walls contain muscle fibers. Magnesium helps

117

maintain normal arterial tone by preventing spasms and tightness of the arterial walls. Thus, magnesium rich foods, such as dill weed, are useful in treating and preventing high blood pressure. Physicians all over the world have found that the regular consumption of magnesium, whether as pills or in the diet, leads to a significant reduction in high blood pressure. In fact, in numerous cases the blood pressure may be normalized just from taking magnesium alone.

5. Dill combats digestive distress and is especially valuable for irritable or spastic stomach. Stomach aches in children is another use. Simply immerse several sprigs of fresh dill weed in a pot of hot water. Drink three or four cups daily, adding honey, if desired. This tea may also be useful in calming colic in children.

6. Dill is good for the memory. Researchers have proven that dill contains substances which help prevent the age associated decline in mental capacity. Interestingly, in civilizations wherein dill weed is regularly consumed, senility and Alzheimer's disease are nonexistent.

Eggplant

Like most of the vegetables consumed in the United States eggplant was introduced to the West by Arabic-speaking merchants, who brought it to Islamic Spain during the 13th century. From there it was introduced into Europe and Italy, where it became a staple food. Today, in parts of Europe and Asia eggplant is an admired delicacy. In America it is a neglected, rarely used food. It seems to sit forever on the produce shelves and must often be disposed of for lack of purchase. This is despite the fact that eggplant has a long history in America since it was first introduced by the Spaniards in the 16th century. While indigenous Americans eat it only rarely if ever, it remains a primary food for those with Mediterranean or Asian ancestry.

Eggplant is tasty and nutritious. It is a good source of minerals and contains a fair amount of B vitamins, notably folic acid, pyridoxine, and biotin. It is an excellent source of potassium, containing nearly 500 mg per cup. Furthermore, eggplant provides valuable curative powers. Recent research points to its anti-cancer effects. In civilizations where eggplant is a staple, such as Greece and Italy, cancer is less common.

Proper preparation of eggplant requires effort. However, if you don't have time to prepare lengthy menus, here is a simple method for getting your eggplant. Simply peel eggplant and slice it. Marinate it overnight in extra virgin olive oil, garlic, salt, and vinegar. Fry it in the morning (or with supper) like potatoes.

Top Eggplant Tips

1. Eggplant lends itself to marinades. Peel and slice eggplant into 1/4 inch slices. Add lemon, vinegar, olive oil, garlic, and spices. Refrigerate and marinate for 24 hours. Then use it in casseroles, stir fry, and meat dishes.
2. Mediterranean dips are an easy and tasty way to regularly consume eggplant. The eggplant is cooked and then blended in a food processor into a paste. Various ingredients are added such as sesame seed paste (tahini), garbanzo beans, extra virgin olive oil, parsley, and lemon juice. Such dips are a healthier, as well as more tasty, alternative to the commercially available bean or cheese dips.
3. Eggplant makes an excellent breakfast vegetable. Prepare the eggplant overnight by marinating it in olive oil, lemon juice, garlic, and vinegar. Cook it in a skillet in a bit of oil or butter along with eggs or meat.
4. Like the Greeks, eat eggplant with hamburger, lamb, and/or feta cheese. It aids the digestion of meat and enhances flavor.
5. Eggplant and olives go well together. As an excellent appetizer prepare an eggplant based dip, recipes being available in Grecian or Middle Eastern recipe books. Pit and slice large black or green Greek olives; place on a relish tray with sliced vegetables. Dip olives and vegetables in eggplant dip; it tastes good and makes you feel great.
6. Before buying gently squeeze the eggplant to be sure it is firm. If it is spongy, do not buy it. Check also for color; fresh eggplant should be a uniform purple color without brown or rust spots.

Top Eggplant Cures

1. It has been in vogue to avoid eggplant, because it belongs to the nightshade family, the thinking being that nightshades cause allergic reactions and/or arthritis. Don't fall prey to this thinking. Allergic reactions

to eggplant are rare. For instance, allergic reactions to citrus, wheat, and even carrots are considerably more common than allergy to eggplant. There are no contraindications for eating eggplant, unless you noticeably become ill from eating it. The lemon you might squeeze on the sautéed eggplant is a more likely aggravating cause of the allergy and/or arthritis than the eggplant itself, as allergic intolerance to citrus is common.

2. If you have sluggish bowels or constipation, eggplant is an ideal remedy. It contains substances which help lubricate the intestinal lining, plus it is rich in fiber. If you eat eggplant every day, it is bound to improve elimination and will aid in the healing of irritated membranes.

3. If hemorrhoids are a problem, eat eggplant at least every other day. By softening the stool and healing damaged membranes, the fiber and chemicals in eggplant help diminish hemorrhoids and prevent their recurrence.

4. If there is a family history of cancer, eggplant must be on the daily menu. This plant has a prolonged folk history as an anti-cancer vegetable. Recent research confirms that it possesses chemicals which inhibit tumor development, although the exact nature of these chemicals remains unknown.

5. Eggplant is an ideal remedy for combating irritable bowel as well as Crohn's disease and ulcerative colitis. This is because it contains a substance similar to mucous, the natural protective substance lining the healthy colon wall. Bowel diseases are partially due to a deficiency in this protective mucous coating. The coating prevents the colon wall from becoming damaged or infected. Eggplant helps rebuild this protective lining, improving bowel and digestive function.

6. For heart disease patients eggplant should become a regular part of the diet. Eggplant contains a variety of substances which help prevent fat accumulation in the arteries. What's more, this vegetable contains chemicals which prevent damage to the heart and arteries from stress and toxic chemicals. It is no coincidence that wherever in the world eggplant is eaten regularly heart disease is rare.

7. If you suffer from digestive difficulty, eat eggplant often. It is one of the easiest of all foods to digest and, therefore, is invaluable for those with a history of allergies or digestive problems. Furthermore, eggplant improves the digestibility of other foods, including meats and fatty foods.

8. If you wish to lose weight, eat eggplant with meals as often as possible.

It is extremely filling plus it contains certain substances, which help speed the burning of fat.

Eggs

From the beginning of time humans have consumed eggs from a wide range of creatures. The primitives routinely gathered eggs, regarding them as a delicacy. Apparently, the pharaohs first produced eggs on a commercial scale.

Eggs are a health food. They are one of Nature's most concentrated sources of nutrients. Ensminger calls eggs a "marvel of nature" and describes them as "one of the most complete foods known...." Cooper, in *Nutrition in Health and Disease*, scores them second only to milk as a source of quality protein. She also notes importantly that they provide a greater amount of the critical growth factors, vitamin A, vitamin D, and riboflavin, than milk. Arlene Stadd describes in *Eggstra! Eggstra!* that eggs contain at least 13 vitamins, which is more than virtually any other food. Furthermore, they are one of the few foods containing naturally occurring vitamin D. Because of the enormity of nutrients they contain, as well as their unique balance of nutrients, numerous authorities have described eggs as the "perfect food."

Eggs have been unfairly maligned. If there is a problem with them, it is related to the way they are produced or a consequence of allergy. However, if you are fortunate enough to tolerate eggs without allergic tendency, they will become one of the most versatile of all foods.

In the recent past eggs served an immensely valuable role in human nutrition. This is illustrated by the fact that commercial production of eggs before WW II in the United States alone reached several billion dozen per year. This was a time when the National Research Council demanded that in order to meet basic nutritional needs Americans should consume at least one egg per day. This was also a time when heart disease was a rarity relative to today's incidence despite the daily consumption of eggs by millions of Americans. Remember also that this was an era wherein eggs were not only a regular breakfast food but were also used as appetizers, in desserts, and in a wide range of baked goods. During the 1930s - 1950s the number of Americans who went a day without consuming an egg or a portion thereof were few indeed, and, yet, it was an era wherein heart disease was relatively rare.

The primary reason for avoiding eggs is paranoia over cholesterol. It has been heavily publicized that eating eggs or other foods containing cholesterol increases the risk for heart disease by elevating the level of blood cholesterol. This is simply untrue. Recent research proves that dietary cholesterol is not strongly linked to heart disease nor is it the cause of high cholesterol. Here are the latest facts. While Americans have conserved on cholesterol consumption and reduced dietary fat intake, heart disease is still on the rise. What about the French paradox? Compared to the United States and Canada, heart disease is relatively rare in France despite the consumption of a high fat diet and the daily intake of such food as full fat cheese, heavy cream, fatty meats, olives, and eggs. Dozens of foreign societies continue to eat foods rich in saturated fat and cholesterol without ill effect. The Eskimos are an excellent example. While eating the standard ration of whale or seal blubber, they ingest a greater amount of cholesterol in one meal than diet conscious Americans may consume in a week. The point is don't become deranged, paranoid, or upset concerning the much maligned cholesterol molecule. It is a part of food, and it can't do any harm. Quite the contrary, failing to consume it is harmful, because it is required by the body for a variety of functions and is a needed component of human nutrition.

Interestingly, eggs are extremely low in saturated fat, plus they contain rich supplies of lecithin, a phospholipid which reduces the levels of harmful fats within the bloodstream. So, if you wish to combat fat accumulation within the arteries, eat lecithin rich foods, and eggs are the richest common source.

Eggs are supremely rich in protein and boast the highest protein quality and digestibility of any food. Virtually 95% of its protein content is assimilated, a feat accomplished by no other food. Even the yolk is high in protein, containing some 18% by weight, which makes it higher in protein than beans or rice. In fact, by separating the yolks from the whites, the protein balance, that is the balance of essential amino acids, is disrupted, and the protein is no longer complete. The fat is found exclusively in the yolk and consists primarily of phospholipids and cholesterol. Interestingly, yolks contain unique fat-protein combinations, including lipoproteins, the latter being invaluable for transporting cholesterol throughout the body. It's no wonder that scientific research recently reinforced the fact that eggs not only fail to raise cholesterol levels but actually help decrease abnormal cholesterol counts by boosting levels of the lipoprotein known as HDL (commonly known as good cholesterol). HDL cholesterol is the primary lipoprotein responsible for keeping cholesterol levels in check.

A powerhouse of vitamins and minerals, eggs are found top on the list of most food charts for nutrient content. Not surprisingly, they are the number one dietary source of natural cholesterol. They are singularly the top source of lecithin and, therefore, choline and inositol. They are second only to cod liver oil (which is more accurately described as a food extract rather than a food) and animal liver as a source of vitamin D. They contain a good supply of vitamin A and are one of the rare animal food sources rich in vitamin E. They contain a lifesaving quantity of vitamin B_{12}. They are super-rich in thiamine, and three eggs provide over a milligram of natural thiamine. Rich food sources of riboflavin are rare, but eggs are one of those few. Folic acid and biotin are also plentiful. Eggs also supply minerals, particularly phosphorus, iron, and zinc.

Top Egg Tips

1. Always cook eggs with onions and garlic if possible. These condiments aid in the metabolism and digestion of the cholesterol in the yolk, plus, they accelerate the metabolism of cholesterol, as well as choline and inositol, in the liver. In short, eggs become an even better food when combined with garlic and onions.
2. Cook eggs as often as possible in the soft mode, that is with the yolk still liquid. Not only are soft eggs easier to digest than hard boiled eggs, but this method of cooking also preserves critical nutrients in the yolk, which are readily destroyed by excess heat.
3. Be aware that allergy to eggs is relatively common, affecting some 20% of the population. If you react negatively to commercial eggs, you may fare better with farm fresh fertile eggs. They are the type of eggs that you buy from the local private farmer, where the eggs are fertilized by the rooster. The chickens feed randomly in the barn yard or weed beds, eating seeds, insects, and who knows what else. In other words, they consume their natural forage.

A few farmers collect duck eggs, and allergy to this type of egg is relatively rare. Duck eggs, which, by the way, are delicious, are the best option to choose in the event of egg allergy. Egg Beaters, that is synthetic eggs, are not an option.

4. Some individuals are allergic only to egg yolks and can tolerate the whites. If you react to eggs, try cooking only the whites.

5. Most people believe that white and brown eggs are the same, but this isn't true. According to Loretta White's *The Good Egg* brown eggs contain larger yolks and are richer in vitamins and minerals than white eggs.

6. Never wash eggs until they are ready to be used. The water removes the natural protective coating, which serves as an antibiotic; this coating, therefore, prevents spoiling. However, do wash them just prior to use, as this may remove accumulations of bacteria or chemicals.

7. If you have trouble beating eggs stiff for baking or food preparation, it may be simply because the eggs are too fresh. Crack the eggs and remove the whites. Place the whites in a covered container and refrigerator for 24 hours. Then try beating them.

8. Egg shells are porous. Be sure to keep eggs covered in the refrigerator, hopefully in their original carton. If not, they will tend to absorb odors from other foods, and this may tarnish the taste.

9. If you wish to keep eggs fresh indefinitely, dip them in a heavy fat such as liquefied tallow or coconut oil. The oil will fill the fine pores in the egg and block oxygen entry, since it is the oxygen which eventually spoils eggs.

10. If making hard boiled eggs, be sure to pierce the end of each egg with a pin before heating. This will depressurize the egg and prevent it from cracking during cooking.

11. If you wish to make an omelet that looks like the master chef's, separate the yolks and whites; beat each separately, fold together, and then cook. The omelet will cook more uniformly.

12. Don't serve eggs in silver lined vessels, and don't eat them with silverware. The sulfur in the eggs leaches the silver into the food.

13. Save eggshells; they are an ideal fertilizer, providing much needed calcium. Grind them and place the powder in potted plants or in the garden. Your plants will be healthier and more nutritious because of it.

14. Eggs won't make you fat. They only contain 75 calories each. The

only effect they can have is to help normalize weight, and, to reiterate, they do not cause obesity.

15. The digestibility of egg whites can be enhanced by beating them. Whip eggs aggressively before adding to recipes or when making omelets.

16. Always cook eggs on low or medium heat. If they are cooked rapidly on high heat, they will become tough or chewy, plus, the high heat destroys much of the nutritional value.

17. Contrary to popular belief, just because an egg contains a blood spot doesn't mean its fertile or inedible. The spot forms when a blood vessel on the yolk bursts during the yolk's formation. It is entirely safe to use.

18. Eggs can be frozen but not in their shells. To freeze beat the eggs gently, just enough to blend yolks and whites. Place in plastic freezer containers.

Top Egg Cures

1. If you wish to begin the day with plenty of energy, eat eggs for breakfast. Eggs are utterly rich in nutrients, and there are few foods which match their nutritional supremacy. They provide much needed protein for balancing blood sugar and maintaining energy.

Cravings for sweets and caffeine will be diminished as a result of eating eggs for breakfast. Nervous energy will be calmed by the high content of choline and inositol, plus increased energy will be generated as a result of the egg's rich supply of B vitamins such as biotin, folic acid, pyridoxine, choline, and thiamine. Some individuals are allergic to eggs, and in this instance eating them may make you feel tired.

2. If you are constantly hungry between meals, eat eggs as a filling and nutritious snack. Cook a batch of hard boiled eggs; eat an egg or two as a between meal snack. This will settle the appetite and balance the blood sugar.

3. Diseases of the nerves are usually associated with a deficiency of fats, specifically lipids. The lipids are needed for the development of the outer coating of the nerves, known as the myelin sheath. Cholesterol is the major component of this sheath. This illustrates the importance of eating eggs, the richest readily available source of cholesterol. The egg prescription is particularly valuable for those suffering from multiple

sclerosis, ALS, myasthenia gravis, spinal cord degeneration, diabetic neuropathy, paralysis, and peripheral neuropathy. This is because cholesterol, choline, biotin, and inositol, which are abundant in eggs, are required for the repair of the various cells of the nervous system. The myelin sheath, which degenerates in nerve diseases, consists largely of cholesterol, choline, and inositol.

4. If you have heart disease, high blood pressure, or hardening of the arteries, you must eat eggs. Does this shock you? It shouldn't, since these diseases are caused by nutritional deficiencies of such nutrients as B vitamins, zinc, calcium, copper, choline, inositol, biotin, niacin, pyridoxine, folic acid, and potassium, all of which are found in eggs in dense amounts. The fact is eggs are the perfect food turned vitamin supplement for heart disease patients and in no way cause heart disease. If they do, why are the South African egg farmers free of heart disease, despite eating four eggs daily? Why was the heart disease incidence in the United States so low in the 1930s and 1940s, when eggs were among the most popular American foods? In 1952, when the incidence of heart disease was still relatively low, government nutritionists mandated that an egg a day was necessary for optimal health. The egg prescription was heavily publicized in an effort to prevent disease. Eggs are far from a cause of heart disease, rather, with their plethora of nutrients they help prevent it and may even be regarded as part of the cure. Recently, a deficiency of folic acid was determined to be a primary cause of heart disease. This is because folic acid deficiency leads to the build-up in the blood of a toxic chemical known as *homocysteine*. The heart and arteries are readily damaged by this chemical. Eggs are one of the best sources of folic acid. Therefore, for individuals with heart disease, eliminating eggs could be dangerous.

5. If there is a side effect, it is allergy to eggs, which afflicts some one of five Americans. If you suffer from this dilemma, eating eggs may result in certain symptoms such as upset stomach, heartburn, gas, diarrhea, bloating, colitis, fatigue, rash, itching, irritability, depression, swollen joints, or joint pain. The allergic individual may more readily tolerate farm fresh fertile eggs versus the commercial variety. Such eggs may be purchased from the local farmer or from specialty markets. However, in many instances the allergic sensitivity is so extreme that eggs must be avoided entirely. If you need the nutrients in eggs, and who doesn't, duck

126

eggs, which can only be purchased from private farmers, may be the answer. Allergy to them is relatively rare.

6. An old folk remedy for eggs is that they may cure baldness. True, they are rich in nutrients needed for building hair and other protein. However, there is little proof that applying eggs topically is the answer. Yet, eggs do make an ideal hair conditioner. If you have a child (or adult) with unmanageable or coarse hair, try an egg yolk and vinegar conditioner. Shampoo the hair and use the conditioner as follows: apply a mixture of the yolk of one extra large egg and one teaspoon of apple cider vinegar (beat mixture well before applying). Let stand for ten minutes and then rinse. Repeat daily until the stiff or unmanageable hair is calmed.

7. Who would ever think that an egg could be used to cure a cut? An old folk remedy is to rub the inside coating of an egg shell (i.e. the membrane) on a cut or wound. According to the prescription the wound will heal readily without infection or scarring. While this was never tried in my clinic, the remedy is sound. The inner lining of the egg shell is normally sterile, so it must contain a yet to be discovered antibiotic. Plus, albumin (egg white) has been documented to induce healing both for wounds and on burns. In fact, egg white has been utilized successfully in burn treatment throughout the world and is a common prescription in foreign countries.

8. Individuals who benefit greatly from eating eggs include invalids, hospitalized patients, nursing home patients, and those with impaired digestion. Cooper notes that eggs are "easily digested by almost everyone." The fat in egg yolks is among the most easily digested of any type, since it exists in an emulsified form. This means it is essentially predigested. The emulsification is a consequence of the high lecithin content in eggs, as lecithin greatly accelerates fat digestion and absorption. However, individuals with digestive problems may be allergic to a variety of foods, including eggs. In this instance opt for organically raised eggs or perhaps duck eggs.

9. High cholesterol is regarded as the plague of modern civilization. However, millions of Americans have abnormally low cholesterol. Low blood cholesterol levels may be more dangerous than high levels. This is because low cholesterol is a marker for cancer, as well as neurological diseases, such as multiple sclerosis, Alzheimer's disease, and Lou Gehrig's disease. It is also a warning sign of collapse of the hormone system,

particularly the female hormone and adrenal systems. The fact is the death rate rises precipitously when cholesterol levels plummet below 150. If your cholesterol level is abnormally low, particularly if it is below 150, eat eggs and other cholesterol rich foods on a regular basis. Other foods naturally rich in cholesterol include liver, muscle meat, salmon, sardines, caviar, herring, crab, lobster, shrimp, butter, cheese, and milk. Remember, cholesterol is a necessary nutrient and is, in fact, essential to our existence. It is essential, because a litany of life-giving molecules are produced from it. Vitamin D, estrogen, testosterone, and adrenal steroids are all synthesized in the body from cholesterol. Bile, without which fat itself cannot be digested, is also derived from cholesterol. A low fat, low cholesterol diet is the antithesis of what should be consumed in the event of neurological and hormonal disorders or for that matter virtually any disease.

Fennel

Fennel is both a vegetable and spice belonging to the parsley family. Usually, the term fennel signifies fennel seed, which is actually the fruit produced by this plant. Fennel seed is rarely consumed in American cooking, although it is commonly used in certain European countries, particularly Germany, England, and France. However, fennel stalk can be purchased in specialty markets and some grocery stores. It looks a bit like celery (its from the same family), only with more delicate leaves. However, the taste is entirely different, being sort of licorice-like. Fennel stalk can be eaten raw, cooked in stir fry, or added to soups.

Fennel has an ancient history as a medicine and is currently popular in Europe and the Middle East, where it is administered most extensively. Hippocrates and Dioscorides prescribed it as a diuretic and digestive tonic. In the Medieval times it was respected as a fat burner, while it purportedly built muscle. It has been relied upon for thousands of years to stimulate milk production in lactating mothers. Fennel tea, as well as oil of fennel, was/is a popular European remedy for cough and respiratory diseases. In England it is administered to reverse obesity. Currently, it is used in Saudi Arabia as a kidney tonic, digestive aid, immune stimulant, and metabolic aid. In Africa it is used for diarrhea and stomach ache as well as for menstrual irregularities. Jamaicans rely upon fennel to combat

128

the common cold. In North America the Cherokees found it invaluable for colic and gas in babies.

The fruit of fennel contains the greatest concentration of therapeutic components, mainly as fats. There are two categories of fats: crude fats, which are non-volatile, and essential oils, which are volatile. The crude fats include saponins, which are cholesterol-like molecules, essential fatty acids, and a large amount of antioxidants, notably vitamin E. Incredibly, fennel contains 75% of its vitamin E as *gamma-tocotrienol*, making it higher than virtually any other substance tested. This substance is regarded as the most powerful antioxidant of the vitamin E family.

The mineral content of fennel seed is impressive, and it is particularly rich in calcium and potassium. It also contains large amounts of magnesium and phosphorus.

Fennel essential oil is a convenient means to gain the benefits of this plant. Oil of fennel may be of greater therapeutic value than the fruit (i.e. seeds) for a variety of conditions, mainly because it is a concentrate of the active components. Be aware that commercial fennel oil is often of low quality or it may be adulterated. For a guaranteed pure fennel oil free of chemical contaminants use Oil of Fennel by North American Herb & Spice Co. The fennel oil by this company is carefully tested to ensure it is free of adulterants.

Top Fennel Tips

1. Don't just use fennel seed. Buy the stalks. Cut them and use as a tasty raw vegetable. Or, add to soups and stir fry.
2. Fennel seed is an excellent contribution to any spicy meat dish. Simply add whole or ground seeds to the meat during cooking. Fennel lends itself especially well to fatty meat such as lamb, roast, and regular ground beef.
3. When making cheese dips, add fennel. Simply mix the seeds into any soft cheese dip. Sprinkle over cream cheese; add to yogurt. Be sure to use the whole fat dairy products. Not only are they more nutritious but the added fat also enhances the digestion of the fennel seeds.
4. Fennel adds to the taste of virtually any fish dish. Sprinkle fennel seed over fish when baking. Add a few seeds to fish soup or chowder.
5. Fennel is an excellent addition to sweet bakery. Here, it adds a licorice like taste, and it is commonly used overseas for this purpose. Fennel oil

may also be used in bakery, but only a small amount is necessary, as it imparts a powerful flavor.

6. Fennel may be used as a garnish on a variety of dishes; it adds a sweet licorice-like finish. In particular, garnish any cream soup with a few fennel seeds.

Top Fennel Cures

1. If you suffer from an upset stomach, indigestion, or intestinal gas, eat fennel. Slice fennel stalk and eat several slices. Or, make fennel tea. Add a teaspoon of fennel seed to a cup of hot water. Let steep for 20 minutes and drink.

2. According to James Duke, PhD, author of the *CRC Handbook of Medicinal Herbs*, fennel oil is a top remedy for hookworm infestation. Apparently, the oil exerts specific action upon this worm, killing it and/or driving it out of the body. For hookworm or, for that matter, any worm infestation, take oil of fennel, five drops three times daily. Follow this dosage for two or three weeks. Oil of fennel is a fairly strong substance, so only modest amounts are needed. Use it only when needed, or, for maintenance take small amounts, like 5 to 10 drops, on a daily basis.

3. For spastic colon fennel is ideal. Take oil of fennel, 5 drops twice daily in juice or water. Fennel, particularly the oil, contains potent chemicals which relax spastic muscles, that is it eliminates cramps, while strengthening the normal bowel functions. Use both fennel seeds and stalks in cooking as much as possible.

4. For sluggish kidneys fennel is the remedy of choice. Researchers note that fennel, particularly the oil, markedly stimulates the flow of urine. Furthermore, this diuretic action is long-lasting, up to 24 hours after each dose. It is not an uncomfortable urination but is instead an improvement in the natural flow of urine. Oil of fennel also increased the excretion of noxious substances through the urine. Because of these actions oil of fennel would be invaluable in the prevention of kidney stones. In fact, since ancient times fennel oil has been used to dissolve kidney stones.

5. Lactating mothers who are failing to produce enough milk desperately need fennel. Drink fennel tea every morning. For a more powerful milk stimulant take fennel oil, 5 to 10 drops twice daily. Use also fennel seed as well as the stalk.

6. To improve digestion, drink fennel tea every morning. Simply pour boiling water over a teaspoon of fennel seed. Let steep for one hour and drink warm or re-heat. Or, take oil of fennel, 2 to 5 drops with juice or water with breakfast.

7. Fennel, particularly the oil, is invaluable for colic and stomach aches in children (or adults). Make fennel seed tea and mix it with juice or milk. Fennel oil is fairly potent, so use only a small amount, like one or two drops. However, it should not be given to newborns. Commercial and aromatherapy grade fennel oil are not meant to be used internally. Oil of Fennel by North American Herb & Spice Co. is pure fennel oil without additives or contaminants, as proven by assays, and, thus, it is edible.

Filberts

It is commonly believed that filberts are the same as hazelnuts, but they are not the same. While they are closely related botanically, they are indeed different nuts. Filberts are the fruit of a tree, which originates in Europe and Asia, while hazelnuts are the fruit a Native American wild bush. I have picked wild hazelnuts, and they are delicious. However, the taste is different from that of commercial filberts, plus they are usually inordinately small. Filberts are the supermarket variety, and these are mostly imported, primarily from Turkey. A fair amount are grown in the United States, especially in Oregon.

Filberts are among the most nutrient dense of all foods. They are one of the richest food sources of vitamin E. One cup provides an incredible 28.5 mg of the nutrient. Filberts are also packed with immense quantities of calcium, phosphorus, magnesium, potassium, and iron. They offer a greater amount of potassium per ounce than most vegetables, and four ounces provides about the same amount of potassium as a banana. In the nut family filberts are so rich in calcium that only almonds supercede them. Incredibly, they offer a greater amount of phosphorus per ounce than milk. This is important, since few foods besides milk products contain both calcium and phosphorus in high concentrations. The fact is both almonds and filberts can be blended to make a milk substitute and are used for this purpose in the event of milk intolerance.

Filberts are one of Nature's finest sources of monounsaturated fatty

131

acids, the same type found in olive oil. Filbert oil is not only a nutritious fat but it is also a gourmet treat. In France award winning restaurants use it to enrich the flavor of sauces, salads, and entrees.

The vitamin E content of filberts makes them exceptionally valuable. This is because top vitamin E sources are few, and the only common sources of this nutrient in the American diet are nuts and the germ of grains. Eggs, salmon, and spinach are also commonly eaten, and their vitamin E content may represent a significant source, depending upon the quantity eaten. Unfortunately, millions of individuals avoid eating nuts, seeds, and eggs, as well as salmon, for fear of the fat content. Yet, what these individuals often fail to realize is that fat soluble vitamins, such as vitamin E and vitamin D, are found almost exclusively in fatty foods. Furthermore, the vitamin E found in the non-fat sources, such as spinach, is difficult to absorb, unless that food is eaten with fat Perhaps this is why it is traditional to pour bacon fat on spinach salad, although extra virgin olive oil (possibly with warm feta cheese) is the superior choice; bacon fat cannot be recommended. Fat blends with fat, and fat in the diet provokes the absorption of dietary vitamin E. When fat is consumed, it instigates the liberation of fat digesting enzymes, which are essential for vitamin E absorption. Plus, dietary fat urges the liver to produce bile, a substance which is mandatory for the digestion and absorption of vitamin E or, for that matter, any other fat soluble vitamin.

This is yet another condemnation against the low fat diet. Not only does such a diet fail to provide sufficient amounts of vitamin E, but it also creates the scenario for the vitamin's failed absorption. This means that a meal of beans and brown rice with dark green leafy vegetables, while containing a fair amount of vitamin E, will fail to achieve the bottom line: absorption of vitamin E into the blood. Perhaps this is why vegetarians often have major warning signs of vitamin E deficiency: pale, pasty skin muscular fatigue, and irritability. Even if they take supplemental vitamin E, vegetarians must be sure to consume it with a fatty meal.

It is important to comprehend the fat connection to optimize dietary vitamin E. Here are some luscious examples. Sweet potatoes contain a good amount of vitamin E, but be sure to eat them with butter. Spinach is the richest vegetable source, so pour extra virgin olive oil on spinach salad, or sauté it in butter or oil. Salmon contains vitamin E, so be certain to cook it in its rich natural juice. Roast filberts and almonds in coconut fat, hazelnut oil, or extra virgin olive oil. The roasting process breaks down the fiber in the nuts, which aids in vitamin E absorption, although some of the vitamin E is destroyed by heat. The added fat is also beneficial, since it provokes an increase in the secretion of bile and digestive enzymes, both of which are needed for vitamin E absorption.

Top Filbert Tips

1. If you make your own bakery, try adding filberts to the recipes. Add chopped filberts to breads, rolls, and muffins. Filbert flour serves as a unique means of fortifying grain flour. It is exceptionally dense in vitamins and minerals, particularly vitamin E, niacin, phosphorus, and calcium. Imagine having the nutritional benefits of the nutrient density of nuts in powdered form. Added to flour it greatly increases the vitamin and mineral content of baked goods.

Filbert flour is perhaps the top food source offering condensed amounts of vitamin E. If you eat enough of it, you may well avoid any need for vitamin E supplements. Filbert flour, a specialty item, may be ordered from Gourmet Natural Foods (see Appendix B).

2. If you are a popcorn fiend, try cooking it in filbert oil. It makes the most luscious buttery tasting popcorn you will ever taste, without the butter. This is the perfect popcorn oil to use for individuals who cannot tolerate butter.

3. Buy filberts fresh in the shell. The shell helps prevent the sensitive oils in the nut from turning rancid. Crack extra quantities of the nuts, and store in the freezer. Freezing also prevents rancidity.

4. Raw filberts are quite tasty, but they are also luscious roasted. Fresh filberts may be roasted in an oven. They may be dry or oil roasted. To roast in oil use a large baking pan and add heavy oil such as clarified butter, coconut oil, hazelnut oil, or extra virgin olive oil. In a preheated oven (300 degrees) heat oil for 10 minutes and then add nuts. After cooking for 20 minutes with reduced heat (200 degrees), dust with sea salt. Roast until nuts brown slightly; avoid over-cooking.

5. Filbert (hazelnut) oil is highly nutritious and is a superb source of vitamin E. Use it for roasting nuts, making popcorn, or cooking French fries. Filbert oil is an excellent oil for stir fry, and it is ideal on salads.

Like olive oil, filbert oil is primarily monounsaturates. This type of oil is known for its positive effects upon the cardiovascular system. The regular intake of monounsaturates significantly decreases the risks for cardiac diseases of all types, including coronary artery disease, congestive heart failure, mitral valve prolapse, cardiac arrhythmia, and hypertension. Monounsaturated oils are certainly superior to commercial vegetable oils, which are primarily polyunsaturates. Opt only for filbert oil which is processed by chemical and heat-free extraction, in other words that which is cold-pressed. Filbert oil is almost always labeled as hazelnut oil.

6. Filberts make a great addition to pie crusts. By adding filbert flour the starch content of the crust is reduced, while the protein and vitamin content is greatly increased.

Top Filbert Cures

1. Filberts contain the nutrients needed to rescue women from menstrual problems. Women who suffer from ovarian cysts, painful menses, menstrual cramps, irritability, depression, and sore breasts should eat filberts on a daily basis. Filberts supply significant amounts of much needed nerve tonics, such as calcium, magnesium, potassium, and phosphorus, plus vitamin E, which help relax the uterine muscles. Vitamin E also helps reverse soreness and swelling of the breasts, as manifested by a condition known as *fibrocystic breast disease*. According to the *Journal of the American Medical Association* vitamin E alone arrests this disease. Filberts are a top source of this vitamin. To get enough of the vitamin to combat fibrocystic breast disease, eat at least one cup of filberts daily.

2. Men who suffer from impotence should eat large amounts of filberts on a regular basis. The rich content of vitamin E will revitalize the sex glands and improve pelvic circulation. Vitamin E brings much needed oxygen to the sex glands, and this leads to a normalization of function.

3. If you wish to fall asleep like a baby, eat filberts just before bedtime. A large handful will usually suffice, but eat more if desired. The rich content of calcium, magnesium, and phosphorus nourishes and calms the nerves. These minerals help induce a state of balance and relaxation within the nervous system. Thus, restlessness, irritability, anxiety, agitation and, of course, insomnia are eliminated.

4. Heart disease responds to the filbert prescription. In fact, filberts are a

134

perfect food for the heart. They contain virtually all of the nutrients needed to optimize the function of the heart and blood vessels, including calcium, magnesium, potassium, selenium, niacin, biotin, folic acid, vitamin B_6, pantothenic acid, thiamine, and vitamin E. The vitamin E content alone is sufficient reason to add filberts to the daily menu. The potassium content is particularly valuable for high blood pressure patients, especially those taking diuretics, which destroy potassium. Filberts offer the benefit of larger amounts of potassium per serving than bananas, plus they are free of sugar.

5. If you lack energy, filberts may give you a boost. These nuts provide an immense density of B vitamins. The rich supply of niacin, folic acid, pantothenic acid, thiamine, and biotin helps accelerate metabolism and boosts energy. The increase in vitality is often immediate. Eat a handful of fresh filberts whenever you feel exhausted, and expect energy levels to climb.

6. If you suffer from cold sensitivity or if your extremities are constantly cold, you desperately need to eat filberts. Their rich content of monounsaturated fats and vitamin E will induce dramatic improvements in circulation.

7. Filberts are an ideal food for diabetics. Individuals with diabetes are usually severely deficient in potassium, calcium, magnesium, and vitamin E, and filberts would help correct these deficiencies. Filberts are high in protein and fat, while being low in sugar and starch. Thus, they create no strain upon the pancreas and, in fact, enhance pancreatic function. Plus, their rich vitamin E content helps prevent the major plague of diabetes: circulatory disease.

Garlic

Garlic is probably the most well known supermarket cure. History proves that it has always been the top cure. The ancient Egyptians regarded it as a cure all, and the tomb builders consumed it regularly as a strength tonic. Known for worshipping just about anything, if the ancient Egyptians had a food incarnate, it was garlic. They even used it in mummification. In ancient Greece garlic was used both as a food and medicine. Grecian physicians advocated it for a wide range of ailments, including intestinal infections, lung disease, infected wounds, toothaches, nerve disorders, and apparently heart disease. Like the Egyptians, the Romans gave garlic to laborers and soldiers specifically for enhancing strength and endurance. The Prophet Muhammad, the world's greatest naturalist, successfully applied it topically for neutralizing venomous bites. He also noted that garlic should be consumed to protect against exposure to summer sun. Indeed, modern scientists know that garlic is invaluable for fighting the ill effects of excessive sunlight, since its sulfur and selenium molecules help neutralize the toxicity of ultraviolet radiation. During the Middle Ages garlic was used for a wide range of disorders, including lung afflictions, heart disease, infections, and snake bites. In 17th century England it was used to successfully defeat the plague. In the 19th century Pasteur determined that it obliterated microbes. In the 20th century British physicians administered it for treating infections as well as gangrene. In fact, the British, as well as the Germans and Russians, used it for treating wound infections during both world wars. Today, garlic has become the world's most frequently prescribed medicinal herb.

As indicated previously garlic is known for its ability to increase strength and endurance. This may largely be a result of its plethora of sulfur compounds, which are needed for protein and hormone synthesis. The synthesis of uncountable human proteins and enzymes are dependent upon dietary sulfur. Garlic is essentially a sulfur supplement.

Since ancient times it has been recognized that garlic can prevent serious diseases, especially communicable diseases. The Talmud, one of the most ancient of all holy books, mentions garlic as a parasite killer. The Romans used garlic to ameliorate respiratory infections, particularly tuberculosis. In the Middle Ages it was applied topically and taken internally to fight the plague. More recently, in the early 1900s, American mothers successfully utilized garlic to combat flu epidemics by hanging garlic necklaces on their children. The fact is garlic possesses potent natural antibiotic activity against a wide range of organisms. This property makes it useful for virtually any type of infection, including lung, liver, urinary tract, blood, bone, and intestinal infections.

Another great attribute of garlic is that, in contrast to prescription antibiotics, microbial resistance to it is rare. In fact, garlic, that is raw garlic, is one of the few substances capable of killing antibiotic resistant microbes. These drug resistant organisms are one of the major plagues of modern civilization and are the bane of modern medicine. No doubt, such infections have reached epidemic proportions. In fact, according to *Hippocrates* magazine, some 130,000 individuals die every year from drug resistant microbial infections. Pharmaceutical companies offer little hope for any improvement in this dilemma. They admit that it is impossible to synthesize drugs fast enough to keep pace with the rate of microbial resistance. In other words, the likelihood for creating any "magic bullets" is nil. This makes it evident that only natural antibiotics can be relied upon to bring relief. In terms of killing power garlic is perhaps the cadillac of all natural antibiotics, and microbial resistance against it is rare.

Garlic is also effective against a type of organism for which antibiotics are impotent: yeast. Scientific studies document how raw garlic kills a variety of yeasts, and it is particularly active against the notorious Candida albicans. In fact, garlic is more active against this yeast than any other substance tested, including Nystatin and caustic agents such as gentian violet. One study showed how it even outperformed amphotericin B, one of the most powerful antifungal agents known. The garlic, in a raw form, effectively killed *Cryptococcus*, a type of fungus that infects the brain and spinal cord.

Parasites are immune to standard antibiotics, but they are vulnerable to garlic. Raw garlic kills the majority of parasites, including amebas, tapeworms, roundworms, pinworms, flukes, trichomonas, and Giardia.

Garlic kills bacteria. Researchers have thoroughly documented how raw garlic kills unusually hardy bacteria such as Salmonella, E. coli, Shigella, staph, strep, Proteus, and mycobacteria, the latter being the type that causes tuberculosis.

A plethora of scientific research has been published regarding garlic's effects upon circulation. Researchers note how it decreases the stickiness of the blood and lowers blood pressure. The positive results may be dramatic; in as little as 90 days garlic supplements have been found to lower blood pressure by as much as 30 points. Other research documents how it increases blood flow to the internal organs as well as the extremities.

Garlic relaxes the nerves and blocks stress, and this certainly aids in the reversal of hypertension and heart disease. It thins blood and mobilizes fat. It also blocks cholesterol and triglyceride synthesis in the liver. Cholesterol and triglyceride levels may be lowered or normalized simply via the regular consumption of garlic. If the cholesterol levels are abnormally high, garlic may induce as much as a 30% reduction within just a few weeks. To achieve this effect at least three cloves of garlic must be consumed daily. Furthermore, garlic raises the good HDL cholesterol and preserves this valuable cholesterol molecule by preventing its oxidation. In searching for the reason that the French or Mediterranean people have such low rates of heart disease, there is no need to pursue the obscure. It is probably the garlic, the olive oil, and the herbs that are responsible.

Cancer meets its match with garlic. Raw, cooked, and supplemental garlic have all been proven useful both in the test tube and in humans. According to researchers at New York University Medical Center individuals who regularly consume garlic have a significantly lower rate of stomach and colon cancer than non-eaters. Here is an even more astounding statistic: studies performed at China's Medical Research Institute (Tianjin, China) show that cancer deaths in countries where garlic is a staple are nearly 10 times lower than elsewhere. In particular, the incidence of cancers of the digestive tract drop significantly wherever garlic is consumed. Other research points to a significant reduction in cancer of the esophagus, colon, lungs, skin, and breast in regular garlic users.

There has been much speculation regarding the mechanism of action of garlic's anti-cancer effects. Some believe it is related to various anti-cancer compounds found in large amounts in garlic, particularly its innumerable sulfur-bearing proteins. Others attribute the effect to certain anti-tumor trace minerals; garlic is rich in selenium and germanium. Yet, it may be more simplistic than this. The fact is garlic, particularly when eaten raw, outright kills cancer cells.

Top Garlic Tips

1. For optimal benefits consume garlic on a regular basis. Keep it in the kitchen at all times. Use garlic in raw, cooked, granulated, and powdered forms. Garlic readily lends itself to a wide range of foods and recipes. It is an ideal herb for virtually any meat, egg, or fish recipe, and even if the

recipe doesn't call for it, consider adding it regardless. It also enhances the taste of starches such as rice, potatoes, and squash. Be creative with garlic, as the benefits will be enhanced taste and better health.

2. If recipes call for onions but not garlic, consider adding garlic also. Master chefs know that any recipe that relies on onions lends itself readily to garlic.

3. If social concerns prohibit eating garlic, remember that cooking dissipates some of the odor. Parsley is the ideal cure for garlic breath. Chew a few sprigs after eating raw garlic; the chlorophyll in parsley acts as a natural deodorant, and garlic breath is quickly dissipated if not eradicated.

4. If raw garlic is on the menu, try eating it with fatty foods such as cheese, olive oil, or avocados. The fat minimizes some of the offensive properties. In many European countries it is a tradition to eat garlic with cheese, and this has scientific merit. Because of its fat content, cheese or, for that matter, any other fatty food, helps coat the stomach, reducing the irritating effects of the garlic upon the stomach and intestinal walls. Furthermore, fat helps entrap garlic's volatile oils. This allows the oils to exert their antiseptic powers over a prolonged period both along the gut wall and in the blood. In other words, if you eat raw garlic, be sure to also eat it with some sort of dietary fat. If it is put on salads, add also cheese and/or olive oil. Make garlic dips using sour cream or avocados as a base.

5. Cook garlic often as a side order. Prepare baked heads of garlic as an appetizer at least twice per week. One head of garlic per person is a serving. However, beware of overindulgence. Eat only one serving, because if you eat too much cooked garlic, you will probably develop stupendous gas. To help block the gas attack take digestive enzymes after eating baked garlic.

6. Garlic should be used in any recipe calling for meat, poultry, or fish. Preferably, use fresh raw cloves, but if this is unavailable, granulated, paste, or powdered forms may be used.

7. Buy organic garlic whenever possible. The reason is that commercial garlic is irradiated, a process which destroys much of its nutritional value. Furthermore, commercial garlic may be contaminated with pesticides. Ironically, garlic itself is a pesticide, and microbes fail to grow in it, while pests abhor it. While it seems senseless, supermarket garlic is grown with pesticides, herbicides, and fungicides.

8. Use garlic in meat, fish, poultry, and egg dishes as often as possible. It

not only imparts an excellent flavor in these foods, but it also is a tremendous aid for fat digestion. In particular, if an individual has an intolerance to heavy or fatty foods, garlic should be a dietary mainstay. Garlic helps break the fat molecules into simple compounds which may be readily absorbed.

9. Never refrigerate garlic. When refrigerated, it may retain moisture, which may cause it to mold. It keeps best at room temperature in a ceramic or glass bowl. The peel is protective, so peel only as needed.

Top Garlic Cures

1. If you have a history of fungal infection, raw garlic must be included in the diet frequently. It is one of Nature's most potent anti-fungal agents. One clove of raw garlic per day will aid in the eradication of fungal infection, but more can be eaten, as the benefits will be accelerated by the increased dosage. Raw garlic can be used as a vaginal or rectal suppository, and it is usually highly effective. Be aware that burning may occur. If irritation persists, discontinue use. However, usually it is well tolerated. There is a warning: regardless of the point of application garlic permeates the body. So, even when it is applied topically the body will smell of garlic throughout.

2. Garlic is an emergency medicine and is useful in the treatment of a variety of acute illnesses. Knowledge of how to use garlic in disasters may prove life-saving, especially when no doctor can be accessed. Let's look at some examples.

a) *poison ivy*: crush several cloves of garlic and apply the juice to affected region(s). Cover with gauze and repeat if necessary. The itching and inflammation should dissipate almost immediately. Remove the application after an hour.

b) *food poisoning*: eat a clove of raw garlic every hour until pain and/or diarrhea are resolved. There is a warning: large amounts of raw garlic may cause gastric distress, so use this dispensation only temporarily.

c) *minor burns*: crush several cloves of garlic and drip the juice on the burn. Don't touch open or blistering burns with hands, as this may contaminate the skin with bacteria. Use a dropper bottle to apply the garlic juice.

d) *contaminated cuts*: if there is a deep cut, like a glass or knife cut or a puncture wound, be sure to rinse the wound thoroughly, especially if the wound is contaminated with dirt. For all complicated or deep wounds, see a physician immediately. However, garlic is useful for minor cuts or abrasions. Crush a few cloves of garlic and apply the juice. This will sting, but it will also prevent life-threatening infections from gaining a foothold. There is a word of caution: use garlic only in wounds that are of a mild to moderate nature. Never use it in life threatening deep injury such as a stab or gun shot wound. In the event of a serious wound seek medical help without delay. Never put foreign items in large open wounds. The garlic prescription is for minor wounds, such as cuts, abrasions, insect bites and puncture wounds, in other words, everyday injuries that might occur at home or work or while traveling.

e) *venomous bites*: see a doctor immediately. However, on the way to the emergency room crush several cloves of garlic; apply the maceration to the wound—the venom will be neutralized. Garlic is the primary constituent of cobra anti-venom remedies used by snake charmers in India. When they are bitten, they know that immediate application of garlic will prevent venom poisoning.

3. Acute respiratory disorders, such as chronic cough, croup, or asthma, may respond to a garlic prescription. Make a garlic cough syrup. Crush several cloves of garlic and mix with vinegar and honey. If raw flaxseed is available, add this also. Give a teaspoon of this mixture several times daily until the illness improves or is eliminated. Garlic has been used as an asthma remedy since ancient times.

4. Garlic is the ideal natural medicine for resolving high blood pressure. Use garlic in as many recipes as possible. Consume both raw and cooked garlic on a daily basis. Taking garlic capsules might also help in order to receive a minimal daily dose in case the individual fails to get it in the diet. Be sure to reduce alcohol, sugar, and caffeine consumption, all of which are primary causes of high blood pressure. Because of its tendency to induce the retention of fluid, sugar is perhaps the major culprit. The excess fluid places significant pressure upon cardiac function. In fact, sugar is a greater cause of fluid retention and high blood pressure than salt. Salt is a needed part of the diet, and we cannot live without it. We can live perfectly well without refined sugar.

5. Load up on garlic in the event of major sun exposure. If you are planning a prolonged trip in the sun, take garlic supplements regularly prior to the exposure. About 8 capsules daily of aged garlic provides valuable quantities of sulfur for building up the skin's defenses against the sun. Extra selenium, 200 to 400 micrograms per day, is also protective. Natural beta carotene and vitamin E, taken internally as well as applied topically, are also highly protective against solar rays.

6. If there is a strong family history of cancer, especially colon or breast cancer, consume garlic on a daily basis. Eat modest amounts of raw garlic and use it often in cooking. Achieve additional protection with a garlic supplement. Selenium potentiates the benefits of garlic; take 200 mcg of organically bound selenium daily.

7. If the cholesterol level is uncontrollably high, adding garlic to the diet is essential. Eat it on a daily basis in liberal amounts. Hundreds of scientific studies document how garlic lowers cholesterol levels. One reason is that it inhibits cholesterol synthesis in the liver. It also aids in the digestion and elimination of excess cholesterol as well as triglycerides. Adding garlic to the diet is the most convenient and effective means of achieving a cholesterol reduction. However, garlic supplements also reduce cholesterol levels, and numerous studies show how certain garlic supplements taken over a prolonged period lower cholesterol levels significantly and may even eventually normalize levels.

8. Diabetics should include garlic in the diet regularly. However, there is a warning to heed, but it is a positive one. Garlic increases the efficiency of insulin, while also increasing its synthesis. This means that the need for insulin or oral anti-diabetic drugs will assuredly decrease. The reason for this positive effect could be purely nutritional: eating garlic is like taking a sulfur supplement, and sulfur is a major nutrient required for insulin synthesis. Furthermore, garlic blocks the toxic effects of excessive sugar upon the circulatory system. In essence, garlic is a type of natural insulin.

9. Heavy metal poisoning may be effectively treated with garlic. This is because garlic contains a dense amount of sulfur compounds, which bind heavy metals, that is lead, iron, mercury, arsenic, and cadmium, and remove them from the body. Furthermore, garlic is rich in minerals which antagonize heavy metals, notably selenium, sulfur, and germanium. The symptoms of heavy metal poisoning vary with the type of metal involved, but general symptoms include fatigue, memory loss, hair loss, depression,

apathy, weight loss, skin disorders, numbness of the extremities, headaches, and muscular weakness.

Ginger

Ginger is botanically a tropical plant, and, while no one is sure of its country of origin, it is probably native to Southeast Asia or perhaps India. Ginger has been used as food and medicine since the beginning of history. In ancient India it was regarded as a cure-all. In China it has been used as a food and medicine for tens of thousands of years. Its introduction to the West occurred over five thousand years ago. The ancient Greeks regularly imported it from the Orient, even making their own ginger bread. Marco Polo mentioned ginger as a medicine, as did Vasco da Gama. During the Middle Ages and the Age of Discovery wars were fought over the ginger trade. Then, it was so highly regarded that only the royalty were allowed to eat it. Ginger was planted in the New World by Spanish conquerors. Eventually, it became popular in the continental United States as a spice and medicine. By the early 1900s the use of ginger as a medicine became commonplace; thus, the origin of "ginger ale."

Recent studies document how ginger possesses potent anti-cancer actions. In particular, it contains a compound known as *beta ionone*, which slows tumor growth in experimental studies. The secret to achieving this anti-cancer benefit is the regular, that is daily, intake of ginger. Ginger possesses a diversity of medicinal actions. It is an invaluable digestive stimulant. It aggressively and effectively cures a wide range of digestive disorders. Pharmacology books written as late as the 1940s listed it as the primary cure for digestive disorders. Even then it was known that ginger increases the flow of all of the digestive juices, including saliva, stomach acid, pancreatic enzymes, and bile. Ginger is particularly valuable for stomach disorders, especially nausea, heartburn, stomach aches, and bloating. It is a virtual guaranteed cure for intestinal gas as well as belching. It enhances appetite and optimizes absorption. Ginger is particularly useful for nausea, and regardless of the cause, it usually obliterates it. However, be aware that nausea may be a signal of serious disease, so if the condition is unresponsive, see a physician.

Ginger's greatest versatility as a grocery store food is a result of its powers as an internal and external antiseptic. It is unique, because it possesses both antibiotic and antiinflammatory capacities. This means that it kills microbes and also reduces inflammation, swelling, and irritation. Whether applied topically or consumed internally, ginger speeds the rate of healing of virtually any damaged or infected tissue.

Ginger may be administered directly on wounds or it may be taken internally. For digestive disorders eat it raw or cooked; add it to as many foods as is possible. Its greatest efficacy is liberated when it is juiced, and in this manner larger dosages may be administered.

Top Ginger Tips

1. Use fresh ginger in just about everything. Add to soups, and use it in seafood and fish preparation. This spice greatly enhances the flavor, but it also strengthens the resistance against disease—immediately.
2. Powdered ginger is acceptable to use when preparation time is limited and if fresh is unavailable. Unfortunately, commercial ginger is sprayed with pesticides. Urge your grocery store to carry pesticide free non-irradiated ginger, powdered as well as fresh.

Perhaps the best usage for powdered ginger is in baking. However, when cooking stir fry, meat dishes, and casseroles, nothing supercedes the taste and nutritional benefits of fresh ginger.
3. Wash ginger thoroughly and remove the skin. This will aid in removing pesticide residues.
4. Ginger is an excellent flavoring for cookies and other bakery. Both fresh and dried ginger may be used. When recipes call for cinnamon and/or cloves, be sure to also add ginger. These spices blend well together and greatly enhance the health value of the bakery.
5. The best way to prepare fresh ginger is to grate it. This helps liberate the juices and volatile oils. It also enhances the nutritional value and taste. Be sure to grate it just prior to use, since ginger loses much of its curative properties with time, especially after it is peeled.
6. Ginger keeps well when refrigerated, but it may mold, especially if kept in a plastic bag, because plastic bags retain moisture. In order to prevent molding, store ginger in a paper bag or in a covered ceramic or glass container.

Top Ginger Cures

1. For an upset stomach, fresh ginger root is the best remedy possible. Ginger stops pain and reduces inflammation. It has a predilection for the stomach and directly increases the flow of gastric juices, while soothing inflammation.

Recently, it has been discovered that chronic disorders of the stomach, including heartburn, pain, and ulcers, are caused by infection of the stomach lining. The most frequent culprit is an organism known as *Helicobacter pylori*. It is so named, because it possesses a curved shape. At one end of the curve exists a sort of tentacle, which latches firmly into the stomach lining. Once this organism "roots in" it is difficult to eradicate; essentially, it evades immune defenses.

Infection of the stomach lining by Helicobacter leads to inflammation, pain, and, eventually, ulceration. Doctors can diagnose the existence of this organism through a variety of sophisticated tests. The regular consumption of ginger helps in the destruction of this organism, since ginger is a natural antibiotic and since it speeds the healing of damaged tissue.

2. If you suffer from dizzy spells, eat ginger root for a rapid cure. While the reason is unknown, ginger is a specific cure for dizziness due to non-pathological causes. Perhaps it is because ginger contains a variety of natural chemicals which accelerate blood flow, or perhaps it is due to some direct effect of ginger upon the nervous system. Whatever the reason, the important issue is that it works, often immediately and dramatically.

3. If you have a headache and it seems to be caused by something you ate, try fresh ginger root as an internal as well as topical remedy. The ideal method is to chew fresh ginger and hold the macerated portion under the tongue for as long as possible. This method will deliver the active ingredient directly into the bloodstream by passage through the thin layer of tissue under the tongue. Also, place slices of fresh ginger on the temples or base of the neck. Replace every two hours. Or, eat ginger—the milieu of chemicals in it help reduce inflammation throughout the body, particularly within the gut, the latter being inflamed during migraines. Many "migraineurs" know how upset their stomachs become during or prior to a migraine attack. Perhaps it was something that was eaten which

provoked the attack. In any event, if food/beverage is the culprit, the inflammatory reaction within the intestines must be treated, and ginger is the remedy of choice.

4. If you have diarrhea and nothing seems to stop it, ginger root is an excellent remedy to try. If the diarrhea is severe, it may be necessary to consume a considerable amount of ginger, and the only way to do this is by juicing it. Drink as much as two cups of ginger juice daily until the diarrhea abates. If a juicer is unavailable, mix crushed ginger with honey and eat as much as possible. For best results avoid solid foods until the diarrhea is resolved. The broth of salty soups may be tolerated.

5. Indigestion is the plague of today's civilization. If you suffer from digestive disturbances, bloating, and/or indigestion, eat raw ginger. Or, add several thin slices of raw ginger in hot water. Sip on ginger tea until the discomfort disappears.

6. Millions of individuals suffer from a tendency to become sick from rapid motion such as occurs in flying or boating. Motion sickness is readily cured by ginger root. Numerous scientific studies, including several published in such prestigious journals as the *Lancet*, have documented how ginger proved to be the superior cure, working better than pharmaceuticals such as Dramamine.

7. If you can't seem to break the cycle of a cold or the flu, ginger may come to the rescue. Add sliced fresh ginger to a pot of hot water and drink ginger tea; several cups daily would suffice. Add it to soups or broths, and, if you can handle the heat, chew on fresh ginger throughout the day.

8. Ginger is an excellent heat producing food. This is of value for those suffering from cold sensitivity. Interestingly, it also combats sensitivity to heat, since it helps dissipate excess heat. Thus, it an excellent tonic for preventing heat exhaustion and/or heat stroke. So whether the weather is too hot or too cold, ginger tea is an ideal beverage. Simply add sliced or shredded fresh ginger to boiling water. Let steep for a few minutes and drink. Make home-made ginger ale with the remaining tea. Serve over ice; add a small amount of honey, if desired.

9. Use ginger to break a fever. It is a powerful agent for inducing sweating, and sweating helps cool the body through evaporation. Furthermore, ginger helps break fever by accelerating the immune response against the infectious agent. If the organism dies, the fever will break.

10. Ginger is an ideal remedy for arthritis. It contains a variety of chemicals which reverse inflammation, including bioflavonoids, vitamin C, enzymes, peroxidases, curcumin, and essential oils. The fact is ginger, with its uncountable antiinflammatory chemicals, superceded antiinflammatory drugs, such as aspirin and indomethicin, in clinical trials. In a study performed in Denmark all patients taking ginger reported that they had "better relief of pain, swelling, and stiffness than with the intake of NSAIDs." Remarkably, 80% of the patients improved dramatically after suffering interminable pain for decades. What's more, there were no side effects related to ginger, while the side effects from taking the drugs alone are extensive, and some of the side effects are fatal. For instance, thousands of Americans die every year from bleeding ulcers induced by various antiinflammatory drugs, notably aspirin, Indocin, Motrin, Voltarin, Naprosyn, and Clinoril.

Modern medicine's method of treatment for arthritis is an utter failure. Nothing significant has been accomplished in over 100 years. Sir William Osler, America's "Father of Medicine," elucidated this fact prophetically when he proclaimed, "When a patient with arthritis walks in the front door, I feel like leaving out the back door." Ironically, ginger was listed in the pharmacopoeia probably within Osler's library as an effective antiinflammatory drug as well as a digestive tonic. Perhaps even more ironically, modern research conducted in Japan and China, as well as the United States, proves ginger not only prevents ulcer formation but is also an outright cure. If you are taking powerful antiinflammatory drugs, it would be advisable to include ginger in the diet on a daily basis in order to protect the body against ulcer development.

Grapes

Grapes have been regarded as a health food since ancient times. Lately, the potential of grapes as a health aid has resurfaced largely because of the intense publicity touting the health benefits of wine. Yet, commercial varieties of grapes, as well as commercial wines, are relatively devoid of nutrients. Grapes are mostly sugar and water. The primary ingredient of wine is alcohol. Wild grapes are another matter; they are rich in nutrients, particularly bioflavonoids. Dark skinned grapes are the most nutritionally dense of all commercial grapes. The skin of these grapes contains large amounts of bioflavonoids. Grape skin is one of the top sources of potent disease-fighting bioflavonoids such as *resveratrol* and *quercetin*. After accounting for the bioflavonoids and the fiber in the skin, the remainder of the grape is sugar, although the seeds are nutritionally dense and contain oil as well as the highly regarded flavonoids known as proanthocyanidins. Grapes contain respectable amounts of potassium, manganese, and chromium but are relatively low in other minerals.

It is unfortunate that grapes, one of God's greatest foods, have been so thoroughly contaminated. They are consumed by the ton for the making of alcohol (wine). They are sprayed repeatedly with pesticides; untold tons of these chemicals are dumped on vineyards every year. They usually retain a residue of pesticides. Much of this is on the skin, and careful washing will remove it.

In ancient times grapes and grape extracts were used for a variety of ailments, including fatigue, memory loss, indigestion, diarrhea, constipation, hemorrhoids, kidney disorders, high blood pressure, and heart disease. The "grape cure" was popularized during the early 1900s, particularly in Europe. This was obviously prior to pesticide contamination. Grapes were regarded as a remedy for detoxification of the body; the reversal of a wide range of diseases was claimed. There is a scientific basis for these claims. According to Blumgarten's *Materia Medica* grapes contain organic acids, which are gentle but effective digestive stimulants. These acids increase salivary flow and enhance the secretion of digestive juices. Blumgartner notes that tartaric acid, a main component of grapes, particularly sour grapes, improves urine flow. This explains the former use of grapes for preventing or reversing kidney stones.

Modern research confirms the value of the grape remedy. Researchers publishing in *Science* magazine discovered that grapes contain a compound, known as resveratrol, which exerts strong anti-cancer properties. The researchers found that this natural chemical halted the progression of experimental human leukemia and blocked breast cancer formation in mice. Illinois investigators determined that grapes contain a substance which impedes tumor growth by some 98%.

The rich flavonoid content of grapes may account for its value in heart disease. Studies show that extracts of grapes have potent effects upon the arteries, causing relaxation and improved blood flow. Thus, grape extracts may be helpful in preventing spasticity of arteries, which is a major cause of blood clots as well as heart attacks. At the University of Toronto researchers determined that resveratrol, that powerful grape flavonoid, was the most potent compound tested for preventing excessive blood clotting. Resveratrol, in relatively small amounts, inhibited blood clotting by 50%, making it comparable to aspirin but obviously less toxic.

Many people believe that drinking wine is the best way to gain the benefits of grapes. Millions of Americans currently drink a few or several glasses of wine per week under the guise that it provides cardiovascular protection. However, research by Dr. John Folts debunks this theory. Dr. Folts, director of cardiovascular research at the University of Wisconsin, found that it is the natural chemicals in grapes, not alcohol, which are cardioprotective. Folts, the discover of the aspirin/heart disease connection, found that grape flavonoids were more effective than aspirin in preventing heart disease. Realizing the power of grapes and the toxicity of alcohol he made a profound conclusion: if possible, take a pill of dried grape flavonoids, not just the seed but the whole grape, as the ideal heart disease protection. Thus, research makes it clear that it is the natural medicines, such as grape flavonoids, that offer the best and safest protection, not the drugs. Alcohol is a drug.

Grapes are one of the most readily digested of all foods. They are an ideal fruit for children and may be used to satisfy sweet desires instead of candy, pop, or juice. They are a good food for individuals with sensitive stomachs or digestive disorders, as they are gentle on the digestive tract and require little energy to digest. Grapes are extremely high in sugar, and this fact may limit their consumption in certain individuals, particularly diabetics and hypoglycemics as well as individuals with fungal infections.

Commercial varieties contain relatively few vitamins, although fresh grapes are a fair source of vitamin C. However, they are one of the best fruit sources of chromium and manganese, both of which are needed for blood sugar control. They are also a good source of potassium. However, the main nutritional value is found in the flavonoid content. While it may be difficult to get therapeutic levels of flavonoids from commercial grapes, a special substance known as *sour grape* is a particularly nutritious grape extract. It is made from young wild-growing grapes before they sugar. These grapes are grown in virgin soil free of chemicals; no pesticides are used. Sour grape is extremely dense in flavonoids, including resveratrol, ellagic acid, quercetin, epicatechin, rutin, and catechin. Plus, it contains naturally occurring Pycnogenol. Collectively, these flavonoids are known as *polyphenols*. Sour grape is also an exceptional source of organic acids, notably tartaric, gallic, and malic acids. These acids help balance the pH of the body, plus they act as digestive and urinary tonics. In contrast to commercial grapes sour grape is high in trace minerals, particularly chromium, potassium, iron, germanium, manganese, and calcium. The type of calcium in sour grape is readily absorbed. This natural grape extract is available as *Red Sour Grape* capsules. It is the top source of naturally occurring polyphenols. To order call 800-243-5242.

Grape syrup is another extremely tasty traditional grape product. It is made from the entire grape, so it is a grape concentrate. Grape syrup is an excellent source of calcium, chromium, potassium, manganese, iron, and flavonoids. It is particularly high in the all-important flavonoid resveratrol. Grape syrup is partially fermented, so it is readily digested. Thus, it is an excellent sweetener for children and individuals with sensitive stomachs. See Appendix B.

Top Grape Tips

1. If you buy commercial grapes, wash them thoroughly. They are almost always contaminated with residues of pesticides, which are readily removed by vigorous washing. Wash with cold water or soak in a surfactant or a similar non-toxic substance. Surfactants make water wetter, allowing the water to penetrate dirt, grime, chemical residues, and oil and expedite its removal. Simply soak grapes in a solution of water and a small amount of surfactant for 10 minutes, and then rinse thoroughly.
2. Another option is to buy organically raised grapes, which can be carried upon demand by supermarkets. One of the most well known brands is Pavich's, and this company guarantees that their grapes are chemical-free.

3. Remember that raisins are dried grapes. While they are high in sugar, they are richer in nutrients than fresh grapes and are relatively rich in iron, calcium, phosphorus, and potassium. The fact is raisins contain twice as much potassium as bananas. Yet, the high sugar content prohibits them as a food for many individuals, particularly diabetics.

4. Grapes are primarily sugar, and this means that they are poorly tolerated by diabetics. They are also taboo for individuals with low blood sugar or fungal infections. Small amounts on an occasional basis may be tolerated. To build tolerance for natural sugars, take HerbSorb. This natural herbal supplement contains several herbs, notably fresh fenugreek, cumin, black caraway, and coriander seed, which aid in regenerating the function of the organs which process and digest sugar. HerbSorb assists the function of the pancreas, liver, and intestines. Patients with poor sugar tolerance routinely improve after taking this formula.

5. Imagine having all the nutritional and curative benefits of grapes without the sugar. Red Sour Grape is made from a type of grape which grows in the mountains of various Mediterranean countries. For centuries it has been utilized as a natural medicine, primarily as an aid to digestion and a remedy for heart disease. It is called sour grape, because it is essentially devoid of sugar. Instead, it is loaded with a great array of nutrients, containing far more vitamins and minerals than any type of fresh grape, whether commercial or organic. Sour grape contains premium quantities of naturally occurring quercetin, perhaps more than any other food concentrate. According to Terrence Leighton, professor of biochemistry at the University of California-Berkeley, naturally occurring quercetin is one of the "strongest anti-cancer agents known." He describes how it essentially halts genetic damage, that is toxic damage to our chromosomes, from various poisons and chemicals, plus it blocks the spread of cancer once it develops. Yet, there are other reasons why sour grape is invaluable as a food and medicine. When this type of grape powder is produced, the seed, as well as the skin, are retained. Thus, it is rich in proanthocyanodins, newly popularized as *Pycnogenols.* In contrast to the Pycnogenol supplements found in health stores, sour grape powder provides Pycnogenol-like substances in an entirely unprocessed form. Truly a whole food, it contains everything excellent about grapes without the negatives.

6. Purple grape juice, such as Welch's, is a sort of natural medicine, if you can handle the sugar. It is rich in bioflavonoids such as anthocyanidins and ellagic acid. Recently, it has become popular to consume these substances by drinking wine. However, a small glass of purple grape juice is superior to wine as a health aid and contains a more dense supply of the curative bioflavonoids than wine.

7. Be aware that commercial grape products are usually highly contaminated. The contaminants include pesticide, fungicide, and herbicide residues plus solvents. The latter are used in the extraction of the active principles from grape seeds. Thus, virtually all of the grape seed supplements are laced with solvent residues. Red Sour Grape is invaluable, because it is made by a totally natural process and is free of synthetic chemicals.

8. Imported grape syrup is the most nutrient dense natural sweetener available. It is the only syrup containing high amounts of flavonoids. Plus, it contains abundant amounts of minerals. You'll love it on cereals, on toast, in yogurt, and in anything else requiring a sweetener.

9. For a super-nutrient rich dip combine the imported grape syrup with your choice of nut butter. Spread on crackers or toast for a luscious treat. This fine imported grape syrup is only available via mail order (see Appendix B).

Top Grape Cures

1. If you can't control a child's (or adult's) sweet tooth, have them eat grapes. Buy organic red, purple, and green grapes and let the sugar addict feast upon them. This is a far superior sweet fix than candy or other junk foods. Eventually, the sugar addict will develop a taste for fresh fruits and vegetables and will abhor the taste of synthetic sugar.

2. If your joints are aching, try eating grapes, especially red or purple varieties. The skins of grapes, as well as the seeds, contain certain bioflavonoids which fight inflammation and swelling. These chemicals are known technically as proanthocyanidins. A truly natural extract, Red Sour Grape is a superior and more convenient means of receiving proanthocyanidins in a concentrated form. Because of its extremely high concentration of bioflavonoids, it is an ideal food/remedy for combating joint disease.

3. If your child has an upset stomach, feed him/her sour grapes. The tartaric acid in sour grapes is a tremendous stimulant for digestion and helps obliterate stomach pain, especially in children. Or, use Red Sour Grape as the grape source. Simply open the capsule and add to meals or beverages: two or three capsules daily.

4. If you have difficulty digesting fruit, especially citrus fruit, grapes are worth trying as an alternative. They are one of the most readily digested of all fruit. Unfortunately, ripe or sweet tasting grapes are high in sugar. This is important, because some individuals, especially those with weakened immunity or yeast infections, are intolerant to sugar, and even natural sugar upsets their systems.

5. Red Sour Grape makes the perfect energizing tea. Simply empty two or three capsules into boiling hot water and let steep for 20 minutes. Drink while hot with honey, cream, or, preferably, drink it plain.

6. High blood pressure will likely respond to the grape prescription. Eat sour red skinned grapes and wild purple grapes if they grow in your locale. There is a warning: in susceptible people sugar can cause water retention, and grapes are full of it. If you are sensitive to sugar go easy on the grapes and use instead Red Sour Grape. Take two or three capsules three times daily; for stubborn conditions double this dose. The grape prescription may be so effective that the need for medications may be reduced or eliminated. Be sure to engage upon this regimen while under a doctor's care. Dietary changes are crucial; stop eating sugar, drinking alcohol, and, if you smoke, quit.

7. Researchers have determined that bleeding disorders are often caused by bioflavonoid deficiency. This is because a lack of bioflavonoids leads to fragility of tiny blood vessels in the body known as capillaries. These microscopic blood vessels essentially burst in the event of bioflavonoid deficiency. If you suffer from a condition manifested by a tendency to bleed easily, such as nose bleeds, easy bruising, stroke, hemorrhoids, uterine bleeding, blood in the urine, or bleeding in the stool, consume foods rich in bioflavonoids. Such foods include colored grapes, strawberries, tangerines, papaya, mango, black currants, blackberries, blueberries, dark colored vinegars, and bright colored herbal teas. There is a warning: blood in the stool or urine may herald cancer. Be sure to have such symptoms evaluated by your physician.

8. Miscarriages are a type of capillary hemorrhage. The benefits of

bioflavonoids, as well as vitamin C, in curing this condition are immense. In a study involving over 1,000 women suffering from miscarriages fully 90% of women placed upon vitamin C/bioflavonoid rich diets successfully gave birth. Furthermore, miscarriages are often caused by a condition known as toxemia, which is manifested by fluid retention and high blood pressure. In the near East sour grape is used to eradicate high blood pressure. Take Red Sour Grape, two capsules three times daily. The positive effects upon high blood pressure, capillary fragility, and toxemia are likely due to its unusually rich content of the bioflavonoid quercetin, which researchers have found to be an effective blood pressure normalizing agent.

9. If you have a family history of cancer, Red Sour Grape is a must. As mentioned previously researchers have determined that resveratrol, the main pigment of red grapes, may be the most powerful naturally occurring anti-cancer agent. Preventively, take two Red Sour Grape capsules three times daily. Also, buy organically grown red grapes and eat a bunch or two every week.

10. Red Sour Grape is an ideal remedy for individuals with kidney problems. It is a tremendously valuable tonic for the urinary tract; tartaric acid, its main constituent, has an extensive folk use as a stimulant to urine flow as well as a kidney stone preventive. For maintenance take two capsules twice daily.

Grapefruit

Grapefruit is perhaps the cadillac of all citrus fruit. Like other citrus fruit, grapefruit was brought to America by Spanish traders. Originally, citrus trees were brought to Spain via Arabic-speaking traders, who procured them from Persia and India. With the ideal climate of the Mediterranean, citrus trees flourished in Spain, and from there were disseminated throughout the Mediterranean and then to the New World.

Grapefruit is beneficial as a supermarket food, because it is relatively dense in nutrients, while containing less sugar than other citrus fruit such as tangerines or oranges. This makes it the citrus fruit of choice for individuals who must follow a low sugar diet. Grapefruit is relatively rich in vitamin C and contains a considerable amount of folic acid. A single large grapefruit provides nearly 100% of the RDA for vitamin C. Pink grapefruit provides beta carotene, which is indicated by its color, while white grapefruit is devoid of it. Interestingly, red/pink grapefruit is rich in another newsworthy carotenoid: lycopene. This substance, which is responsible for the reddish color, is an invaluable anti-cancer compound.

Both white and pink grapefruit are among the few fruits which contain good amounts of folic acid. A tall glass of fresh squeezed grapefruit juice contains about 60 to 90 mcg, fully 15% of the minimum daily requirement. Think about it. If you drink a large glass of grapefruit juice with each meal, you meet all of your minimum vitamin C and a large portion of the folic acid needs. Contrast this to three glasses of a soft drink, which scores zero for vitamin C and folic acid. In fact, it is minus zero, since sugar, as well as NutraSweet, destroy folic acid and vitamin C. Grapefruit is also exceptionally rich in bioflavonoids. Most of the bioflavonoids are entrapped within the white pulp, so in order to liberate them it is necessary to juice the grapefruit; extra pressure on the rind when juicing will liberate the bioflavonoids. A tall glass of fresh squeezed grapefruit juice may contain 200% or more of the RDA for vitamin C, while in 8 ounces of supermarket juice (as found in the milk-carton container) you are guaranteed at least 100% of the RDA. So if you have a craving for grapefruit juice, you are probably craving vitamin C. This is particularly true of men, especially those who are under stress or who have hard labor jobs. A recent study indicated that men require as much as 200 mg of vitamin C just to meet the minimum bodily needs. That is over three times the government's so-called minimum daily requirement. The urge for grapefruit might also represent a craving for bioflavonoids, which aid vitamin C metabolism and are also necessary for maintaining the health of the circulatory system. Those suffering from a disorder of the circulatory system or who develop the warning signs of bioflavonoid deficiency, such as easy bruising, varicose veins, spider veins, nose bleeds, and hemorrhoids, should eat grapefruit or drink fresh grapefruit juice on a regular basis.

Grapefruit contains surprisingly large amounts of minerals. One medium fruit supplies nearly 50 mg of calcium and about 30 mg of magnesium. Its potassium content of 385 mg makes it rival bananas as a top source.

Allergic reactions to citrus fruit are relatively common. No one knows for sure why so many individuals develop negative reactions to them, but what is certain is that tens of millions of Americans are allergic to them. This is unfortunate, since citrus fruit is among the most nourishing of all foods. Research conducted on my patients shows that allergy to lemons and limes is most common followed by oranges and pomegranates. Allergic reactions to grapefruit were uncommon compared to the other fruits. In fact, some individuals who are allergic to citrus are able to occasionally tolerate grapefruit as well as tangerines.

Top Grapefruit Tips

1. Request chemical free grapefruit from your grocer. Some of the major supermarket chains now carry pesticide-free, i.e. organic, varieties, but if they don't, you can request it. Unfortunately, most growers spray large amounts of pesticides on their trees, and residues are absorbed into the fruit. This is both wasteful and dangerous: grapefruit contain their own pesticide and do not need to be sprayed. Furthermore, natural pesticides, such as garlic and cayenne, work equally well without the toxicity. In fact, certain pesticide formulas containing garlic, cayenne, or other herbs are now available. Help make the market more secure for yourself and your offspring by demanding chemical free fruit. Use natural substances as pesticides around the home, and avoid the use of chemical pesticides, which damage both the environment and your health.

2. Commercial grapefruit should be washed thoroughly to remove pesticide residues. Soak the fruit for five minutes in a water-surfactant solution. Remember, always wash the outside of the fruit before peeling or cutting in order to remove both chemicals and microbes.

3. If possible, make fresh grapefruit juice and drink it right away. However, if this is not possible, the best alternatives are the fresh squeezed varieties packaged in containers that protect them from light, for instance, the type available in milk cartons. Light, particularly fluorescent light, destroys certain vitamins, notably vitamin C, vitamin A, and riboflavin. Another healthy variety is fresh frozen grapefruit juice, the type, of course, with no sugar added.

4. Grapefruit lends itself well to virtually any type of salad. Add it often to fruit and vegetable salads, and it will enhance the taste while providing much needed vitamin C.

5. Make use of the inner rind of grapefruit. This white pulpy substance is essentially concentrated bioflavonoids. Bioflavonoids are invaluable for strengthening connective tissue and blood vessels. They are needed to fight inflammation, swelling, and redness, and they strengthen immunity. Eat the white pulp outright, or remove it, and save it for use later in soups, stir fry, or casseroles. However, be sure to use only organically grown grapefruit for this purpose.

6. Another method for retaining the power of grapefruit bioflavonoids is to save the inner rind from summer grapefruit by drying it and storing it in the freezer. To prevent colds or help combat them when they occur, add several teaspoons of the dried rind to a pot of hot water. Add also ginger, cloves, and cinnamon sticks. Drink several cups daily for a tea rich in vitamin C, bioflavonoids, and natural antibiotics.

7. Don't throw the rinds of grapefruit in the garbage. The rind and pulp may be useful, as the natural citrus oils they contain possess a plethora of valuable attributes. They are deodorizers; place rinds in the refrigerator for a few days to absorb odors. Then, dispose of them through the sink's garbage disposal to help deodorize it. Or, leave the rind on the kitchen counter or in the bathroom to absorb noxious fumes and combat foul organisms.

8. When eating grapefruit halves don't use sugar or honey on them. Sweeteners actually make grapefruit taste bitter. Instead, sprinkle sea salt on them, and this will actually enhance the natural sweetness.

Top Grapefruit Cures

1. Grapefruit and grapefruit juice are remedial for physical exhaustion. This power-packed food contains naturally occurring potassium in a highly absorbable form. The potassium gives the body a sudden surge of energy. Plus, grapefruit is supremely rich in vitamin C, and natural vitamin C creates energy. Both physical and mental fatigue are symptoms of potassium deficiency as well as vitamin C deficiency. The rich potassium content may also prove valuable in the event of mental exhaustion, especially that caused by stress, since potassium is required for the conduction of nerve impulses, and this mineral is depleted by stress.

2. If you have heart disease, you must eat grapefruit regularly. Grapefruit

is rich in citrus pectin, which has been proven to help lower cholesterol levels and prevent fat from being deposited in the arteries. Because pectin is a chelating agent, it also assists mineral absorption, and the minerals are the body's most crucial heart attack defense mechanism. The vitamin C content of grapefruit is critical, as this nutrient is required to maintain the health of the circulatory system. The fact is the arteries, as well as the heart muscle, degenerate in the event of vitamin C deficiency.

3. For individuals suffering from inflammatory disorders, such as arthritis, fibromyalgia, migraines, bronchitis, and joint disease, grapefruit should be the ideal cure. It is rich in substances which are required to heal the joints such as vitamin C, folic acid, and bioflavonoids. However, there is a caveat. Allergic reactions to citrus, particularly the pulp and oil, are common in individuals suffering from arthritis, migraines, lung disease, and fibromyalgia. This means that citrus fruits may aggravate or actually cause arthritis. One way of determining if grapefruit is helpful or detrimental is to have an allergy test performed. Another way is simply to eat grapefruit and evaluate the results. If the arthritis seems to worsen, citrus must be avoided. If it seems to improve, then the nutrients in citrus may be needed for healing. If citrus must be avoided, there is no need to lament. Other vitamin/mineral rich fruits, such as kiwi, apricot, and melons, will probably be well tolerated; kiwi in particular possesses antiinflammatory properties.

4. If you are losing visual powers or if you suffer from cataracts, you must eat grapefruit and drink grapefruit juice. The bioflavonoid, vitamin C, and folic acid content will likely improve the vision and help block cataract formation. Eat at least one grapefruit a day or one large glass of grapefruit juice to help combat visual loss.

5. If constipation or diarrhea is a problem, grapefruit will probably help. The pectin softens the stool and increases its natural bulk. In addition, grapefruit pectin helps enhance digestion by stimulating bowel action. Furthermore, regarding diarrhea, grapefruit contains citrus oils, which are, in fact, natural antibiotics. These oils are found in especially high concentrations in the seeds and rind. If diarrhea strikes, eat only the rind and seed for the natural antibiotic effect.

6. If your skin is aging excessively, grapefruit might be the answer. Grapefruit contains a plethora of potent antioxidants, which are found in the fruit as well as the seeds and inner rind. If you desire the anti-aging

benefits of grapefruit, all three must be eaten. There is a word of caution: if the rind is eaten, be sure the grapefruit is organic, that is free of pesticides, because the rind is where the pesticides are concentrated.

7. Easy bruising may respond to grapefruit. This is because bruising is commonly caused by a deficiency of vitamin C and bioflavonoids, and grapefruit contains both in rich amounts. The most effective means to use grapefruit for bruising is to drink freshly squeezed grapefruit juice on a daily basis. Be sure to grind as much of the inner white pulp into the juice as is possible, since this pulp is rich in bioflavonoids, which prevent blood vessels from breaking.

Honey and Royal Jelly

It is impossible to know when honey was first used as a medicine. Suffice it is to say that its usage dates before recorded history, and, therefore, its medicinal use spans literally tens of thousands of years. Primitive humans collected honey and valued it immensely. King Solomon apparently recommended it for strength and good health. The Greeks found it such an effective tonic that they dispensed a honey based drink to the Olympic athletes prior to competition. Hippocrates was an ardent fan of honey, recommending it for wounds, ulcerations, boils, and various skin disorders. Galen, who lived during Roman times, found that honey helped cure poor eyesight. Prophet Muhammad recommended honey for a wide range of illnesses, especially infections and digestive ailments. During the Middle Ages Arabic-speaking physicians dispensed it combined with rose petals as a cure for tuberculosis. The tombs of the Pharaohs contained honey, still in an edible form. No other food could have survived intact.

Propolis, another bee product, was apparently used in mummification. Like honey, it is a natural preservative. Honey has long been known for its preservative actions. Royal jelly, which is the food of the queen bee, was consistently used by the ancients as a skin tonic and wrinkle remover. Yet, the question is can substances, such as honey, bee propolis, and royal jelly, preserve and lengthen our lives? Interestingly, epidemiologists have determined that of all professions the bee keeper is the longest lived. Virtually all ardent bee keepers, especially those living in foreign countries, live past 80 and many reach the age of 100 years plus.

These life expectancy results are easy to comprehend when studying the chemistry of honey and other bee products such as royal jelly and propolis. Royal jelly is the most nutritionally dense of all bee productions, containing significant amounts of protein, fatty acids, vitamins, and minerals. While honey is primarily sugar, it is probably not the latter which accounts for its life-enhancing effects. Honey, in its native state, contains a wide range of substances, including enzymes, vitamins, minerals, organic acids, pollen, and natural antibiotics. It's antibiotic actions may largely account for its health benefits. Remember the honey in the tomb? All other Egyptian offerings had decomposed thousands of years prior, but the honey remained intact and edible. The reason is that microbes are unable to live in honey and, therefore, cannot decompose it. The ancient Egyptians knew of honey's antimicrobial action and administered it topically for infected wounds. Today, prominent medical journals, such as *Infection* and *British Journal of Surgery*, report that honey is the superior substance tested for stubborn infected wounds. In particular, as reported in *British Journal of Surgery,* individuals suffering from antibiotic resistant skin infections are virtually universally cured by honey applications. The Journal reports how 58 individuals with disastrous wound infections were completely cured by the honey applications, which induced normal healing while sterilizing the wounds. Only one patient failed to be cured, meaning that the honey induced an unprecedented 98% cure rate. One reason for this response was the fact that honey sterilized the wounds, killing all bacteria and parasites. Recently, it has been determined that honey also exerts antibiotic actions when taken internally. Researchers have determined that the growth of caustic bacteria, such as staph, strep, E. coli, Shigella, and Proteus, is inhibited after honey is eaten. In some cases honey partially or completely destroyed the organisms. This benefit is probably a combination of direct action against the organisms, plus honey helps stimulate immunity against the them.

No one knows for sure precisely how honey is made, nor is its exact composition understood. What is known is that it contains well over 180 substances, and many of the chemical structures remain unidentified. The raw material for honey is primarily nectar, which bees collect from various plants. Some honeys are made almost exclusively from the nectar of one type of plant, such as buckwheat, clover, or tupelo, while others, such as wild flower, are made from innumerable plant nectars.

Just why honey possess such immense antiseptic powers remains largely unknown. One reason honey is an effective topical antiseptic is that it dehydrates the wound site, therefore, preventing microbial growth. Microbes require moisture to become activated. While researchers have found a variety of natural antiseptics in the honey, including hydrogen peroxide, they still cannot entirely account for its unusually potent actions. What is certain is that it is one of the safest and most useful of all natural medicines, plus it has a wonderful taste.

It becomes obvious from this information that honey is a complex medicinal food which only Nature can produce. It will never be synthesized, nor will any drug ever duplicate its powers. Obviously, if it is processed and adulterated, its curative powers will be diminished significantly.

Royal jelly is also a complex substance, containing hundreds of different compounds. It is exceptionally rich in vitamins, minerals, fatty acids, and amino acids; in fact, it is so rich that it supercedes virtually any food source. For instance, royal jelly is several times richer in biotin than meat or nuts, and is denser in amino acids than eggs or milk. It is by far the top source of pantothenic acid. It is also the best naturally occurring source of steroid hormones, which may be useful in the formation of such important compounds as natural estrogen, testosterone, progesterone, vitamin D, cortisone, and DHEA (all of which are steroids). The estrogenic compounds formed as a result of royal jelly consumption are non-toxic.

It is always a good idea to get as many vitamins as is possible in food. In other words natural sources are superior to the synthetics. This is particularly true of riboflavin. The very best sources of riboflavin are relatively uncommon: royal jelly, saffron, brewer's yeast, and desiccated liver. These are rarely consumed. However, royal jelly is the top natural source, and it is readily available. The problem is if the royal jelly is processed, the riboflavin is destroyed. *Royal Kick* is the highest grade of royal jelly available. Extracted without heat or chemicals, its riboflavin content is preserved. Thus, Royal Kick is an excellent natural supplemental source of this nutrient. Royal Kick is also rich in naturally occurring pantothenic acid, a key vitamin needed for energy production. Furthermore, it is unique as a royal jelly supplement, because it is the only one fortified with extra pantothenic acid. Researchers found that the potency of royal jelly is doubled by adding pantothenic acid. Royal Kick is also fortified with natural vitamin C in the form of acerola cherry extract, making this an ideal anti-stress formulation. To order call 800-243-5242.

Top Honey/Royal Jelly Tips

1. Honey's active ingredients are destroyed by heat. Unfortunately, it may be difficult to find unheated honey in the supermarket. However, select comb honey as the first choice. It is heated to a lesser temperature than the clear pasteurized honey. This becomes obvious, since high heat would melt the wax of the comb. Raw honey, that is honey which is not heated or is heated only gently (enough to get it out of the hive), is the most useful type in terms of healing powers.

2. If the honey you buy is excessively thin, consider exposing it to the air. Evaporation will occur, and the honey will thicken. Thick honey is easier to use as a paste for applying on wounds and injuries.

3. If possible, buy unfiltered honey. This type of honey contains pollen, which adds to its nutritional value. Plus, honey pollen, when consumed regularly, strengthens immunity and combats allergies. One word of caution: a small percentage of individuals may be allergic to pollen or honey. If you develop a rash, itch, cough, or other symptoms after eating honey or pollen, desist from using it.

4. Experiment with several types of honey. Each honey is different in taste and curative powers. Honey's nutritional value, healing powers, and taste are entirely dependent upon the plant source. This means that there are thousands of honey tastes and medicines. Amazingly, honey is the most diverse natural medicine in the world.

5. If you see "Honey for Sale" signs while traveling in rural areas, always investigate the situation. Find out what type of honey it is and how it is processed. If it is unheated and unfiltered or if it is heated to no more than 100 degrees, consider purchasing it. Remember, every type of honey is different, and there is no way to test it without trying it.

6. Use honey primarily as a natural medicine and as a condiment. Don't consume honey in excess. Just because it is natural doesn't mean you can eat it by the ton. Remember, North Americans are the top consumers of

sugar in the world. Currently, sugar consumption has reached unbelievably high levels: some 150 pounds per person each year. The fact that honey is natural might cause an individual to believe that it can be eaten profusely. Don't replace one sugar fix with another.

7. Avoid cooking honey or using it in bakery, since heat destroys its healing properties. Use it raw for the best benefits. If you wish to cook with sugar, use raw cane sugar, which is not adversely affected by heat.

8. Royal jelly may be an invaluable food supplement if it is pure and unaltered. Its quality varies greatly. This quality and price is measured by the content of a steroid known as DOCA (10-hydroxy decanoic acid). *Royal Kick* premium-grade royal jelly contains the highest possible DOCA content, about 6.5%, which makes it the most potent grade available. Without a high content of this active ingredient, royal jelly is rather impotent.

Top Honey/Royal Jelly Cures

1. Apply honey to burns of all types, even serious ones. Honey dramatically speeds the healing of burns. Its application would prove lifesaving in hospitals for the treatment of severely burned patients, if they would use it.

Honey saves lives, because it prevents the loss of fluids and electrolytes from severe burns. In other words, it halts the oozing of fluids that results from destruction of the skin layers. Furthermore, it sterilizes the burn area, entirely preventing infection. What's more, the likelihood of scarring in wounds is diminished, and, in some cases as a result of honey applications no scars are seen.

Raw honey provides optimal burn healing attributes, because it contains a variety of antibiotics and enzymes not found in pasteurized honey. The enzymes exhibit potent curative powers, stimulating wound healing, killing microbes, and inhibiting scar formation. The rich enzyme content of honey may largely explain the 10-fold increase in healing rate seen in burns treated with it.

The aforementioned was accented in 1991 by Dr. M. Subrahanyam's study on the treatment of minor burns with honey published in the prestigious *British Journal of Surgery*. Patients were either treated with

163

honey or the standard anti-burn drug, sulfadiazine. Incredibly, 91% of the patients treated with honey showed complete sterility of wounds within a mere seven days, and nearly 90% had complete wound healing within two weeks. In contrast, only 7% of the drug treated burns were sterile in a week, and healing was also sluggish, with only 10% being healed in the two week period. Scarring, as well as pain, was significantly reduced as a result of the honey applications. Thus, there was a dramatic difference between honey treatment and traditional therapy. It is a travesty that, despite the disparaging nature of these results, the value of honey for burn treatment in the Western world remains unknown. The use of honey for burns was first elucidated by the Prophet Muhammad in the 7th century A.D., and its efficacy has been proven repeatedly since ancient times.

2. For diarrhea honey is a front line remedy. If treated early in its course, honey is virtually a guaranteed cure for diarrhea, helping to reduce the frequency of stools usually within 24 hours or less. If the diarrhea is unrelenting, use large amounts of honey, perhaps a quarter cup three or four times daily. Be sure to avoid all solid foods.

3. Honey is an ideal remedy for chronic cough. Simply mix 2 tablespoons of honey with one tablespoon vinegar or lemon juice. Take this mixture 4 to 6 times daily or until cough or irritation dissipates. If the cough continues or worsens, see your doctor immediately. Usually, however, mild cough is entirely eliminated with this simple remedy. For stubborn coughs mix honey with oil of oregano (see Oregano section).

4. Honey is the perfect food for malnourished individuals, especially those suffering from either weight loss or intestinal malabsorption. Honey is predigested, which means that it is gentle upon the digestive tract and is readily absorbed. For an ideal malabsorption drink, mix one fourth cup raw honey in 10 ounces of goat's milk. Blend and drink for an incredibly tasty, digestible, and nourishing beverage. For superior nutritional value add to this 3 tablespoons of Nutri-Sense protein drink mix. Nutri-Sense more than triples the nutritional value of any drink. Readily digested by virtually anyone, especially those with chronic disease, Nutri-Sense provides a broad spectrum of minerals, vitamins, and fatty acids in the original unprocessed state. It is truly a top notch food supplement and is incontestably superior in therapeutic efficacy for aiding individuals with maldigestion, malabsorption, weight loss, and failure to thrive versus the typical "synthetic" protein mixes. Goat's milk and honey make an ideal

medium for Nutri-Sense. However, in the event of goat milk allergy or sugar intolerance, mix Nutri-Sense in juice—tomato, V-8, and grapefruit juice all work well with it.

5. Honey is a tonic for the cardiovascular system. According to Dr. Thomas of Edinburgh, Scotland, honey has a marked effect in improving cardiac function in the event of a weak heart. Even in an emergency setting Dr. Thomas, whose findings were published in the *Lancet*, found honey invaluable and life-saving. Furthermore, he notes that it helped cure a case of severe pneumonia when all else had failed. It took two pounds of pure honey to save the patient's life.

6. Infected wounds notoriously respond to the honey prescription. Simply apply raw honey to the wound and cover with a sterile dressing. Repeat the application every 12 hours. Usually, significant improvement will be observed within 24 hours or less. If the wound fails to heal or if it worsens, see your physician immediately.

7. Don't hesitate to use honey as the preferred antiseptic for everyday injuries such as minor cuts, abrasions, burns, sores, boils, etc. It is infinitely superior to common medicine cabinet cures such as iodine, Mercurochrome, and hydrogen peroxide.

8. In the case of anorexia honey is the ideal food to administer. It requires no energy to digest and, in fact, provides much needed energy to a weakened body. For adolescents with anorexia nervosa a tablespoon of raw honey three times daily will assuredly regenerate the appetite and bring a quick resolution to this serious disease. An excellent tonic for anorexia nervosa is to add two tablespoons of raw honey to a quart of goat's milk. Add three tablespoons of Nutri-Sense (see Appendix A) and blend, adding water to achieve desired thickness. Consume the entire mixture daily until the appetite returns. This nutrient dense shake is ideal for stabilizing weight. To enhance the regeneration of appetite and normal weight add a few capsules of Royal Kick premium-grade royal jelly to the shake (see Appendix A). Royal jelly, especially when combined with pantothenic acid, is a highly effective treatment for anorexia. It regenerates defective appetite by rebuilding the function of the digestive tract and by normalizing the function of the hormones which control digestion. Interestingly, if the appetite is excessive, royal jelly normalizes it, and, if it is feeble, royal jelly invigorates it. When combined with pantothenic acid, as in Royal Kick, royal jelly greatly stimulates digestive function, revitalizing the entire digestive system.

9. Fatigue is readily ameliorated with royal jelly. If you suffer from sluggishness, fatigue, muscular weakness, or poor exercise tolerance, try Royal Kick, 2 to 4 capsules every morning. It seems to work universally for all energy-related problems.

Horseradish

Horseradish is regarded as a condiment or spice, but this has not always been the case. In ancient times it was used strictly as a medicine. It is believed to have originated in England or perhaps Hungary or Western Asia. It developed its current reputation as a food primarily in Germany during the Middle Ages. The Germans and Danes were the only Europeans who actually ate it. The strong flavor and aroma of horseradish is due to its volatile oil content. The oil possesses a cyanide containing substance called *allyl isothiocyanate*. However, do not fret. This type of cyanide is organically bound and, therefore, non-toxic. To its plus, this natural cyanide is toxic to one type of "organ:" cancer cells. Evidence exists that the regular consumption of horseradish may dramatically decrease cancer risks. In other words, the horseradish can do no harm and can only help. If you grate or prepare fresh horseradish, the volatile oil will be lost, and, thus, its healing attributes are diminished. Immediately immerse the grated root in vinegar or lemon juice, or, even better, a few drops of olive oil. The added oil will absorb the horseradish's volatile oils and prevent their loss in the air.

As a condiment horseradish is usually consumed with protein, notably beef. This makes sense, since horseradish is rich in enzymes, which aid in protein digestion. Mixed with vinegar, lemon juice, and chopped cilantro it makes an invaluable condiment for meat. It may also be mixed with sour cream or yogurt, which not only helps diminish the overpowering taste but makes it easier to use as a dip for meat.

As a medicine, horseradish supplies powerful inflammation-fighting chemicals. These chemicals include essential oils, enzymes, and vitamins. Furthermore, horseradish is relatively rich in vitamin C. According to Ensminger a tablespoon of the fresh herb contains over 12 mg, which makes it richer than most fruits and vegetables, including corn, peas, cabbage, beet greens, blueberries, cherries, and grapes.

Traditionally, horseradish has been used to fight swellings, joint pain, arthritis, and stiff muscles/joints. It may be taken internally or applied directly to the painful, swollen, or irritated region. However, it has also been used as a stimulant for sluggish kidneys. Herbalists record that horseradish obliterates water retention due to kidney problems. The prescription is to boil an ounce or more of chopped fresh horseradish in a pint of water. The residue is drunk, three or four tablespoons at a time, over a 48 hour period.

Top Horseradish Tips

1. Use horseradish as a condiment whenever eating roast beef as well as steak. Mix it with sour cream for an easy and tasty recipe for dipping meat. Horseradish aids in the digestion of meat. This is because it contains meat digesting enzymes and also helps increase the flow of digestive secretions.
2. If fresh horseradish is unavailable, buy ground horseradish, which is available in small jars at most supermarkets. This is convenient for adding to sauces.
3. It is common to eat horseradish with shrimp as a normal part of the recipe for red sauce. However, use it also as a condiment for fish. It particularly lends itself to fatty fish such as salmon, sardines, herring, mackerel, and trout. The horseradish enzymes will aid protein digestion, and the volatile oils stimulate the digestion and absorption of fish oils. Make a large batch of red sauce and keep it available for use whenever fish or seafood is on the menu. Remember, horseradish is a powerful preservative, so, like mustard, it remains fresh for long periods.
4. Use horseradish as you would use mustard. Spread it on sandwiches or hamburgers for a tangy and invigorating taste.
5. Horseradish is rich in vitamin C. During ancient times it was relied upon to prevent scurvy. In Northern Europe it was one of the few sources of this nutrient that could be made available all year long. This is because the vitamin C content in horseradish remains relatively constant even if the root is stored without refrigeration. This fact is further proof of the unusual medicinal powers of this root.
6. Horseradish remains fresh indefinitely. Always buy the fresh root, and

only use the commercially prepared variety as the last option. This is because the active ingredients of the root are rapidly lost as soon as it is processed.

7. Add horseradish to tuna, chicken, salmon, beef, or egg salad. This will impart a pungent flavor, plus horseradish contains preservatives, which help prevent microbial growth.

Top Horseradish Cures

1. If you have sluggish kidneys or suffer from water retention, horseradish is a remedy of choice. Grate one tablespoon of fresh horseradish and crush it with a mortar and pestel; mix with one tablespoon of apple cider vinegar. Add the mixture to a pint of boiling water, and let steep four hours; be sure to cover to prevent the escape of the active ingredient. Strain pulp and drink.

2. Aching, stiff, or swollen joints are no match for horseradish. Mix freshly grated horseradish in butter or coconut fat, and apply to the affected site(s). Cover with gauze. Apply a fresh dressing every 12 hours until pain/swelling ceases.

3. Hot as it is, horseradish is actually a cure for indigestion and heartburn. This is largely because horseradish provokes the proper flow of digestive juices. The increase in digestive juices leads to complete digestion of the food, and heartburn, as well as indigestion, are erased. Furthermore, horseradish is exceptionally rich in enzymes, which assist the digestion of fat and, particularly, protein. This may be why the herb has become so popular for meat dishes. Amazingly, this meat digesting function became known in ancient times before anyone ever conceived of the existence of meat digesting enzymes. Europeans seemed to realize this instinctively.

4. Hoarseness and cough have been cured over the centuries with horseradish. Simply mix the grated herb with honey and perhaps vinegar, and eat several tablespoons per day until the condition is resolved.

5. Cancer may find its match in horseradish. This herb contains two anti-cancer compounds: allyl-isothiocyanate and peroxidase. The former is a cyanide containing compound, which exerts specific toxicity against cancer cells. Peroxidase, an enzyme which reverses cellular degeneration, is one of Nature's most potent anti-cancer substances.

6. Horseradish is a tonic for congestive heart failure. It strengthens the heart and impels the kidneys to remove excess fluid. While congestive heart failure is a serious disease and must be treated under a doctor's care, eating horseradish will assist in the cure.

7. For poison ivy, hives, eczema, or dermatitis, pack the involved region with a horseradish compress. Grate one or two tablespoons of horseradish. Crush with mortar and pestel; mix with honey, or mix in a fatty base such as lanolin, coconut fat, or butter, and apply to the involved region. Repeat as necessary, but discontinue use if redness or inflammation persists. Allergic reaction to horseradish is rare, but this herb does increase local circulation, and this may lead to redness or temporary irritation.

8. Lice or scabies finds its match in horseradish. This is largely because of the immense amount of sulfur in the herb, and sulfur is toxic to lice as well as the scabies mite. Follow the previous recipe, and apply the mixture to the involved region. If applying on hair, be sure to avoid contact with eyes. If horseradish juice enters the eyes, flush thoroughly.

9. Horseradish is perhaps best known as a remedy for stuffy sinuses. Obviously, as is attested by anyone who has eaten it, horseradish dramatically opens sinus passages. If you are plagued with clogged sinuses or chronic sinus infections, eat horseradish every day for at least two weeks. This alone usually eradicates the dilemma.

Kiwi Fruit

By its name it might be thought that the kiwi fruit originated in the land of the Kiwi bird: New Zealand and Australia. Rather, it is originally a Chinese plant, and it was known as late as 1906 as the Chinese gooseberry. This name is the result of the fact that, like gooseberries, kiwi fruit grow on vines and have a hairy surface. After being introduced to New Zealand early in this century, it rapidly became a staple food and valuable commodity. New Zealanders renamed it in order to assist their marketing efforts.

While its originators were unaware of it, kiwi fruit is a tremendously valuable health food. It is relatively low in sugar compared to most fruits, while being packed with curative vitamins, minerals, and enzymes. One large kiwi fruit contains a greater amount of vitamin C than a cup of strawberries, an orange, or half a grapefruit. This means that kiwi fruit is an excellent source of vitamin C and contains a greater amount of this nutrient than the majority of fruit. In fact, it is so rich that it would be more nutritionally correct to consider a kiwi instead of an orange per day when attempting to meet minimal vitamin C needs; for instance, a medium-sized orange contains 60 to 80 mg, while a four ounce kiwi contains 100 mg. Kiwi is also a top source of folic acid and beta carotene.

Although few people realize it kiwi fruit is a top source of dietary fiber. There is a greater amount of fiber in three kiwi fruits than a bowl of bran flakes, and the fiber content is increased dramatically if they are eaten with the skin on.

Kiwi fruit is a highly effective digestive aid, because it contains a powerful enzyme called *actinidin*. In fact, pureed kiwi makes an excellent tenderizer if used in a marinade for meat. The enzyme is so powerful that simply rubbing a half kiwi fruit on meat will tenderize it. Another reason kiwi aids digestion is that it is an extremely rich source of potassium, a mineral which is needed to stimulate the flow of digestive juices.

Top Kiwi Tips

1. Never add fruit to gelatin; the gelatin won't solidify, because the enzymes in kiwi will digest it.
2. Use kiwi fruit in meals containing meat; it greatly aids in the digestion of dense protein such as milk, meat, eggs, and poultry.
3. Kiwi is an ideal fruit for breakfast. Not only does it taste good, but it is also easy to digest, which is important for those who find it difficult to eat breakfast. When nothing else seems to be tolerated, try eating kiwi fruit with some protein, for instance, a boiled egg. Kiwi fruit improves appetite, and soon the individual will desire a more complete breakfast as a result of consuming it regularly.
4. Whenever eating heavy food, such as nuts or meat, eat an organic kiwi for dessert. The digestive enzymes in the kiwi fruit will greatly aid in the digestion of the protein-rich meal.
5. If possible, buy kiwi when they are in the hard state. Once they become soft they have lost much of their curative, that is enzymatic powers. If the

fruit can be easily dimpled, don't buy it. Fresh kiwi are so hard that they are difficult to dimple.

6. Much of the enzyme content of kiwi is found just under the skin. If the kiwi is washed thoroughly, it may be eaten entirely, including the skin. This will also provide much needed fiber.

7. Kiwi fruit is an excellent addition to cottage cheese; use it instead of pineapple. While pineapple is nutritious, kiwi is actually richer in vitamin C, potassium, and enzymes.

Top Kiwi Cures

1. Along with papaya, kiwi is a top fruit for combating indigestion. Sour stomach, stomach ache, and heartburn may all be successfully treating by eating one or two unripe kiwi. The more sour or unripe the fruit is the more aggressive will be the anti-heartburn action. If you have a tendency to have a sour stomach, eat a kiwi fruit for dessert.

2. Kiwi is an excellent remedy for inflammatory disorders. The enzymes in kiwi act as antiinflammatory agents. If you suffer from an inflammatory disease, such as arthritis, fibromyalgia, polymyositis, migraines, lupus, or psoriasis, eat kiwi on a daily basis.

3. Kiwi may be the answer for colon disorders, particularly irritable bowel syndrome, Crohn's disease, ulcerative colitis, and diverticulitis. Digestion is impaired in all of these disorders. Kiwi fruit is valuable, because it is readily digested, and it tremendously aids in the digestion of other foods. Furthermore, the enzymes in kiwi help reduce the swelling and inflammation which typically occurs in the aforementioned disorders. If you suffer from inflammatory bowel disease, eat a kiwi fruit with every meal. Be sure to select fruit which are firm. These are highest in enzymes and are also sour in taste.

4. Constipation meets its match with kiwi fruit. Not only is it loaded with fiber, but it also contains a dense amount of digestive enzymes, which are needed to promote healthy elimination. Kiwi is far from a harsh laxative; it simply helps normalize digestion and assimilation. If you suffer from severe constipation (less than one bowel movement per day), eat a kiwi fruit with each meal, and be sure to eat the skin (but wash it thoroughly before eating).

5. Individuals suffering from inflammation of the joints and muscles

171

should consume kiwi regularly. The enzymes found in kiwi could prove a boon for individuals with arthritis or fibromyalgia. These enzymes are also valuable for combating low back pain, hip pain, and sciatica. Eat two firm kiwi fruit daily, preferably on an empty stomach. The latter will optimize the absorption of the fruit's antiinflammatory enzymes.

Oatmeal and Oat Bran

Interestingly, the first known reference to oats in human literature refers to their use as a medicine. They are rather a late development in humankind's history of commercial grains and were apparently first cultivated a mere 2,000 years ago. Oats were introduced in America during the early 17th century, when they were planted on the Elizabeth Islands.

Oats are easier to digest than the majority of common grains such as wheat and rye. Oatmeal has been a mainstay in the American diet since the 1800s, but it has fallen out of vogue recently. The once famous oatmeal breakfast recently became an antiquity for the modern generation of Americans. However, oats are making a comeback, primarily as a result of publicity on the value of oat bran in lowering cholesterol levels. In fact, because of this publicity, oat bran became a panacea, and during the late 1980s people were gulping it down by the ton in every form from Cheerios to oat bran muffins. Then, in 1990 a scientific study was published in the *Journal of the American Medical Association* indicating that oat bran was impotent in lowering cholesterol levels. The results of this study were publicized nationally, and interest in oat bran, as well as oatmeal, plummeted irreversibly. There is a slight rebound in interest, because the gist of the research does indicate positive effects. For instance, research conducted at the University of Kentucky's College of Medicine clearly shows that oat bran has a mild but significant cholesterol lowering effect. This makes sense, since all types of bran reduce blood cholesterol levels. Yet, a cholesterol lowering effect is certainly not the primary reason for eating oats. They are a good source of nutrients—protein, fatty acids, vitamins, and minerals—and that is what makes whole oats and, particularly, oat bran so valuable.

Oats are a good source of thiamine and vitamin E. However, virtually all of the thiamine and vitamin E is found in the bran and germ. Thus, it is more correct to describe oat bran rather than oatmeal as a top source of nutrients. This means that oat bran cereal, which is available commercially, is the best type to eat in order to achieve the greatest nutrient density per serving. Oat bran is unusually rich in magnesium, phosphorus, and iron. It contains a fair amount of riboflavin, but, in contrast to other grains, such as wheat and rice, it is virtually devoid of niacin. A diet heavy in oats may lead to niacin deficiency especially if a considerable amount of corn is eaten which is also deficient in niacin. This deficiency is represented by dry, scaly skin, sore or inflamed tongue, dry mucous membranes, dermatitis, fatigue, memory loss, irritability, depression, mental confusion, diarrhea, and nausea. High cholesterol and/or triglycerides are also a sign of niacin deficiency, as is heart failure. The main problem with oats and corn is that both lack sufficient niacin and tryptophan. Tryptophan is an amino acid, which can be converted by the body into niacin. Growth, energy, strength, and mental prowess cannot be sustained by a diet deficient in niacin and/or tryptophan. This type of diet is common in the South, where niacin deficiency is endemic.

Oat bran cereal is available commercially as Mother's Oats made by Quaker Oats. The best way to eat oat bran cereal is to serve it hot combined with foods which boost the niacin, tryptophan, and protein content. In order to fortify oats, add whole milk, which is rich in tryptophan, an amino acid that is deficient in oats. Eating oat bran cereal topped with milk along with a couple of eggs would suffice in providing a nutritionally complete meal, since eggs are inordinately rich in niacin and contain large amounts of tryptophan.

Oats may be commonly sprayed with pesticides; ideally, buy organically grown oat bran or oatmeal. For information on a high quality organically grown oat bran see Appendix B.

Top Oat Tips

1. If you enjoy oats, make your own oat fortifying foods. What I am warning you about is the fact that commercial oat-based foods often contain much more than oats, and the other ingredients are undesirable. The additives include sugar, hydrogenated oil, refined vegetable oil, and artificial flavors/colors. As a result, the health benefits of the oats are

obliterated. It can be enjoyable to cook your own recipes and, most importantly, you can make the recipes healthy by controlling the quality of the ingredients in the baked goods. Make your own oatmeal breads and cookies using oatmeal, oat bran, pure butter, raw sugar, eggs, and other quality ingredients. Always soak oats in the cooking liquid overnight.

2. Oatmeal is a healthy cereal, and it is an ideal cereal for children. Get children accustomed to an oatmeal breakfast in preference to commercial boxed cereals. Top the freshly cooked oatmeal with a small amount of pure raw honey and whole milk or cream. Add cinnamon and raisins, if desired. This is certainly superior to commercial cereals, which are usually laced with white sugar, corn syrup, food dyes, artificial flavors, synthetic iron, and other undesirable ingredients.

3. Oat bran cereal is the oat cereal of choice for adults and is ideal for children as well. It is significantly richer in nutrients than regular oatmeal. This is because the bran, which is the outer coating of the oat grain, is the region of the greatest nutrient density. Being lower in starch than oatmeal, oat bran is exceptionally rich in protein, fat, vitamins, and minerals. It is a top source of minerals and is one of the richest sources of magnesium known.

4. If you must sweeten the oatmeal, add raisins or currants. Don't add molasses, white sugar, or brown sugar. That will make the meal excessively high in carbohydrates, which will upset body chemistry. High carbohydrate breakfasts place great stress upon the adrenal glands. If the adrenals are continuously battered via high carbohydrate load, a variety of symptoms will likely arise, including blood sugar disturbances, uncontrollable appetite, headaches, irritability, muscle spasms, joint pain, cold extremities, heartburn, dizziness, moodiness, agitation, and fatigue. By itself, oat bran is sweet enough. Ideally, add no sugar, but, instead, top the cereal with cream, whole milk, and/or cinnamon. If you must add sweeteners, use a bit of honey or grape syrup.

5. If you make homemade baked goods, fortify the recipes with oat bran. This will enhance the nutritional status of the bakery, making it more filling and less starchy. Preferably, add Nutri-Sense, which more than triples the nutritional quality of the bakery (see Appendix A).

6. Remember, oat products contain gluten, a protein which is difficult to digest for certain individuals. If oats are poorly tolerated, this may be an indication of gluten intolerance, a condition which afflicts millions of Americans. In this instance, all gluten containing grains must be avoided,

a category which includes wheat, rye, barley, spelt, and oats. Oats are also rich in phytic acid, a substance which is in reality a type of fiber. Phytic acid interferes with the absorption of trace minerals, particularly zinc and calcium. Due to the phytic acid content, a high intake of oats can lead to trace mineral deficiency. Soaking oats ovenight in the cooking liquid with seasalt and two tablespoons of yogurt can eliminate this problem.

Top Oat Cures

1. Oat bran is at least part of the answer for high cholesterol levels. Though there has been some controversy regarding its effects, the gist of the evidence indicates that when it is used as a regular component of the diet it may reduce cholesterol levels by as much as 15%. Oat bran is an excellent source of a type of roughage known as soluble fiber. This type of fiber tends to bind to excess cholesterol molecules, preventing them from being absorbed. Furthermore, oat bran is a decent source of vitamin B_1, choline, inositol, and vitamin E, all of which have been shown to lower cholesterol levels.

2. Oat bran is a superior type of bran for ameliorating constipation than is wheat bran. The latter may actually aggravate constipation, as a consequence of wheat allergy. Allergic reactions to wheat lead to the destruction of the gut wall, and the result is sluggish bowel function. If you suffer from constipation, try fortifying flour with oat bran when making baked goods. Also, eat a large helping of oat bran cereal for breakfast. For another superior fiber source top the cereal with a tablespoon of Nutri-Sense, which is high in several types of edible fiber (see Appendix A). However, in the case of allergic intolerance or gluten sensitivity even oat bran may aggravate digestive disturbances and induce constipation.

3. Oat bran may aid in the cure of moodiness, irritability, and depression. This is because it is a rich source of thiamine and magnesium, both of which are needed for optimal mental function. These nutrients are required for the manufacture of neurotransmitters, the chemicals responsible for the transmission of messages within the nerve cells. Niacin and tryptophan are also needed for enhancing neurotransmission, but these are lacking in oats. That is why it is important to fortify the oat

bran by adding whole milk, which is rich in both niacin and tryptophan. Further fortification can be achieved by adding a tablespoon of Nutri-Sense, which is incredibly rich in niacin—far more than is found in milk. Three heaping tablespoons of Nutri-Sense contain as much as 40% of the minimum daily requirement for this vitamin.

4. Many individuals claim that without eating starch or cereal with meals, they cannot get full. Instead of eating white flour-infested toast or bagels with breakfast, eat a bowl of oat bran cereal. The bran is lower in starch and higher in protein than any other commercial cereal, plus, because it is rich in fiber, it is quite filling. To make it even more filling and nutritious, top the cereal with a tablespoon of Nutri-Sense, which is rich in chromium, the blood sugar regulating mineral. The fiber, vitamins, and minerals in the oat bran/Nutri-Sense combination will create a sensation of fullness and help prevent overeating. What a power-packed, nutrient-rich cereal this is, full of iron, magnesium, chromium, thiamine, pyridoxine, pantothenic acid, choline, inositol, niacin, and vitamin E.

5. Oat bran is a good source of iron and contains a greater amount of this nutrient than oatmeal. For women with iron deficiency anemia a breakfast consisting of oat bran and eggs, both of which are rich in iron, is ideal for gradually replenishing iron stores. To aid in iron absorption consume a large glass of citrus juice with this breakfast; the citric and ascorbic acids accelerate iron delivery from the intestines into the bloodstream.

Olives and Olive Oil

God alone knows how long the olive has been used as food and medicine. What is known is that humankind cultivated olives even before recorded history. It is believed that Abraham used olives and olive oil as medicinal aids. Cured olives were left in the pharaohs' tombs as food for the afterlife. The Greeks mention olive oil as a medicine useful for a variety of ailments. Some olive trees still alive in the Mediterranean are said to have been "born" before Christ. The olive is mentioned prolifically in the Bible, and the Qur'an devotes an entire chapter to it.

Spain and Italy are the major producers of the olives and olive oil available in America. Lesser amounts are produced in China, Australia,

Greece, and the United States. Fortunately, the ancient traditional method is still used to cure olives and extract the oil, and, thus, few if any noxious chemicals are used. Ensminger notes that the method of extracting olive oil in the Mediterranean remains traditional: heavy mechanical presses are used to extract the oil without heat or chemicals. It may be filtered, but there is no other refining or adulteration. This is extra virgin olive oil only.

In dozens of countries, notably Spain, France, Greece, Crete, Lebanon, and Italy, olives and olive oil are staple foods. Here, the health benefits of olives and olive oil have been known for untold centuries. An Italian chef or a villager in Spain, Greece, or Lebanon is unimpressed by the latest "breakthroughs" on the health benefits of olive oil. Tell the foreigner that olive products block heart disease and he/she will probably laugh, as if to say, "We don't even have heart disease here despite living to an old age—we already know about our olives." The fact is on the island of Crete, where olive oil is essentially drunk instead of eaten, the heart disease incidence is nil. The people of Crete have the highest consumption of olive oil in the world and one of the lowest rates world wide of degenerative disease. Obviously, olives and olive oil are largely responsible. The French, who enjoy excellent health, eat olives and consume large amounts of olive oil. This certainly could explain the comparatively low incidence of heart disease and cancer occurring in France.

Olives and olive oil are primarily fat, although olives contain a small amount of protein. The fat is chiefly monounsaturates, although a significant portion, nearly 20%, may be saturated. Both of these types of oils are highly digestible and readily absorbed into the blood. Interestingly, despite their oil content olives are low in calories; a handful contains a mere 100 calories. Contrary to popular belief, they are not fattening.

The primary nutritional value of olives is the result of their fat content. The fatty acids in olive oil serve as fuel and assist the function of the internal organs. This is particularly valuable for organs with a rapid metabolic rate, that is those which have a high demand for fuel such as the heart, kidneys, brain, thyroid gland, adrenal glands, liver, thymus, pituitary, and pancreas. Fats are the perfect food for providing fuel calories for the internal workings of the cells. The fact is the cells and organs of the body thrive on the type of fats found in olive oil.

177

Top Olive and Olive Oil Tips

1. Don't give up French fries; cook them in extra virgin olive oil. Cut washed potatoes into fries. Using a skillet heat olive oil (use about a half inch layer) on medium-low heat until hot; add fries and cook until slightly browned, turning if necessary. Remove and place on paper towels for a few moments. Serve hot with all-natural ketchup (note: Westbrae, a health food supplier, makes an excellent tasting sugar free ketchup known as *Unketchup*. Do not save or reuse the oil.

2. Use olives on salads. The fat in olives provides fuel calories for creating energy and strength, and these calories, for instance, cannot be provided by raw greens. Furthermore, the olives provide the fat necessary to provoke the secretion of bile, which is required for the absorption of fat soluble vitamins, carotenes, and phytochemicals.

3. If possible, purchase olives which are preserved in vinegar. This is because vinegar helps prevent vitamin loss from the olives, plus it inhibits microbial growth. Perhaps the best reason is that vinegar gives the olives a zesty taste.

4. If you think the olive oil in your cupboard is extra virgin, think again. Unfortunately, labels cannot be trusted, and just because an oil is labeled extra virgin it is no guarantee of purity. The purity of olive oil is a measure of how much acid it contains. Extra virgin olive oil contains very little acid, less than 1 %, while refined olive oil contains much more. In the past export governments carefully measured the acid level, and any oil measuring greater than 1% couldn't be deemed pure (i.e. extra virgin). Unfortunately, a variety of unscrupulous companies are artificially reducing the acidity of the oil, meaning that poorer quality oils are passing as extra virgin. Practically, this means that extra virgin olive oil may contain as little as 10% cold pressed/extra virgin oil, the remainder being heat or chemically extracted oil. If possible, demand in writing a guarantee from the manufacturer that their oil is unaltered and 100% pure extra virgin olive oil. There is one simple rule that you can use to procure an original oil; select the oil with the deepest green color you can find—this is a reasonable assurance of purity and a lack of processing.

5. To determine if the oil you buy is extra virgin perform a taste test; this is how connoisseurs evaluate oils. Place a teaspoon of the oil on the front of the tongue and hold between tongue and palate. Good quality oils have

a sweet taste, which is detectable only across the tongue horizontally and on the top of the palate. Poor quality or rancid oils are tasted vertically, that is they tend to induce a burning taste that runs into the sinuses, nose, and, particularly, up and down the throat. Pure, extra virgin oils are generally free of aftertaste, but poor quality ones may leave a bitter taste that lasts for several minutes.

6. Once the olive oil you purchased is opened, be sure to refrigerate it. Although it is more stable than other vegetable oils, olive oil can readily become rancid, and refrigeration impedes this process. One way to thoroughly block rancidity is to add antioxidant essential oils. Both oil of oregano and oil of rosemary are ideal. Add a few drops of each to each liter of olive oil, and this will significantly impede rancidity.

7. Use olive oil in cooking, but don't overheat it. Never heat it on high temperature. Use at the most medium-low heat.

8. If you can't digest fat, you can probably digest olive oil. It is certainly the most digestible of all oils. One reason is that it contains large amounts of *lipase*, an enzyme which digests fats. In a sense, olive oil is the perfect fat, because it digests itself.

9. Don't overuse olive oil. It is a rather precious substance, and small amounts go a long way. Use at most a few teaspoons when sautéing food. If you are deep frying, use the least amount possible. When you are done frying if you measured correctly, there should be little oil residue left in the pan. The oil should be discarded after use.

Top Olive Cures

1. Use olives and olive oil as a source of fuel for the body's energy needs. They are ideal for individuals suffering from fatigue, whether mental or physical. The fatty acids in olives are utilized to created energy in the muscles, so olives and olive oil are ideal fuel foods for athletes.

2. Olives make a great between meal snack. They are filling and are certainly far more nutritious than traditional snacks, which are generally high in sugar and starch. Because olives are filling, they help prevent binging on snacks such as pretzels, chips, cookies, doughnuts, and candy.

3. Olives are a top source of salt. Remember, salt is a nutrient, and some individuals require a regular intake of high salt foods for maintaining the

function of the adrenal glands. If you crave salt or if you have weakened adrenal function, you may thrive on salty snacks (see the *Self-Test Nutrition Guide*, i.e. The Adrenal Failure Syndrome). The reason is that with adrenal failure no matter how much salt is consumed, it is readily lost in the urine and, thus, must continuously be replaced. This is because the hormone which helps the body retain salt, *aldosterone*, is lacking.

4. Olives are one of the easiest of all foods to digest. If you suffer from a sensitive stomach, food allergies, or irritable colon, eat olives on a daily basis. Because of their rich content of monounsaturated oils, olives aid digestion and stimulate liver function. They also aid in the production of bile, which is needed for fat digestion.

5. Extra virgin olive oil is an excellent remedy for dandruff and may even be of value in hair loss. Rub the oil into the scalp at night; apply a night cap. Wash off the oil with shampoo in the morning. Repeat this treatment daily for at least one week.

6. If you can't seem to get full, eat a handful of olives with each meal. The olives provide fat, which creates satiety. Olives are an ideal between meal snack for individuals suffering from sweet cravings, uncontrollable appetite, or blood sugar disturbances.

Don't be concerned about the fat content. Ironically, people eat a wide range of salty snacks, loaded with processed fats, without concern. Yet, they often worry about the fat content of natural foods such as olives and nuts. Olives are certainly superior to less nutritious and more fattening snacks such as chips, cookies, microwave popcorn, and pretzels, all of which contain added fat.

7. If you desire the finest complexion in the world, eat olives regularly. Olives provide the types of oils needed for a Mediterranean complexion. For the finest skin ointment rub a fine grade of extra virgin olive oil on the face at night and leave on while sleeping. Wash off in the morning. Better yet, take it internally; two tablespoons of pure extra virgin olive oil every day.

Onion

Even garlic fails to overcome the position of onion in history. Worshiped by the ancient Egyptians and honored in the Bible, the onion is perhaps the most universally utilized spice known to the human race. Alexander the Great relied upon onion rations for giving his troops strength and stamina during battle.

Onions were first cultivated in the Middle East. From here they were disseminated throughout the world. They were introduced to the Americas by Columbus, who planted them in the West Indies.

Onions have been utilized as a natural medicine by virtually all civilizations. In some ancient civilizations they served as a primary food. This versatility is due to the fact that they are easy to grow and have a long shelf life. Onions are an invaluable tonic for the body and are highly digestible. In fact, onions are a digestive aid and are particularly valuable for aiding in the digestion of meat and fat.

Onions contain a good supply of nutrients and are high primarily in sulfur and potassium. A mere half cup contains 130 mg of potassium. Raw onions are also a respectable source of vitamin C. Depending on the size, one onion may contain as much as 20 mg of vitamin C. Green onions are unique, because they contain a large amount of vitamin A, which is concentrated in the green shoots as beta carotene. Green onions also provide considerable amounts of folic acid and far more vitamin C than regular onions. Depending upon the size a single green onion contains as much as 8 mg of vitamin C. A cup of chopped green onion tops contains 80 mcg of folic acid, which makes them richer in this nutrient than other highly touted sources such as cabbage, Brussels sprouts, lettuce, tomatoes, and cauliflower.

Top Onion Tips

1. Don't buy onions which have soft spots. This means they are rotten and are contaminated by bacteria or fungi. Make sure they are firm throughout. Some onions may feel firm but show evidence of mold growth; even though it appears to be on the outside, the onion is likely rotten throughout.

2. Onions should never be stored in plastic bags, as plastic retains moisture, and this leads to spoilage. Refrigerate onions only after they are cut, since refrigeration also causes them to retain moisture. Moisture provokes the growth of molds, which cause the onions to spoil.

3. Red onions are usually the mildest or sweetest variety, although some yellow onions, such as Maui and Vidalia, are mild in taste. Yellow and white onions are the strongest tasting varieties.

4. The curative properties of onions are found largely in the volatile oils, the substances which make us weep. Try to utilize the entire onion, once it is dismembered, or use it within a few days. Onions also absorb odors from the refrigerator, and this spoils the taste.

5. Use fresh onions, either sliced or diced, in all meat dishes, especially beef, turkey, chicken, or salmon entrees. Onions liberate a variety of substances which help keep the meat fresh by inhibiting bacterial growth. One way to avoid food poisoning at a picnic is to add plenty of chopped onions to all meat or poultry dishes. Plus, be sure to include onions in salads, since vegetables may also transmit infection.

6. Green onions are a neglected delicacy which should be consumed more often. They are a more dense source of nutrients than bulbous onions, plus they offer a totally different taste. Use them raw on salads and diced in stir fry or casseroles.

7. The best tasting and most nutritious onions are relatively small in size. They should be no bigger than the size of a large lemon. These onions tend to have a richer flavor and are less fibrous than huge onions, plus they are easier to chop and grate than the larger sizes. The smaller onions, particularly red and green varieties, contain a greater amount of vitamin C and also contain a wealth of beta carotene. Unfortunately, nutrition isn't usually a consideration when onions are harvested, and they may grow to be excessively large. The point is that older onions tend to be less sweet, less juicy, more bitter, and more fibrous than the younger varieties. Always choose small onions for superior taste and nutrition.

Top Onion Cures

1. Red, green, and yellow onions contain chemicals known as bioflavonoids, which block inflammation and decrease swelling. This means they are an ideal food for arthritics. There is a word of caution: some arthritics are allergic to onions, and in this instance the arthritis could get worse on the onion prescription. If no allergy exists, eating an onion per day may well keep the joint pain at bay.

2. Onion juice is the perfect anti-burn remedy. Simply crush enough onion to cover the burn either with the pure juice or with the macerated onion. Cover lightly with gauze, and repeat as needed until pain, swelling, and blistering dissipates. The burn will heal more readily and with less likelihood of scarring as a result of the onion bandage. Onion juice also helps speed the healing of minor cuts and abrasions.

3. Onions thin the blood, because they interfere with the formation of blood clots. Thus, they are an excellent remedy for circulatory disease, specifically hardening of the arteries, heart disease, coronary artery disease, congestive heart failure, stroke, and diabetes. Individuals suffering from impaired circulation and/or heart ailments should eat onions, both raw and cooked, every day.

4. Recently, it has been documented how onions act to thin mucous in the respiratory passages such as the nasal mucosa, sinuses, and bronchial tree. This is no surprise to anyone who handles onions in the kitchen—that acrid chemical that arises from them and causes the eyes and nose to run is the same one responsible for opening up clogged passages. The chemical is useful, because a variety of respiratory disorders, notably asthma, bronchitis, chronic cough, and sinusitis, are associated with thickened mucous and congestion of the respiratory membranes. The volatile oils in raw onions, which are liberated when they are cut, open clogged passages and liquefy mucous. Furthermore, these oils are natural antiseptics and are capable of killing a wide range of microbes. The caustic nature of onion juice proves useful in the event of microbial infection. The fact is regular consumption of onions is highly effective in preventing the onset of infection, particularly respiratory infections such as bronchitis, colds, flu, pneumonia and sinusitis. In order to prevent lung infections it is important to keep the mucous liquefied. This allows the natural immunity of the lungs to remain highly active as a result of a phenomenon known as ciliary action. The cilia are tiny hair like projections, which are located on the cells that line the bronchial tract. The cilia are in constant motion, driving foreign substances away from the vulnerable inner portions of the respiratory passages. If bacteria get into the bronchial tubes or lungs, it is the cilia which drive them out. The cilia function optimally if the mucous is liquid, and their motion stagnates if mucous thickens. Onion oils and juices keep the mucous thin and help maintain normal ciliary motion.

5. Cancer is associated with thickened blood. The thick blood not only diminishes oxygen and nutrient supply to the tissues, but it also increases the likelihood for the spread of tumors. By thinning the blood naturally, the tendency for tumors to spread is significantly reduced. Onions also contain a powerful anti-cancer substance known as quercetin. This is only found in onions which have color, that is yellow and, particularly, red onions. Harold Newmark, a professor at Rutgers University, notes that quercetin inhibits the growth of bowel cancer, but it probably works for other cancers as well. It is believed that quercetin blocks the genetic damage that leads to cancer. If you have cancer, eat onions on a daily basis, and if you wish to prevent cancer from striking, onions should be on the daily menu.

6. Hepatitis has reached epidemic proportions in the United States and has become the major cause of liver disease world-wide. There are a variety of types of hepatitis, which is defined as inflammation of the liver. Hepatitis may be caused by excessive eating (particularly high sugar consumption), chemical toxicity, infection, and alcohol consumption. The latter is itself a form of chemical toxicity. Besides alcohol, drug overdose and drug reactions, whether prescription or illicit, is the major cause of chemical hepatitis. Pharmaceutical drugs are a primary cause of hepatitis. Incredibly, millions of individuals develop drug-induced hepatitis each year. For instance, as many 100,000 individuals develop hepatitis from the drug acetaminophen alone, and this is a non-prescription substance. If you suffer from drug-induced hepatitis, regularly include large amounts of onions in the diet. Drink onion juice, one cup or more daily.

Onions are the ideal remedy for hepatitis. To achieve optimal effects juice the onions. The juice of two or three onions is a virtual cure for hepatitis, especially infectious hepatitis. Drink the juice every day until the hepatitis is cleared.

7. Gallbladder disease may also respond to the onion cure. Onions are capable of dissolving stones and certainly prevent gallstone formation. If you have gallstones or gallbladder disease, eat at least one whole raw onion daily. In order to aggressively dissolve the stones drink a cup of onion juice twice daily. For an even more powerful gallbladder remedy add the juice of radishes and parsley. Black radish and onion juice is the most powerful type for dissolving gallstones.

8. Onions are an ideal remedy for individuals troubled with irritable

bowel syndrome, spastic colon, or constipation. This is because they contain bioflavonoids, which act directly upon the intestinal walls to decrease swelling and inflammation. Furthermore, dried onions, as well as shallots, contain a considerable amount of fiber, which helps regulate bowel function. Dried onions and shallots contain up to 10 times more fiber, protein, and bioflavonoids than fresh onions. Additionally, they have a mild laxative action, just enough to help but not enough to make things worse.

9. Onions are an ideal food for individuals with lung disease, particularly asthmatics. This is especially true of red onions, which contain large amounts of quercetin, a bioflavonoid useful in combating inflammatory lung disorders. Furthermore, onions contain volatile oils, which soothe irritated bronchial tissues, while opening clogged nasal, sinus, and bronchial passages. There is a word of caution: asthmatics often suffer from food allergies, and allergy to onions is a possibility.

Oregano

Oregano, one of the most well known spices, is also one of the world's finest natural medicines, that is if it is true oregano. Virtually everyone is familiar with oregano, largely because of its popularity in pizza, spaghetti, and other Italian fare. However, few people realize that the oregano found in the supermarket, as well as that used by the local pizza palace, may not be truly oregano. Rather, as described by food technologists Drs. Taintu and Grenis, it is usually derived from a plant known as Mexican oregano. The latter is a type of sage brush which is entirely unrelated to oregano.

The confusion about oregano is due to the fact that there are some 40 species of oregano-like plants. However, only a few of these are true oregano species—and all true oreganos grow wild. Furthermore, the terms marjoram and oregano have been used synonymously, adding to the confusion. Thus, the oregano which is available in the supermarket is either Mexican sage or a mixture of marjoram, sage, and perhaps oregano.

The medicinal properties of oregano were largely discovered by the ancient Greeks, who used it extensively as a medicine. However, the Babylonians also described it in their clay tablets as a primary cure. This

185

ancient medicine goes back even further than recorded history. According to Dr. H. Baser, Dean of Pharmacognosy at Andalou University, the use of oregano as an ancient medicine dates to virtually the beginning of human history. A queen's grave, carbon dated to be 50,000 years old, found in what is now known as Iraq, tells the real story of oregano. With the queen were several medicinal plants, and one of them was oregano. This is the oldest record of any aromatic plant ever.

The ancient Greeks were exceptionally fond of oregano, finding it pleasurable for its aroma, taste, and curative properties. They described dozens of medicinal uses for it. They applied the crushed leaves of the fresh plant on sore, swollen joints and sore muscles. When taken internally they discovered that it eradicated parasitic and bacterial infections. They relied upon it for respiratory disorders and digestive complaints. It was the remedy of choice for poisoning and venomous bites, plus it was used both to heal wounds and prevent infection. For battle wounds and injuries it was applied as a pain killer and antiseptic. They found it dependable as a cure for infestations by lice, scabies, and worms. In short, they found that it rejuvenated health regardless of the disease. This explains why they named it *origanos*, meaning "delight of the mountains." Have you ever wondered why the ancient Greeks had such powerful physiques? Perhaps it was the oregano.

The wisdom of the ancients was recently put to the test. A patient of mine suffered a spider bite caused by a brown recluse. After applying pure oregano oil, the massive inflammation of the bite was cured in less than 72 hours. No tissue damage or toxicity resulted. In fact, the oregano oil induced the most rapid and complete cure of a spider bite I have ever seen.

The Romans continued the prolific use of oregano and popularized it in Europe. In the 16th century Europeans used oregano for disinfecting contaminated rooms. By simply placing it in the rooms, the air was sterilized. Before refrigeration bunches of oregano were hung in dairies to prevent microbial growth in milk. Oregano was widely used during the 16th and 17th centuries for conditions such as stomach aches, heartburn, headache, diarrhea, poor appetite, chronic cough, poisoning, water retention, liver disease (including jaundice), tuberculosis, spider bites, scorpion bites, snake bites, and even rabies. It was administered as a dependable anti-diarrheal, even for cholera. For fevers it induced sweating and helped break them quickly. Cavel may have been the first to explain oregano's impressive antiseptic properties. He found that the essential oil of oregano is such a potent antiseptic that it sterilized sewage.

Recent research lends proof to the ancient uses of oregano, particularly its reputed antiseptic powers. A variety of research points to an amazing fact: oregano oil is so potent that a tiny amount, less than even one percent, is enough to successfully combat microbial infections. Incredibly, research published in Greece in 1995 found that a one in 50,000 dilution was enough to partially stymie bacterial growth. A one in 4,000 dilution totally eliminated the organisms. In Italy scientists discovered that of all spices evaluated oregano was the most effective for killing bacteria. Cuban researchers found oregano capable of inhibiting the growth of a wide range of microbes, including Salmonella and E. coli. According to Mexican investigators oregano was the most powerful herb of some fourteen tested in killing Giardia, a noxious intestinal parasite. Furthermore, research published in Switzerland indicates that oregano in relatively small concentrations is capable of inhibiting the growth of virtually all types of fungi and/or yeasts, including Candida albicans. Other researchers found that of all spice oils tested oil of oregano was the most potent for inhibiting microbial growth.

Oregano, that is the wild variety, is rich in nutrients. It is a top source of vitamin E, containing primarily the highly touted gamma tocopherol, which has recently been shown to be a more powerful antioxidant than the type found in the typical vitamin E pill. By weight, it contains more niacin than meat. As a source of trace minerals it is hard to match. Oregano is several times richer in iron than meat and is a better source of calcium than milk, cheese, or dark greens. Impressively, oregano is 16 times higher in calcium than milk and 7 times higher in iron than liver.

Iron is needed to build blood and provide energy, but too much iron can be harmful. Researchers have determined that artificial types of iron, like the kind added to commercial foods or found in iron pills, accumulates in the body, causing organ damage. While synthetic iron may be harmful, oregano contains naturally bound iron, which is entirely safe for human consumption.

Like virtually all other herbs/spices the active ingredients in oregano are found in the oil, which is contained throughout the plant, primarily the leaves. By weight it is 2% or more oil, making it one of the most oil rich herbs known. Oregano oil exhibits perhaps the most potent antiinflammatory and antibiotic properties of any herbal oil known. Carvacrol, a type of phenol, is the name of the active ingredient. This substance is some 20 times more potent than synthetic phenol. For more detailed information about the medicinal properties of wild oregano read Dr. Cass Ingram's *The Cure is in the Cupboard: How to use Oregano for Better Health* (Knowledge House, 1997).

Top Oregano Tips

1. Oregano is one of Nature's finest preservatives. This effect is largely due to its potent antiseptic powers. Add ground oregano to meat, particularly ground beef or lamb. This will help prevent the growth of noxious microbes, plus it adds greatly to the flavor.
2. Add oregano, either fresh (chopped) or dried, to feta cheese. Together, cheese and oregano produce a powerful taste. Plus, the oregano helps neutralize any mold in the cheese. Chopped onions, oregano, feta cheese, and olive oil makes a fantastic appetizer for crackers and/or bread; add cherry tomatoes and turn it into a salad.
3. Ground or fresh oregano makes a tasty and nutritious addition to eggs. The oregano aids in the digestion of egg protein as well as cholesterol. This may be particularly valuable in the event of egg intolerance. It is possible that the eggs will be tolerated better by simply adding oregano. Chop fresh one or two tablespoons fresh oregano along with the tops of green onions into an omelet or fold into scrambled eggs. For a superior taste use crushed wild oregano, which is available as the supplement *Oregamax.* Simply open one or two capsules and add to the eggs.
4. It is difficult to get high quality fresh oregano, unless you grow it yourself. This is because the commercially available type is weak in medicinal and nutritive powers compared to the wild variety. If you plan on growing the herb in the garden, get European or English seeds; this type of oregano is more pungent and, therefore, contains a richer supply of the active ingredient.
5. As mentioned previously oregano lends itself well to ground meats. In particular, crushed wild oregano, as in Oregamax, is an ideal herb for

hamburger. Not only does it add flavor, but it also helps keep the meat free of infection. With the concerns over the transmission of infectious disease from ground beef, it makes sense to add natural preservatives. In essence, oregano prevents hamburger from spoiling, because it inhibits the growth of potentially toxic bacteria. Its effects are so dominating that after adding it to hamburger, the shelf life increases significantly. Add a tablespoon of oregano for every pound of hamburger. For added flavor, mix three or four cloves of diced garlic, or, if fresh garlic is unavailable, use one half teaspoon garlic powder.

6. Use oregano for any cheese containing dish. Traditionally, it tastes good on pizza, but it also adds a rich taste to cheese dip, sour cream, and feta cheese.

7. It has been recognized since ancient times that spices and herbs help prevent the spoilage of food. Now it is known that the volatile oils of these plants inhibit the growth of the microorganisms responsible for inducing spoilage. If packing food for travel or picnics, add a drop or two of oregano oil. A potent antiseptic, it helps protect the food from spoiling, while adding a pleasant, pungent flavor.

Top Oregano Cures

1. Colds and flu meet their match with oregano. This is because carvacrol, the active ingredient in oregano, exhibits significant anti-viral activity. The activity is potentiated by other natural antibiotics such as garlic and onion extract. Oregamax is an herbal supplement consisting of crushed wild oregano. It is combined with synergistic herbs such as *Rhus cariaria*, garlic, and onion. According to the *Journal of Ethnopharmacology* plants of the Rhus genus possess significant antiseptic powers. This may be explained by the fact that they are a rich source of flavonoids, gallic acid, and tannic acid. The tannic and gallic acids exhibit significant anti-bacterial, anti-fungal and anti-viral actions (tannic acid is the substance in regular tea that accounts for its healing properties). The combination of these herbs makes an ideal remedy in the event of colds or flu. If cold or flu strikes, take Oregamax as soon as possible; two or more capsules every hour is the ideal dosage. The more that is taken the more quickly will be the response. To accelerate the cure use oil of oregano, two drops

under the tongue several times daily. Continue until all cold/flu symptoms disappear. The Oregamax/oil of oregano prescription is highly effective. I have seen colds utterly defeated in less than a day and in some cases in a matter of minutes through using wild oregano.

2. Psoriasis and eczema may respond to oregano, especially the wild mountain grown variety. Rosenberg and colleagues of the University of Tennessee discovered that psoriasis and eczema are often caused by microbial infections. These infections occur both within the body, usually in the intestines and mucous membranes, as well as within the skin. Dr. Rosenberg, who is a medical professor at the university, discovered that the lesions of psoriasis and eczema frequently contain yeasts as well as bacteria, including strep and staph. If the organisms are killed internally or externally, the psoriasis improves. If you have eczema or psoriasis, take Oregamax, three capsules twice daily. Take also oil of oregano, several drops twice daily in juice or water. Note: Oregamax is an herbal product possessing natural antibiotic actions and exerts strong activity against fungi as well as bacteria. It is particularly active against yeasts, which are a main cause of psoriasis and eczema. Oregamax is made by North American Herb & Spice Company.

The essential oils in oregano are the active ingredients which are responsible for killing noxious microbes. It is most effective when taken internally, although topically application is advised, especially in mild-moderate cases. For severe cases destroy the organisms from the inside out for a more systemic and effective therapy.

Oil of Oregano made by North American Herb & Spice Co. is made from wild oregano. It is produced by natural methods without the use of chemicals/solvents. Chemical processing destroys the active ingredients. It is also the only liquid oregano oil which is emulsified in extra virgin olive oil. The emulsification process greatly aids in the absorption and tolerance of the oil. When taken internally, oregano oil is a tangy, peppery substance. Some individuals do find it extra hot. If you are unusually sensitive, take a small amount and work up to the recommended amount. Apply the oil once or twice daily until the lesions are eradicated. However, the best usage is internal, because that is where the fungus resides. Take 5-10 drops of oil of oregano twice daily in juice or water. Take also a drop or two under the tongue several times daily. Continue until the lesions are eradicated. As with all remedies if irritation occurs or if the lesions worsen, discontinue use.

3. If you suffer from bloating or gas after eating, use oregano with meals. Since Grecian times, oregano has been administered as an effective remedy for digestive complaints. Use fresh oregano in salads and stir fry, and garnish meat dishes with sprigs of oregano. In addition, take two or three capsules of Oregamax with meals.

4. Diarrhea meets its match with oregano, and, if it is consumed regularly, it is also useful for preventing diarrhea. If you suffer from chronic diarrhea or if you are vulnerable to developing bouts of diarrhea, you must use oregano regularly in the diet. Take several capsules of Oregamax three or four times daily. Combine this treatment with the raw honey protocol found in the honey section. Be sure to drink plenty of fluids. If the diarrhea fails to improve, see a doctor.

Oil of oregano is of tremendous value for reversing diarrhea. Usually, its action is quite rapid. A famous New York City talk show host's experience dramatically illustrates this. The talk host, who has interviewed me several times, received a call from his sister, who suffered unrelenting diarrhea for several days: nothing stopped it. He advised her to try the oil of oregano by taking two drops under the tongue (it is absorbed immediately this way). Impressively, the diarrhea was halted in less than two hours.

5. Fungal infection, particularly candidiasis, responds positively to the oregano prescription. Research published in the journals *Microbiology* and the *Journal of Food Science* notes that oregano possesses significant antifungal properties. Fungal infections are virtually epidemic in America, largely because of the overuse of antibiotics, which encourage fungal growth. Furthermore, the consumption of refined sugars dramatically encourages fungal growth in the body. The vast majority of Americans consume large amounts of refined sugars. It is no wonder that fungal infection represents the most common type of chronic infection seen in doctors' offices today.

Patients suffering from fungal infections should eat large amounts of oregano. However, the wild type of oregano possesses the greatest antifungal powers. If you suffer from internal fungal infection, take Oregamax on a daily basis. Depending upon the severity of infection, take 2 to 3 capsules of Oregamax three or four times daily. For skin fungal infections in addition to taking Oregamax use also oil of oregano topically. Rub the oil liberally into the involved regions. For athlete's foot apply the oil and immediately cover with a sock, as this helps hold the active ingredients against the skin. Take 1 or 2 drops of the oil under the tongue twice daily.

6. Oregano is the ideal herb for reversing lung disorders, particularly bronchitis, asthma, and sinusitis. This positive action is largely because oregano contains volatile oils, which open clogged sinus and bronchial passages. These oils, if inhaled directly, help sterilize the sinus passages. Use fresh oregano in as many recipes as is possible. Take Oregamax, two or three capsules twice daily. Inhale the oil directly from the bottle (or place a drop on tissue paper and inhale).

7. Oil of oregano is the perfect remedy for toothache. It penetrates readily into the gums and teeth and rapidly eases pain. It may be administered several times daily and is non-toxic. Another benefit is that while it eradicates the pain, it also kills infection. This makes it the perfect remedy for pyorrhea, infected teeth, or abscesses. It may also be applied before and after invasive dentistry. By doing so, the risk for serious infection is diminished dramatically.

8. Oregano is a superb remedy for intestinal gas, whether arising in the upper or lower intestine. Fresh oregano may give some relief. However, wild oregano, that is Oregamax, usually resolves this dilemma rapidly and is especially effective in halting foul smelling intestinal gas. Simply take two or three capsules of Oregamax with meals for one or two weeks. Then, take one capsule with meals as a maintenance.

9. Oil of oregano is an ideal remedy for childhood respiratory disorders, including asthma, chronic cough, sore throat, ear aches, and croup. For any type of congestion or constricted breathing simply rub a liberal amount of the oil on the chest at night until the breathing insufficiency or cough dissipates. For greater effect, directly inhale it from the bottle. Oregano oil contains volatile antiseptic agents, mostly carvacrol and a small amount of thymol, which relax constricted bronchial tubes and sinus passages. These volatile oils are so effective that improvement in breathing is often noted immediately. For ear aches rub a small amount near the opening of the ear and take a drop under the tongue several times daily. For sore throats take it under the tongue. Also, gargle with the oil by mixing a few drops in a glass of salt water.

10. Use oil of oregano to combat any type of skin fungal infection. The oil is highly active against all varieties of skin fungi and is an effective

remedy for athletes foot, toenail fungus, fingernail fungus, and ringworm. Carvacrol, the antiseptic agent in oregano oil, is highly antifungal. Researchers found that a tiny amount, less than 1%, is enough to kill all skin fungi tested. Simply apply the oil to the involved region twice daily.

11. Warts are no contest for oregano oil. For best results take it internally, and apply it topically. Prolonged contact gives the best results. Saturate a a piece of cotton with the oil and affix securely against the wart. Repeat this dressing once or twice daily. Take two or three drops of the oil under the tongue twice daily. Take also Oregamax, three capsules twice daily. For tough conditions take larger amounts.

12. Exhaustion and fatigue respond to wild oregano. The ancients relied upon it as an energizer. For a boost in energy take Oregamax, three capsules twice daily. Take also oil of oregano, two drops under the tongue twice daily.

13. Oil of oregano is the treatment of choice for scratchy, inflamed, and/or sore throat. Many individuals complain of a feeling of mucous or blockage in the throat. The latter may signal fungal infection of the throat, larynx, or esophagus. Researchers have recently determined that fungal/yeast infection of the throat and sinuses is far more common than was once believed. Oil of oregano quickly resolves these symptoms, especially if they are caused by fungus. Take two drops under the tongue twice daily and five drops in juice or water twice daily. Rub the oil on the throat at night for a soothing action. Take also Oregamax, two capsules twice daily. Note: constant feeling of fullness in the throat may also be a sign of cancer. If the condition fails to improve, see your doctor.

14. Oil of oregano is an anti-venom. Apply it to any suspect bite, especially bee stings, spider bites, snake bites, coral stings, jelly fish stings, and scorpion stings. It neutralizes the venom on contact. Repeat the application as necessary.

From this plethora of uses it becomes clear that oregano oil is the essential oil for the future. Keep it handy at all times. Don't travel without it. For extra insurance keep a bottle at home, in the car, and at work. It is beneficial on a daily basis. Just remember to use it.

Be aware of the fact that commercial oregano may not be oregano at all. Much of the shelf spice is labeled "Mexican Oregano." This is derived from a plant of the sage brush family, known botanically as *Lippia graveolens*. Most of the finely ground spice in the supermarket is *Lippia*.

The crumbled or leafy oregano is another problem. It is largely marjoram, and, although it is related to oregano, this plant fails to exhibit the healing properties of pure oregano. Unfortunately, the commercial oil is also faulty. As described by Julia Lawless in *The Encyclopedia of Essential Oils* virtually all of the commercially available oregano oil is not truly oregano oil. Rather, it is derived from either red thyme or marjoram. *Oil of Oregano* by North American Herb & Spice Co. is made from 100% pure oil of oregano derived from the true oregano species, and it is **guaranteed wild**.

Papaya

Papaya was first "discovered" in Central America by the Conquistadores in the late 1500s. From there it was disseminated throughout the tropics. Today, papayas are raised in tropical countries throughout the world and are found in virtually every supermarket.

Papaya is a unique fruit, because it is essentially an enzyme factory. It is chock full of enzymes, which are invaluable for aiding digestion as well as combating disease. The vitamin C content of papayas is particularly notable. Incredibly, one medium papaya supplies approximately 160 mg of the vitamin, nearly three times the RDA. The potassium content is massive. A large papaya contains nearly 1,000 mg, the equivalent of two bananas. The combination of enzymes, minerals, and vitamins makes papaya an antioxidant and disease-fighting powerhouse.

Most people believe that the papaya grows on trees, but this is not entirely true. Instead, it is the fruit of a giant tree-like herb, and, because it is more correctly described as an herb than a fruit, this may account for its unusually potent healing properties.

The papaya resembles a melon, and it may grow as large as some melons, attaining a weight of up to 20 pounds. While its solid content is mostly sugar, it contains a higher amount of minerals than the majority of fruit. Plus, it delivers a considerable amount of fiber.

Despite its sweet taste papaya is relatively low in sugar and is a healthy component of a low sugar diet. The reduced sugar content makes it a superior fruit for children instead of oranges, apples, bananas, or grapes. Diabetics should use papaya to replace other fruits.

As a source of vitamin C, papaya is superior to oranges. In addition, papaya is one of the few fruits which provides significant amounts of folic acid. It is so rich that a large papaya contains a minimum of 60% and as much as 100% of the RDA for this vitamin. Vitamin A is the other primary nutrient found in papayas. Occurring as beta carotene, it is responsible for their yellowish-orange color. A medium sized papaya contains over 10,000 I.U. of beta carotene, which equals the minimum daily requirement for vitamin A. The vitamin A contained in papaya is readily utilized by the body. Thus, you may eat as much of this fruit as desired without concern.

Top Papaya Tips

1. Papaya are often available ripe, but sometimes all you can get are green ones. If they are green, let them sit on the kitchen counter in front of a window. Sunlight may ripen them, and this process increases the nutrient content, notably vitamin C and beta carotene. Be wary of buying papayas which are totally dark green. These papayas are picked in an immature state and may never fully ripen. Thus, they are unfit for consumption.
2. Ripe papayas are slightly soft, in other words, you can dent them with the thumb. Another sign of ripeness is if the skin is partially yellow. If it is completely yellow, it might be overripe.
3. Don't throw the seeds away when preparing papaya. Eat them with the papaya, or save them and freeze for later use. If an acute illness, such as diarrhea, food poisoning, sore throat, or the flu, strikes, they may prove lifesaving.
4. Papaya seeds are a superb addition to home made salad dressings. Combine extra virgin olive oil, vinegar, spices, and a few papaya seeds. Mix in blender until the seeds are thoroughly ground. Pour over salads or hot vegetables.
5. Papaya is an ideal breakfast fruit. Since it is low in sugar, it doesn't cause a major stress upon the delicate adrenal glands, which may be sluggish in the morning. However, be sure to eat protein with the papaya; a couple of eggs or a hamburger patty will suffice.
6. Make papaya sherbet. Simply add papaya, ice, and honey to a food processor or blender and blend until smooth. Pack in appropriate containers and freeze.
7. Don't use papaya in gelatin molds. The enzymes will digest the gelatin and prevent it from solidifying.

Top Papaya Cures

1. Papaya is the ideal aid for indigestion. Use it to combat heartburn, bloating, gas, and stomach ache. Eat one half papaya after meals; be sure to also eat the seeds, as they are loaded with digestive enzymes.
2. If you suffer from constipation, papaya will assuredly help you. In addition to its high fiber content, it is rich in digestive enzymes. The enzymes accelerate the digestion of food, and this ultimately causes an improvement in elimination. Furthermore, papaya's enzymes are antiinflammatory. The enzymes are capable of blocking swelling and irritation within the colon, and this improves its ability to eliminate wastes. By regularly eating papaya the digestion will improve dramatically, and the stools will increase in bulk and frequency.
3. Papaya is also an excellent remedy for diarrhea. Its powers are increased if the seeds and pulp are consumed. Often, when nothing else works, papaya and papaya seeds will slow the diarrhea or halt it.
4. Arthritis may readily respond to the papaya dispensation. Eat an entire fresh papaya with the seeds daily for one week. If the arthritis improves, eat one half papaya daily or every other day as a maintenance. Papaya's enzymes are potent antiinflammatory agents, and their action helps decrease joint pain and swelling.
5. Papaya is an excellent medicine for stomach disorders, including stomach ulcers. Some doctors prohibit enzyme rich foods for ulcer patients on the basis that enzymes might aggravate the ulcer. However, this is untrue, as the enzymes actually act in the opposite manner. One study showed that when papaya was fed to animals who were given high doses of medicines that cause ulcers, like aspirin and steroids, significant protection against ulcer formation occurred. This is because papaya's enzymes speed the healing of damaged tissues. Furthermore, papaya is rich in vitamin A (as beta carotene) and vitamin C, and both are invaluable for healing the intestinal or stomach lining.
6. If you are scheduled for surgery, eat plenty of papaya. The enzymes in papaya, notably papain, help keep the blood from congealing and, therefore, help prevent blood clots. Papain has been employed by surgeons throughout the world for preventing adhesions, that is scarring, a common side effect of surgery. Eat a papaya per day to sail through surgery without side effects. There is one word of caution: avoid

consuming large amounts of papaya if you are taking blood thinners. In this case eat it occasionally, like once per week.

7. Papaya and its seeds are a top remedy for back ache. This is because papain, the papaya enzyme, is an aggressive antiinflammatory and anti-pain agent. For a sore back eat at least one papaya per day, and be sure to also eat the seeds.

Parsley

It would be difficult to find a food superior in curative powers to parsley. This is because it is among the most nutrient dense of all foods.

Unfortunately, today parsley has been classified as a mere garnish, and few people utilize it as a regular part of the diet. While the Romans used it as a food, they did instigate the garnish idea by eating sprigs of parsley at banquets. They used it as a before meal breath freshener.

Parsley, a native of the Mediterranean, has been grown commercially as a staple food for thousands of years. It was used heavily by the Greeks and Romans both as food and to a lesser degree as medicine. Galen dispensed it primarily as a diuretic. Britain's Culpeper recommended it for curing bruising tendencies and dissolving kidney stones. Medieval physicians noted that compresses of parsley were effective in ameliorating arthritis. As late as 1926 parsley was listed in the U.S. pharmacopoeia as a treatment for constipation, kidney disorders, and was even described as an alternative remedy for malaria.

Modern herbalists note that parsley is an effective remedy for virtually any illness. According to Dr. George Schwartz one of its unique components, apiol, is a sedative and may account for the sense of calm resulting from eating large amounts of the herb. He also notes that apiol helps reduce fever. Furthermore, it is a tremendous tonic for the malnourished individual and helps improve appetite, while combating fatigue.

More dense in energy-providing nutrients than the majority of green vegetables, parsley is low in water and high in protein. Incredibly, a cup of chopped parsley supplies nearly as much protein as a cup of corn meal. Dried parsley contains as much as 7 times the protein, vitamin, and mineral content of fresh parsley, and, thus, even small amounts added to food may contribute significant amounts of nutrients to the diet. However, dried parsley is low in vitamin C.

Parsley is immensely rich in vitamins and minerals. On an equal weight basis it contains 3.5 times as much vitamin C as oranges, twice as much folic acid as peas, more riboflavin than broccoli, and nearly twice the potassium content of bananas. Broccoli, which is traditionally regarded as a top vegetable source of calcium, is submissive to parsley, which contains fully twice as much per gram. Parsley is also an excellent source of magnesium, containing over 40 mg per 100 grams. This means that it is a richer source of magnesium than the more traditional sources such as brown rice and whole grains.

Top Parsley Tips

1. If parsley is used as a garnish, eat it. Don't waste this valuable plant. It is a dense source of nutrients; it should be consumed in large amounts and not used as a mere decoration.

2. Parsley must be wash thoroughly in cold water. It tends to hold dirt and sand, which is readily removed by rinsing. Do not use warm or tepid water, since it will become wilted.

3. To help preserve parsley add a wedge of lemon or lime to the storage bin. While parsley is a strong vegetable and doesn't spoil readily, it will discolor with time, and this means that valuable vitamins are lost. Onion and lemon prevent parsley from oxidizing and help preserve the vitamin content. Preferably, use parsley soon after purchase.

4. When serving rice or couscous add chopped parsley. For every cup of cooked grain add 1/4 cup of parsley. This will fortify the grain with much needed vitamins and minerals, as parsley contributes significant quantities of vitamin C, folic acid, beta carotene, vitamin E, vitamin K, calcium, potassium, iron, and magnesium. It is worthy to note that rice and grains are low in iron, calcium, and folic acid, plus they contain no vitamin K or beta carotene. Parsley provides all of these nutrients.

5. Instead of using parsley as a garnish, chop or shred several sprigs and toss it with salad greens. Make a habit of always fortifying salads with parsley, which provides much needed vitamin C, beta carotene, potassium, folic acid, and vitamin K.

6. Make a simple but vitamin rich salad from chopped onions, tomatoes, and parsley. Chop equal portions of each and top with vinegar and perhaps crumbled feta cheese. This is a salad fit for royalty.

7. Buy parsley root, if available, and use it regularly as a vegetable. It makes a tasty and nutritious addition to soups and salads. This root is rich in natural chemicals which exhibit anti-cancer properties.

Top Parsley Cures

1. Parsley is a stimulant for impaired digestion. It enhances the action of the stomach and provokes the secretions of the liver. If you suffer from digestive ailments, such as heartburn, gas, bloating, irritable bowel, or constipation, eat prodigious amounts of parsley with each meal. The digestion will assuredly improve rapidly.

2. Water retention is a common consequence of kidney or heart disease. Is the answer to take a diuretic? The problem is that in these diseases diuretic drugs may do more harm than good, because they cause a number of side effects, including mineral depletion and low blood pressure. Water retention may also be the result of allergic reactions to foods and chemicals. Another cause is the excessive consumption of refined sugar. Regardless of the cause parsley is helpful, because it is a natural diuretic and can be consumed with impunity in the event of fluid retention. Depending upon the severity of the fluid overload eat one or two cups of chopped parsley twice daily. For a more potent effect juice two or three bunches of parsley. Drink this juice undiluted in the morning for at least one week to accelerate the removal of excess body fluids.

3. If you have leg or foot cramps, parsley should be included in every meal. Use large amounts of fresh or dried parsley in soups, stir fry, and meat dishes. Add it to salads and vegetable trays. Because it contains large amounts of magnesium and potassium, the regular consumption of parsley will prevent spasticity or cramping of the muscles.

4. Parsley is the ideal vegetable for women suffering from premenstrual fluid retention. It is effective in reducing the water load, because it stimulates the kidneys to excrete water. Furthermore, parsley is rich in magnesium and potassium, both of which act as natural diuretics. It is ironic that synthetic diuretics, such as thiazides and Lasix, actually

deplete potassium and magnesium from the body. They operate in an unnatural fashion by forcing the kidneys to remove water, and the minerals are washed out along with it. With natural diuretics, such as parsley, the body's potassium and magnesium levels are never diminished, and, rather, they are bolstered.

5. Parsley may singlehandedly cure anorexia and/or emaciation. This is because it is extremely rich in a wide range of nutrients, and the nutrients within it are readily absorbed. If consumed regularly, it will regenerate even the most feeble of appetites. Ideally, consume two bunches of parsley daily to defeat anorexia, weight loss, and/or poor appetite. The most ideal method is to juice the parsley. Drink the juice of two or three bunches of parsley daily until the appetite improves and weight gain is established. Be sure to wash each sprig of parsley thoroughly before juicing.

6. For those suffering with high blood pressure parsley and/or parsley root is a top vegetable to consume. In Germany parsley seed is prescribed for high blood pressure; the seeds are steeped in hot water to form a tea. This remedy must not be attempted with commercial seeds, which contain chemical preservatives that may be toxic. However, if you grow your own parsley, save the seeds for use as a tea for combating fluid retention and/or high blood pressure. Yet, the plant itself is a diuretic. Make a salad from chopped parsley and parsley root. Simply chop a bunch of parsley and dice a few parsley roots. Add tomatoes, onions, vinegar and extra virgin olive oil. Eat this anti-high blood pressure salad once or twice daily.

Peanuts/Peanut Butter

Peanuts and peanut butter are indispensible as a source of nutrients and are one of the most nutrient dense of all foods. Rich in protein, peanut butter contains a greater amount by weight than beef or eggs, although the type of protein in it is less complete than the type found in animal foods. According to Ensminger one pound of peanuts is equivalent in protein power to a 14 oz steak or, amazingly, eight eggs.

Peanuts are a rich source of fuel in the form of saturated and monounsaturated fats. However, they are legumes, not nuts, and, thus, are higher in carbohydrates than true nuts. Even so, peanuts are richer in protein than many nuts, including filberts, Brazil nuts, and walnuts. Because they are nearly 30% protein by weight, peanuts are a more dense source of protein than milk or meat.

The vitamin content of peanuts and peanut butter is even more impressive than the protein content. They serve as a top source of thiamine and pantothenic acid and contain a considerable amount of pyridoxine, niacin, folic acid, choline, and riboflavin. This means that peanut butter is essentially a tasty B complex supplement. Keep in mind that riboflavin is found in large amounts in only a few foods, and peanuts as well as peanut butter are among the best sources. Children are commonly deficient in thiamine, riboflavin, niacin, pyridoxine, and folic acid. Peanut butter is an ideal B vitamin supplement for children, as it provides significant amounts of the aforementioned vitamins in forms that are readily absorbed. However, it is important to note that allergic intolerance to peanuts is relatively common in children; adults may also be allergic to this legume. If negative reactions, such as rash, shortness of breath, headache, and/or upset stomach, occur after eating peanuts and peanut butter, avoid them entirely.

Peanut butter, being a concentrate of peanuts, is listed as a top potassium source, containing by weight as much as three times the potassium content of fresh oranges and is also, incidentally, far richer in this mineral than bananas.

Peanuts are relatively high in the amino acid tryptophan, which is known for its calming effects upon the nerves. In fact, peanuts contain such a large amount of this amino acid that they may be expected to produce a calming effect upon the nerves after ingestion. They make a great snack for the insomniac.

Top Peanut Tips

1. When buying roasted peanuts avoid those cooked in hydrogenated or partially hydrogenated oil. Peanuts cooked in peanut or coconut oil are the best choice, but, unfortunately, they may be difficult to find.
2. The best type of peanuts are dry roasted peanuts. The traditional type

are roasted in the shell, salted or unsalted, and these contain the least amount of additives. Dry roasted peanuts in the jar are popular, but they are usually laced with all sorts of additives such as MSG, corn syrup, dextrose, dextrin, and wheat starch.

3. Ball park style peanuts have recently been popularized, and they received their most extensive exposure as a snack on commercial airlines. The ingredients are nothing but roasted peanuts and salt. This is the ideal peanut snack, nutritious with no sweeteners and no synthetic or harmful additives. Don't worry about the salt. It is good for the adrenal glands, plus it enhances protein digestion, and peanuts are mostly protein.

4. Don't eat raw peanuts. They contain goitrogens, which impede the function of the thyroid gland. More importantly, raw peanuts may contain aflatoxin, a potent poison secreted by a fungus which commonly attacks peanuts. Aflatoxin is destroyed during the heating process, so roasted peanuts and peanut butter made from roasted nuts are generally free of this poison. However, if you regularly eat peanut products, it is a good idea to take selenium (200 mcg) and vitamin E (400 I.U.). Researchers have determined that these two nutrients help block the toxicity of aflatoxin.

5. Concerns over contamination of peanuts by mold is legitimate. The mold readily grows on peanuts, especially if they are stored in a moist environment. This mold produces aflatoxin, one of the most powerful naturally occurring poisons known. Fortunately, there is a simple answer to this dilemma. Oil of oregano and oil of cumin readily kill this mold and may even neutralize existing aflatoxin (see Oregano section).

6. A salted peanut snack helps control blood sugar levels and, thus, defeats uncontrollable sugar cravings that lead to binging on sugary snacks. Peanuts are infinitely superior nutritionally compared to sugar fixes such as candy, cookies, cake, pastries, etc. Unadulterated peanuts are an ideal snack, because they are convenient as well as filling.

Top Peanut Cures

1. If you can't sleep at night, try eating a large handful of salted peanuts. The peanuts provide amino acids and B vitamins, which help sedate the nerves, and the salt relaxes the adrenal glands, which are stressed because of the failure to sleep.

2. Peanuts are an excellent food for enhancing athletic prowess and are certainly superior to candy bars or carbohydrate-based drinks. They supply dense amounts of niacin, thiamine, pyridoxine, and pantothenic acid, all of which are needed to boost energy as well as improve endurance and strength. The fat in peanuts improves muscular endurance; use them as a before training snack.

3. For individuals with failure to thrive or low body weight, peanut butter is an ideal food. During the 1930s it was used in the treatment of malnourished individuals. Peanut butter is rich in a variety of B vitamins which are necessary for cellular growth and repair. It is also high in protein and fatty acids. Thus, it is a perfect food for general nourishment. Be sure to buy peanut butter which is free of sugar or corn syrup, since the sugar destroys B vitamins and protein.

5. Many individuals suffer from bouts of weakness and/or exhaustion throughout the day. This may be coupled with sensations of hunger and perhaps even moodiness, irritability, and dizziness. All of these symptoms are warning signs of blood sugar disturbances and may signal adrenal fatigue. Peanuts are an ideal snack for obliterating these symptoms. Eat a handful for a quick energy and mood boost. They provide plenty of B vitamins, minerals, and fuel.

6. Peanuts are the ideal between meal snack for curbing sugar cravings in children. The fat and protein in peanuts, as well as the B vitamins, will halt sugar cravings by balancing the appetite and strengthening adrenal function. Salted peanuts work the best for this purpose, as the salt gives the adrenal glands a natural boost.

Pumpkin

The pumpkin is an excellent source of nutrition. Unfortunately, it is neglected and rarely used except for pies. This was not always the case. Pumpkin is one of those rare foods which is truly American in origin. While native Americans appreciated its immense nutritional powers for untold centuries, the French explorer Jaques Cartier was the first Westerner to stumble upon it. He found it growing in massive amounts in various native settlements near what is today Montreal.

The Natives made no carvings or effigies from their pumpkins; they ate them. Modern humanity has degraded this immensely valuable food to being a mere ornament; people waste it by the megaton every year.

Pumpkin is pure nutrition. Most importantly, it is a superb source of beta carotene. Fresh pumpkin is also an excellent source of fiber and contains a fair amount of calcium and phosphorus. Furthermore, fresh pumpkin is a good source of vitamin C. Canned pumpkin is a concentrate of this vegetable and, thus, is super-rich in beta carotene and is a good source of folic acid, calcium, phosphorus, potassium, and magnesium.

It is truly a travesty if not outright stupidity that pumpkin, the richest natural source of beta carotene, is dumped in the garbage during the fall season instead of being eaten like the natives did. Ironically, individuals often rely on vitamin pills instead of food as a source of beta carotene. The problem is that synthetic beta carotene is relatively impotent in offering curative benefits compared to the natural kind. Actually, evidence exists that synthetic beta carotene is of little, if any, value. Apparently, the synthetic form fails to perform the critical functions expected of this vitamin. In fact, recent research done in Finland found that synthetic beta carotene did nothing positive to reverse disease and may actually have done some harm, although the latter conclusion is probably exaggerated. On the contrary, beta carotene from food has been documented in hundreds of research studies to not only prevent certain diseases but also to act as an outright cure. Illnesses in which naturally occurring beta carotene has been found useful include acne, eczema, heart disease, hardening of the arteries, cervical dysplasia, leukoplakia, emphysema, chronic bronchitis, arthritis, immune deficiency, precancerous skin disorders, and cancer.

Top Pumpkin Tips

1. When selecting a pumpkin pick the small size. Larger ones are lacking in taste and are too fibrous. The pumpkin rind should be hard, as a soft rind is a sign of immaturity.
2. When making pumpkin pie use fresh pumpkin, if possible. The taste is superior, plus it is richer in nutrients than the canned variety.
3. If cooking fresh pumpkin, always save the seeds. Eat them raw or roast

them in an oven until slightly crisp. The seeds are high in minerals, particularly zinc and phosphorus, plus they contain a considerable amount of beta carotene, which accounts for their green color.

4. Canned pumpkin is an excellent food. Incredibly, one can of pumpkin contains over 70,000 I.U. of beta carotene. Canned pumpkin is also rich in folic acid, potassium, calcium, and magnesium. Opt for canned pumpkin made by various organic growers. Walnut Acres produces a superb canned pumpkin, which far exceeds the commercial varieties in nutritional value as well as taste. For more information see Appendix B.

5. When pumpkin is in season, buy several. Cook and preserve by freezing. In this manner the immense nutritional value of pumpkin can be available throughout the entire year.

Top Pumpkin Cures

1. Pumpkin is the ideal food for healing damaged lungs. It is inordinately rich in beta carotene, which is needed for the utilization of oxygen in the lungs. Eat pumpkin at least once per week or, preferably, daily in order to build healthy lungs.

2. Skin disorders, such as acne, dermatitis, eczema, and psoriasis, may respond positively to the pumpkin prescription. This is largely due to pumpkin's rich amount of beta carotene, a nutrient required for the maintenance of healthy skin cells.

3. Pumpkin is an ideal remedy for heart disease. Its supply of minerals and beta carotene nourishes the heart and blood vessels. Eat pumpkin at least twice per week if you suffer from heart disease.

4. Acne finds its match with pumpkin. Beta carotene is a top anti-acne remedy, and pumpkin is one of the richest natural sources of this nutrient. In fact, canned pumpkin is the most concentrated source of natural beta carotene of all common foods. Eat one or two cans of pumpkin per week to help cure acne or other blemishes.

5. Pumpkin is an excellent remedy for intestinal and/or digestive disorders. This is largely due to its vitamin A (beta carotene) content. Vitamin A is required for the regeneration of the cells which line the intestinal tract as well as the stomach. These cells die every five to seven days, and for optimal health they must be regenerated. Otherwise, disease

may develop. If you suffer from colitis, gastritis, heartburn, constipation, or other intestinal disorders, protect your internal lining with natural beta carotene and vitamin A by eating pumpkin. Be sure to eat pumpkin with dietary fats, because the fat aids in the absorption of beta carotene/vitamin A.

Radishes

The radish is another neglected food in the United States, although it is respected greatly in many other nations. It is a member of the mustard family, which accounts for its tart or hot taste. In America the red radish is primarily used, but, world-wide, numerous varieties are consumed.

The radish apparently originated in the hot climates of the Middle East or perhaps Western Asia. From there it was brought to China, where it has always been utilized as a staple.

Radishes belong to the cruciferous vegetables, a family of plants which possess significant anti-cancer powers. Perhaps this accounts for the reduced incidence of cancer among Orientals, since they are lovers of the radish. It is common for the Chinese and Japanese to eat radishes every day. Not only are raw radishes on their menus, but they also eat steamed or pickled radishes.

Radishes are rich primarily in trace minerals, which they concentrate from the soil. If grown on selenium-rich soil, they are one of the best sources of selenium, a mineral which prevents cancer. States with selenium rich soil are in the minority, and they include South Dakota, Texas, Wyoming, Oklahoma, Arizona, Missouri, California (only certain parts), and Colorado. Radishes also contain a considerable amount of vitamin C.

Top Radish Tips

1. Buy only fresh radishes, not the ones that are already processed, that is the ones in which the tops have been removed. If the tops are in good condition, these may also be eaten, as they are richer in certain vitamins and minerals than the radishes themselves.

2. Eat a variety of radishes, not just the typical red radish. Try also daikon, oriental, and Russian (black) radishes.

3. Use radishes in vegetable trays. They are great for dipping in cheese dip or salsa. Daikon is especially versatile for dipping, as it can be sliced like potato chips.

4. In America we always eat radishes raw, but this is not the case in Europe, where radishes are often cooked. Radishes make an excellent addition to soups, especially chicken or turkey soup. They add a tangy taste, while increasing the nutritional value.

5. Radishes and cheese make a great combination. Cut radishes in half or make large slices and spread with soft feta or cream cheese. Add a hint of garlic and/or onion. The garlic, onion, and radishes aid in the digestion of the cheese, but the main reason for preparing this dish is that it is a tasty appetizer.

Top Radish Cures

1. Radishes are one of the top anti-cancer foods. In particular, they impede the development of intestinal, stomach, and breast cancer. Radishes contain a plethora of anti-cancer compounds and, depending upon where they are grown, may be rich in the top anti-cancer mineral: selenium.

2. Radishes are tremendously valuable for stimulating digestion. This is because they contain a variety of chemicals which increase the flow of digestive juices. Black or Russian radish is a time-honored remedy for sluggish liver function, as this type of radish stimulates the flow of bile. If you suffer from maldigestion and/or liver problems, eat radishes on a daily basis.

3. Head colds, congestion, and sinus problems all respond to the radish prescription. Radishes are rich in volatile sulfur compounds, the substances which give them their hot flavor and which also help open blocked nasal/sinus passages. These substances are similar to those found in onions, another anti-congestion remedy. For eliminating congestion eat a large handful of radishes twice daily. To potentiate this effect, also consume a large slice of raw onion. Regarding congestion the rule is when in doubt "burn" it out with naturally hot foods.

4. Radishes are an ideal food for assisting immunity. They contain a variety of chemicals which possess natural antimicrobial actions. Plus, when grown upon the appropriate soil they are one of the top sources of selenium, which protects the immune system from toxicity. However, regardless of where they are grown, radishes are an aid to immune health. Regular consumption may lead to a significant improvement in the resistance against common microbial infections such as colds, sore throats, ear infections, and flu. If you are vulnerable to the development of everyday infections, it might be a sign of a *radish deficiency*.

5. Constipation meets its match with radishes. Rich in fiber and digestive stimulants, the regular intake of radishes helps regulate bowels. Furthermore, radishes are an excellent source of naturally occurring water, since they are over 90% water by weight. Thus, they help hydrate the body, and dehydration is a major cause of constipation.

6. If a heat wave strikes, eat radishes. Despite their hot taste, radishes actually help the body dissipate heat. They also contain a type of natural coolant and are refreshing, because they are high in moisture. For a Defeat the Heat Salad slice a bunch of radishes, a medium cucumber, and a small onion. Top with vinegar and extra virgin olive oil and salt.

Red Sweet (Bell) Peppers

Did you ever wonder how something as mild tasting as a red sweet pepper became associated with its name? After all, it is not peppery. Black pepper is entirely unrelated to bell peppers. Yet, one of the relatives of bell peppers, cayenne pepper, is hot, and that is how the name arose. When explorers first discovered red hot peppers in the Americas, they named them after the black pepper plant, because previous to the discovery of cayenne the peppercorn was the hottest spice known. In fact, the Spaniards were actually in search of the peppercorn of the East Indies, but they had to settle for America's cayenne instead. It is an oddity that red sweet peppers are far more popular in Europe as a vegetable and condiment than in their continent of origin.

For centuries, red sweet peppers have been consumed as a staple food in Europe, particularly the Balkans. In Romania during the winter months, when fresh produce is unavailable, the populous relies upon pepper paste as a source of nutrition. Red sweet pepper paste and a mildly spicy red pepper paste are a top sources of vitamin C, which explains the instinctive reliance upon it during the winter in the Balkans. The fact is in Romania roasted red sweet pepper paste is the national dish.

Red sweet peppers are nutritional powerhouses. They are three times richer in vitamin C than oranges. They are also inordinately rich in beta carotene, containing some 11 times more than green bell peppers. Red peppers are one of the best vegetable sources of pyridoxine. They are also a good source of trace minerals, especially potassium, in which they are richer than such highly touted sources as bananas, orange juice, and raisins. Perhaps of greater import is their content of non-vitamin nutrients. Red sweet peppers contain a variety of anti-cancer substances such as bioflavonoids and phenolic acids. For instance, they are one of the few rich sources of lycopene, proven in scientific studies to impede the growth of cancer cells. Lycopene is similar in chemical structure to the more commonly known beta carotene. Although it has no vitamin A value, lycopene is actually a more powerful deterrent to cancer than beta carotene. This pigment largely accounts for the peppers' red color. Red sweet peppers are also high in a type of plant sterol, a cholesterol-like substance, which is useful in vitamin D synthesis. Vitamin D itself is an anti-cancer substance.

Top Red Sweet Pepper Tips

1. Red sweet peppers are the ideal snack for children. They are sweet in taste, plus they are highly nutritious. They contain a greater amount of vitamin C than citrus fruit or dark green vegetables. Plus, they are rich in beta carotene, which is found in relatively low amounts in citrus fruit.
2. Red sweet peppers can be added to virtually any cooked dish. They are an ideal addition to stir fry, casseroles, and most any meat dish. Meat based soup is enriched with them. Chop them and add to rice dishes and omelets. Use red sweet peppers in cooking every day; you're health will improve as a result.
3. If possible, eat red sweet peppers along with fatty food. The various carotene pigments and bioflavonoids in these peppers are its most potent curative substances and are of even greater import than the vitamin

content. These pigments exert actions against aging and cancer. Researchers have determined that these fat soluble components are liberated optimally from the peppers if they are consumed with fat. The fat provokes the secretion of bile and pancreatic enzymes, both of which are needed to transport the pigments into the blood.

Make a vegetable plate containing various types of sweet peppers along with slices of avocados and cheese. This is scientific food combining that allows the individual to garnish the optimal nutritional value of the food.

4. Use red sweet peppers as a traveler's snack. Wash the peppers thoroughly and slice them into spears for a refreshing and vitamin rich snack. They hold up well without refrigeration for a short period, maintaining crispness and freshness for up to 24 hours.

5. Use red peppers often as a garnish, but be sure to eat them. Their rich color enlivens the presentation of virtually any entree.

6. Omelets are enriched by red peppers. Finely chop a tablespoon or two of the peppers and add to omelets as well as quiche.

7. Make your own red sweet pepper paste, or you can order it ready made. For a traditional Balkan recipe combine it with several supermarket cures, particularly chunky tomato sauce, sautéed eggplant and onions, and vinegar. It is delicious as a dip for vegetables, chips or crackers. Spread it on bread. Use it as a healthy dip for shrimp or fish. This Balkan dip is especially rich in vitamins A and C, and crackers and chips are not. Thus, it is an excellent way to make dipping nutritious (see Appendix B).

Top Red Sweet Pepper Cures

1. Red sweet peppers are a major fatigue-fighting vegetable. They help combat fatigue, weakness, exhaustion, and listlessness. If you just can't seem to achieve the physical or mental drive you need, try eating an entire red sweet pepper daily. The rich vitamin C, potassium, and vitamin A content is invigorating, and it should boost energy immediately.

2. Daily intake of red sweet peppers helps block cancer. If cancer exists, they should be consumed daily, both cooked and, especially, raw. Red peppers are rich in pigments which impede cancer cell growth. The absorption of these pigments is increased when the red peppers are consumed with a fatty food such as cheese or avocados.

3. Red sweet peppers are an ideal snack for treating the physical strain/exhaustion from a hot day. This is a cooling food, and it provides critical nutrients, such as potassium and vitamin C, needed to defend the body against hot weather. Furthermore, the peppers are mostly water, so their consumption aids greatly in hydration. For defeating the fatigue and weakness caused by excessive heat, eat an entire red sweet pepper and do so repeatedly, if necessary. For greater anti-heat effects be sure to add salt.

4. When the winter strikes, you need extra vitamin C, so rely upon red sweet peppers. They are a more dependable source of vitamin C than citrus fruit, plus they are less likely to cause allergic reactions. Eat a red pepper daily to keep colds, flu, and other winter infections at bay.

5. Sweet peppers are an ideal food for growing children. They provide exceptionally rich quantities of vitamins necessary for growth, including pyridoxine, folic acid, vitamin A (as beta carotene), potassium, phosphorus, and vitamin C. Add slices of red sweet pepper in school lunches along with carrot or celery sticks. Use pepper slices for dipping in cheese dips instead of potato chips.

6. Red sweet peppers, particularly as a paste, are an important cancer preventive. The paste is valuable, because it is a sort of lycopene concentrate. It is interesting to note that the incidence of cancer is quite low in regions such as Romania, Armenia, Poland, Turkey, and Bulgaria wherein pepper paste is a staple. Eat pepper paste, a top source of anti-cancer nutrients such as vitamin C, beta carotene, and lycopene, on a daily basis. Both sweet and spicy pepper pastes are delicious and healthy.

Rice Bran

Rice bran is the outer coating of rice. It makes the difference between white and brown rice. During the manufacture of white rice, the bran, which includes the germ, is removed. Ironically, this is where the vast majority of the nutrients are found; all that is left is the white kernel, which is essentially pure starch.

Rice bran has become available only recently, largely because of the ability to stabilize it. In the past it has been difficult to preserve, because it rapidly turns rancid as soon as it is removed from the rice kernel. This happens, because enzymes in the bran break down the naturally occurring oil in the bran, causing it to spoil. However, processors have developed chemical free methods to halt the enzyme's activity and, therefore, prevent spoilage. Even so, it is rare to see rice bran on the shelves of supermarkets. Rice bran should have more notoriety, since it is the most nutrient packed of all grain-type foods.

The oil in rice bran is extremely rich in essential fatty acids, containing nearly 40% by weight. It is also high in oleic acid, that valuable fatty acid which accounts for olive oil's healing attributes. Rice bran oil also contains a fair amount of saturated fatty acids, which is a plus, since saturated oils help maintain the oil's stability. Furthermore, the vegetable saturates act as valuable sources of fuel for energy production in cells, particularly cells of high energy organs such as the heart, brain, kidneys, adrenal glands, and thyroid gland.

While the oat bran craze has largely fizzled, interest in rice bran has just begun. Researchers at L.S.U. and the University of California-Davis document how rice bran and, particularly, rice oil effectively reduce elevated cholesterol levels in a more dramatic fashion than any other bran.

Rice bran is extremely rich in vitamins and minerals. It is certainly the most nutritionally complete type of grain food. Fractions of the rice found just over the white kernel, known as rice polish, are also unusually rich in nutrients. The bran and polish may be regarded as a type of crude B vitamin supplement, containing a wide range of B vitamins difficult to find in large amounts within food. During the 1930s-50s, before synthetic vitamins became mainstream, the crude rice extract was the treatment of choice for B vitamin deficiency, and it was used effectively for a wide range of conditions. This may be explained by the fact that food charts list the bran and polish as a top source of biotin, pantothenic acid, niacin, thiamine, pyridoxine, folic acid, choline, inositol, and PABA. Only riboflavin and vitamin B_{12} are lacking.

Rice bran is a more complete product nutritionally if it is combined with rice fractions. These fractions are derived from the remaining nutrient rich coating between the bran and the white kernel. Rice bran, rice fractions, and rice germ are all found in *Nutri-Sense*, a nutrient-dense drink mix. Nutri-Sense is fortified with granular lecithin and stabilized ground flax, which makes it one of the most nutritionally complete natural drink mixes available. The lecithin provides essential fatty acids, choline, and inositol, and the flax provides minerals and omega-3 fatty acids as well as protein. This means that Nutri-Sense is a complete meal shake and cereal additive. The nutrients in it are derived exclusively from natural sources. Because of the variety of natural substances it contains, Nutri-Sense is superior as a source of nutrition to rice bran alone. Nutri-Sense contains certified stabilized rice bran.

Top Rice Bran Tips

1. Rice bran is the easiest to digest of all types of fiber. Use it as a fiber supplement by itself, or add it to bakery to fortify the nutrient/fiber content of flour.
2. Be cautious about buying inexpensive grades of rice bran; they are probably rancid. Defatted rice bran is not an option; it is chemically treated, and the vast majority of the nutrients are depleted by the removal of the fat.
3. Rice bran makes an excellent cereal. Simply add a quarter cup of rice bran to boiling water. Cook until it softens. Top with organic butter, heavy cream or whole milk, and perhaps fruit or chopped nuts.
4. Use rice bran/Nutri-Sense to fortify other cereals; simply add a teaspoon or two to the cereal. This greatly enhances the nutritional value by boosting the content of B vitamins and minerals. Remember, commercial cereal is mostly starch, while rice bran is mostly nutrients.
5. On a hurried schedule begin the morning with Nutri-Sense drink mix. This is a convenient way to achieve a rice bran fix. Simply mix 2 tablespoons of Nutri-Sense in a glass of water, juice, or milk. Especially when taken with milk, this will suffice as a breakfast. This is far superior to the typical quick breakfasts that Americans eat such as commercial instant breakfast drinks, pop tarts, bagels, doughnuts, fast food breakfast sandwiches, boxed cereals, as well as the typical protein powders. All of these foods negatively affect the blood sugar, causing a variety of symptoms, include fatigue and mental disturbances. The point is the individual will feel good after taking Nutri-Sense, and that positive sensation will last throughout the day.
6. Use rice bran or Nutri-Sense as a baking enhancer. For most recipes simply cut the flour by one sixth and add bran or Nutri-Sense instead.

7. Use Nutri-Sense as a traveler's nutritional salvation. It is especially valuable for use when traveling overseas, when the food supply is so dubious that eating could cause more harm than good. An individual can literally live on nothing but Nutri-Sense and water for several weeks. However, ideally pack some dehydrated fruit, such as apricots, peaches, strawberries, and prunes, to provide vitamin C.

Top Rice Bran Cures

1. Nutri-Sense is an ideal drink mix for easing constipation and is superior to rice bran. This is because Nutri-Sense contains the bran, which is loaded with fiber, and also ground flax. The flax provides lignans, which lubricate the intestines, increase bulk, and ease elimination. Take three tablespoons once or twice daily in water or juice as a natural treatment for constipation.
2. For individuals suffering from allergic conditions rice bran is the perfect food. Allergy to rice is relatively rare compared to the more common problem of grain allergy. The fact is rice bran, as well as Nutri-Sense, enhance the body's ability to combat allergies, as they supply dense amounts of immune boosting nutrients such as vitamin E, pantothenic acid, pyridoxine, thiamine, niacin, and selenium, the latter being true if the rice is grown on selenium-rich soil.
3. Rice bran is an ideal food for combating fatigue. This is because it supplies an enormous amount of naturally occurring B vitamins. Energy producing B vitamins include thiamine, niacin, pyridoxine, and pantothenic acid, all of which are found in rice bran in dense amounts. Furthermore, rice bran contains large amounts of magnesium, which assists the B vitamins in the production of energy. By consuming Nutri-Sense instead of isolated rice bran the individual achieves the added advantage of dense amounts of choline, inositol, essential fatty acids, and flavonoids, which accelerate energy production within the liver as well as muscles. Remember, fatigue is reversible if the body is supplied with the chemicals it needs.
4. For individuals with failure to thrive, inability to gain weight, sluggish digestion, or anorexia, rice bran and/or Nutri-Sense is the ideal cure. This

is because rice bran/Nutri-Sense offers a complete array of natural B vitamins and trace minerals, which are needed to help regenerate the body. Poor appetite is a warning sign of B vitamin deficiency, particularly thiamine, pantothenic acid, and niacin deficiency. Rice bran, as found in Nutri-Sense, is the top naturally occurring source of thiamine and niacin, plus it is a good source of pantothenic acid.

5. Rice bran is an ideal source of nutrition for athletes. This is because it is abundant in all of the primary nutrients needed for optimizing cellular metabolism, including vitamins, minerals, essential fatty acids, and amino acids. It also contains hormones which exhibit steroid-like actions. For a nutritional boost superior to the synthetic drinks use Nutri-Sense, two heaping tablespoons in juice or milk twice daily.

6. Most everyone would benefit by adding B vitamins to the diet. The question is should we rely on vitamin pills or attempt to increase the consumption of natural B vitamins? Major warning signs of B vitamin deficiency include fatigue, irritability, memory problems, depression, skin problems, muscle weakness, poor digestion, water retention, and poor appetite. It is astonishing that even after taking multiple vitamins and B complex pills the symptoms often remain unresolved. This may be explained by research conducted in the 1930s and 1940s, the era of vitamin discovery. Numerous scientists discovered that natural B vitamin supplements, that is extracts of foods, cured a wide range of diseases and quickly obliterated the symptoms of nutritional deficiency. However, when the scientists administered synthetic B vitamins, the response was inadequate. This gives credence for the use of rice bran or, preferably, Nutri-Sense, as a potent natural B vitamin supplement just as did the discoverers of B vitamins years ago.

Rosemary

Perhaps the most valuable of all herbs, rosemary, is almost unknown in American kitchens. It seems as if the only known use is for lamb.

Rosemary is a type of pine needle from an evergreen shrub. It grows in moderate climates, such as the Mediterranean, near sea-swept shores. Like other evergreens rosemary exudes the typical balmy camphorous odor. This smell is so pronounced that many people find it too intense.

Americans find the taste of many spices disconcerting, rarely eating them. Ironically, spices such as rosemary were a staple food additive for Europeans, which is the ancestry for the majority of Americans. Instead, we seemingly relish a medley of processed foods laced with dangerous food additives such as saccharin, aspartame, MSG, food dyes, and sulfites. Individuals who eat chemically infested foods with gusto often sneer when tasting food containing rosemary or similar aromatic herbs. I myself at first found rosemary a bit overpowering (except, of course, over traditional lamb). Yet, after using it regularly, it became a desired staple.

Rosemary is rich in trace minerals. It is a top source of calcium and is also rich in magnesium, potassium, sodium, and phosphorus. This makes sense if you know how rosemary grows: right out of the rocks. I have seen Mediterranean rosemary; it seems to only grow on rocky soil and often grows right on rocks and boulders. Its favorite rock is limestone, which explains its dense content of calcium and phosphorus. According to the herbalist Michael Tierra the type of calcium in rosemary is very easy to absorb.

The ancients made heavy use of rosemary both as food and medicine. According to some authorities they used so much rosemary in food that it would taste to us like Mentholatum. Lawless describes it as one of the most ancient of all medicines. Since time immemorial it has been known that rosemary strengthens the brain. Its use as a headache cure dates back 4,000+ years. The Greeks used it extensively to enhance the mind and were particularly fond of it as a memory tonic. In Medieval Europe it was famous as an arthritis cure and was used for both mental and nerve disorders.

Currently, rosemary is recommended for high blood pressure and migraines. The *British Pharmacopoeia* lists it as a remedy for depression and circulatory diseases. Chevallier notes in the *Encyclopedia of Medicinal Plants* that rosemary reverses headaches, even migraines, probably as a result of improved blood flow to the brain. Apparently, rosemary contains a substance, notably the flavonoid *diosmin*, which keeps the arterial walls strong. According to Chevallier rosemary protects the adrenal glands from the toxic effects of stress, and this may also explain its beneficial actions in lowering blood pressure and reversing migraines. Jean Valnet, M.D., author of *The Practice of Aromatherapy*, describes an immense list of uses for rosemary, including sore throat,

216

asthma, bronchitis, sour stomach, bad breath, gas, diarrhea, gall bladder ailments, liver disorders, jaundice, bowel infections, colitis, muscular weakness, fatigue, arthritis, migraines, heart disease, menstrual disorders, adrenal fatigue, poor eyesight, infected or slow healing wounds, memory loss, psychosis, and depression. It is important to note that Valnet is one of the world's most renowned herbalists.

The greatest attributes of rosemary are derived from its volatile oil. Rosemary oil is unique, providing a variety of therapeutic agents. Huang notes in *Cancer Research* that the oil is rich in a naturally occurring antioxidant exhibiting "high antioxidant activity." Umek describes in *Planta Medica* that it is "strongly inhibitory" against viruses. Engleberger and colleagues in the *International Journal of Immunopharmacology* write that rosemary oil curtails inflammation and edema. Other research documents how it prevents liver damage due to exposure to toxic chemicals, and French researchers have shown that both the oil and the herb dramatically increase bile flow.

Rosemary oil's antioxidant properties are perhaps most outstanding. This is probably Nature's most potent antioxidant. Incredibly, Inatani found that rosemary oil is four times more powerful than BHT, the synthetic antioxidant used in preserving foods. Research by Singletary at the University of Illinois may explain this action: rosemary increases the production of the liver's key antioxidant enzyme. After treatment of experimental animals with rosemary, levels of this enzyme, known as *glutathione-S-transferase*, rose 400%. That is an incredibly large increase. Few if any other natural compounds boast such a potent action. This enzyme is the liver's most crucial defense against cancer-causing chemicals.

Top Rosemary Tips

1. Use rosemary with feta cheese and as an additive to cheese dips. On a salad add feta cheese, rosemary, and olive oil. Rosemary lends itself to fat, especially saturated fat. Sprinkle it on any hard or soft cheese.
2. Rosemary is a nourishing and tasty addition to cold vegetable dishes, especially gazpacho. Crumble rosemary and sprinkle over vegetable platters.

3. Rosemary is an excellent addition to any fatty meat or poultry. Add it to lamb and beef, especially roasts. When baking poultry, keep the skin on and sprinkle liberally with rosemary.

4. Oil of rosemary makes bathing an exotic experience. Add several drops to bath water. Put a few drops on a sponge or wash cloth and scrub the skin for an invigorating sensation. Add it to shampoos and pump soap to help make skin and hair more beautiful. Rosemary oil is a non-toxic antiseptic. Therefore, there are immense benefits to be derived by regularly adding it to hand soap, dish soap, and other cleansing solutions.

5. Use oil of rosemary to protect the skin from the sun. Rosemary oil is extremely rich in antioxidants, which help block the toxicity of ultraviolet rays. The oil penetrates the skin rapidly and offers protection on and within the skin. Gently rub it on exposed regions, being careful to avoid the eyes.

6. Rosemary oil makes an excellent breath freshener. Simply take a drop or two twice daily under the tongue or in the mouth for an immediate breath freshening effect and for eradicating bad breath.

7. Be aware that commercial rosemary oil is inedible. Much of it is made synthetically from petrochemicals. *Oil of Rosemary* by North American Herb & Spice is produced exclusively from wild rosemary and is from the edible species. Hercules Strength is another rosemary product made from wild rosemary herb. To order call 800-243-5242.

Top Rosemary Cures

1. If you suffer from depression, rosemary is a must. This herb has been utilized as an antidepressant for thousands of years. Current research indicates that rosemary is a fat soluble antioxidant, meaning it protects the fatty tissues of the body from degeneration. The brain is mostly fat, and it readily absorbs antioxidants from rosemary oil. For mild depression take oil of rosemary, 5 drops three times daily. Also, take Hercules Strength, a rosemary/sage herbal, two capsules three times daily. For severe depression take 10 drops of rosemary oil three times daily and one or two capsules of Hercules Strength three times daily. Note: commercial rosemary oil cannot be recommended for internal consumption. This is because the commercial oil may be synthetic, or it may be processed with solvents. However, the type made by North

American Herb & Spice can be consumed as a natural herbal oil. This Oil of Rosemary is free of chemicals and is derived from the edible herb.

2. In the event of weak memory rosemary is mandatory. Take Hercules Strength, two capsules three times daily. Take also oil of rosemary, 5 drops twice daily. Even if the memory is normal, it is useful, because everyone could benefit from a quicker mind.

3. For migraines rosemary is ideal. It possesses significant anti-pain powers, plus it helps improve blood flow. This means that more oxygen is delivered to the brain; with migraines there is a deprivation of oxygen. During a headache crisis take rosemary oil, a few drops under the tongue several times daily. Rub the oil on the forehead or any painful regions. Also, take Hercules Strength, one or two capsules three times daily.

The anti-migraine action may be explained by the fact that rosemary contains natural pain killers. Tierra claims this herb is so effective that it may be used as a replacement for aspirin. Use it as a rub on any painful joint or lesion. Apply it to burns, cuts, or sores. Take it internally to fight chronic pain.

4. Individuals with heart disease may benefit greatly from rosemary. It is a tremendous tonic for the circulation. Its antioxidant action largely accounts for its cardiovascular benefits. The heart and arteries are readily damaged by toxicity, and rosemary blocks toxic reactions within cells. Rosemary also contains flavonoids, which keep the walls of the arteries and veins strong. If you have heart disease or hardening of the arteries, take several drops of oil of rosemary twice daily. Take also Hercules Strength, two capsules twice daily.

5. Epileptics may need to avoid rosemary oil, especially if they are taking medications. Investigators report that rosemary oil may temporarily exacerbate the symptoms. However, the edible herb is certainly safe, and by regularly eating rosemary epileptics may benefit greatly.

6. For sour stomach, indigestion, or heartburn rosemary is a necessity. It quickly calms digestive distress and obliterates the need for antacids. Take a few drops of the oil or a few capsules of Hercules Strength to calm digestive symptoms of any kind. Repeat as necessary.

7. Rosemary is the top tonic for damaged hair or scalp. Add oil of rosemary to shampoo and conditioner; rub oil of rosemary vigorously into the scalp. For seborrhea or severe dandruff rub the oil into the scalp every night before bedtime. Cover with a nightcap and repeat as necessary.

8. If you are highly stressed, use oil of rosemary regularly. Rub it on the chest and let its aromatic fumes sedate the nerves and brain. Also, rub it on the spine or on tense muscles. Take it internally to calm the nerves. To increase your resistance against stress consume Hercules Strength on a daily basis, two capsules twice daily. Remember, rosemary greatly improves adrenal function, and the adrenal glands are the body's coping mechanism.

9. Numerous researchers have undoubtedly determined that rosemary possesses anti-cancer powers. Apparently, if rosemary is consumed regularly, the body develops a sort of cancer resistance. Japanese researchers put rosemary to the test; they tried to induce skin cancer in laboratory animals by applying toxic chemicals to bare skin. However, they found that if rosemary oil was rubbed on the skin, the animals were resistant. If you have a family history of cancer, use oil of rosemary and rosemary herb on a daily basis. Take also Hercules Strength, one or two capsules three times daily.

10. Respiratory conditions may respond to rosemary. Both the herb and the oil are rich in volatile oils, which soothe irritated sinus and bronchial passages. Since ancient times rosemary has been used for a wide range of respiratory diseases, including sinusitis, asthma, bronchitis, emphysema, and pneumonia. Valnet used it successfully for respiratory infections, including sore throats and bronchitis. The oil is an antiseptic, plus it contains substances which prevent mucous build-up and open clogged passages.

Sage

Historically, sage has been regarded as more of a medicine than a food. As an herb and flavoring for food, the current usage was adopted from the current European habit of adding sage to poultry dishes. Yet, for thousands of years sage's only application in Europe and Asia was as a medicine. In fact, its strong and often bitter taste gives evidence for its profound "medicinal" actions.

The medicinal usage of sage arises largely from the Greeks and Romans, who used it for a wide range of illnesses, including lung conditions, infections, snake bites, memory loss, menstrual insufficiency, and intestinal parasites. Dioscorides writings in the 1st century A.D.

noted that sage leaves were an effective antiseptic when applied to wounds. In the 10th century Arabic physicians indicated that sage has the capacity to extend life, perhaps indefinitely. In the medieval times sage was added to food to prevent spoilage. More recently, early 20th century U.S. pharmacy texts recommend sage as an antiseptic for sore throats and wounds. Its powerful properties have been known throughout the ages.

This emphasis on its medicinal properties is not to slight the tremendous value of adding sage to foods. It is perhaps the perfect meat spice, lending itself especially well to poultry. The health reason has been known for centuries: sage prevents meat from spoiling by halting bacterial growth. According to Castleman's *The Healing Herbs,* sage is useful as a food preservative due to its ability to halt rancidity in fats, since it is rich in antioxidants.

Nutritionally, sage is quite dense in minerals, particularly calcium and magnesium. Incredibly, it is four times higher in calcium than cheese. Virtually nothing can match sage for magnesium content, as it contains nearly 500 mg per 100 grams. This means that sage tea is essentially a magnesium infusion. The only common food sources which can compete are almonds and Brazil nuts, which contain 290 and 320 mg respectively. Sage is also an excellent source of vitamin C.

Top Sage Tips

1. Always use sage when cooking poultry, especially the typical supermarket birds, since commercial poultry is frequently contaminated with bacteria. Often, these bacteria are antibiotic resistant, meaning they may cause serious disease. Sage contains compounds which inhibit the growth of these bacteria. Plus, it strengthens an individual's defenses against these organisms. Ideally, purchase free range chicken, which is cleaner microbially, and dress it with sage.
2. Sprinkle sage on the inside of the poultry carcass and add it to dressing. This will help keep the bird and stuffing free of microbial contaminants, plus it greatly enhances the taste.
3. Add sage to soups, especially soups containing meat. Add two or more teaspoons of crushed sage leaves to the soup. After serving, top each bowl with a few fresh sage leaves, if available.

4. Take a bottle of sage with you when traveling. Sprinkle dried sage leaves on salads. This will prevent food poisoning from unclean produce.
5. When preparing meat dishes for travel or picnics, add sage. This is because the natural antibiotics in sage inhibit bacterial growth, plus its antioxidants prevent the meat fats from turning rancid, which may occur when the food is exposed to heat or sunlight.

Top Sage Cures

1. Sage tea is an ideal remedy for sore throat. Make a strong concoction of sage tea, and drink at least three cups daily until the condition improves. Make a super-strong concoction, and use it as a gargle. Add raw honey for an accelerated effect. The finest sage grows in the Mediterranean and is mountain harvested, that is, it is picked wild. *Hercules Strength* is a nutritional supplement containing wild sage. As a convenient alternative to the tea, take 2 capsules of Hercules Strength twice daily.
2. Women with yeast infections should drink sage tea on a daily basis. Drink one cup with every meal. Drink an additional cup before bedtime; sage is an excellent sedative, since it is supremely rich in calcium, magnesium, and potassium, the critical minerals needed for calming the nervous system. In the event of a fulminant yeast infection this calming effect would be utterly invaluable. Incredibly, while the sage calms the nerves, its potent antifungal agents help the immune system in eradicating the infection. Plus, sage contains essential oils, which kill fungi on contact.
3. Sage tea is the perfect remedy for cold sores and canker sores. Sip on the tea, and swish the fluid in the mouth to ease the pain of these lesions and speed healing.
4. Sage is an ancient remedy for gum and tooth disease, plus it helps whiten the teeth. One reason is that sage is rich in a variety of antiseptics which block the growth of dangerous oral bacteria. To make a sage dentifrice simply grind fresh or dried sage and sea salt preferably with a mortar and pestle until finely pulverized. Use on a toothbrush instead of toothpaste. Recent evidence indicates that fluoride based toothpastes may cause fluoride poisoning, particularly in children. Avoid fluoride based toothpastes.

5. Sage is an excellent remedy for colds, flu, or bronchitis. Use the sage as an infusion, that is as a tea. Steep a double handful of sage leaves in a large pot of hot water for 40 minutes. Sip on this tea throughout the day.
6. Modern research has proven that antioxidants, such as vitamin C, vitamin E, and beta carotene, protect the body from aging and prevent the onslaught of degenerative disease. Certain herbs, such as sage and rosemary, contain antioxidants which are infinitely more powerful than the standard vitamin pill. Sage is loaded with antioxidants. Modern research shows that its antioxidants exert a preservative action on tissues. Hercules Strength is a sage/rosemary antioxidant formula made from wild herbs. As a general antioxidant take one or two capsules with meals.
7. If you suffer from a chronic skin disorder, use sage as often as possible. Make sage tea and drink one or two cups daily. Also, take Hercules Strength, two capsules twice daily.

Salmon

Salmon is one of the finest foods available. It is pure packed nutrition.

Salmon is an unusual fish, because it begins its life in fresh water but spends the majority of its existence in the oceans. Eventually, it returns to the continental streams to spawn, but this is a fatal mistake. Lying in wait are commercial fishermen, who net the salmon at their predictable spawning sites.

There is a great deal of confusion regarding salmon, largely because there are so many types. Names such as sockeye, red, Alaskan, coho, pink, humpback, Chinook, Chum, and Atlantic add to the confusion. Perhaps these various names arose, because salmon is one of the few fish which lives part-time in fresh water and part-time in salt water. Let's clarify this terminology as much as possible:

Chum: A fish with pale flesh, this salmon is low in the valuable fish oils but is still an excellent source of protein and minerals.

Chinook: This is the same as the king salmon. It is the largest type of salmon, reaching over 100 pounds. King salmon is the fattiest type of salmon, possessing a deep red firm flesh, although a few varieties may be nearly white in color.

Coho: This is also known as silver salmon and is one of the smallest varieties. It is rarely canned and usually sold fresh. It tends to be low in oil, unless it lives in extremely cold waters.

Pink salmon: this is the same as humpback and is the smallest and least oily of all salmon. Its flesh is bland looking or barely pink.

Sockeye: This is the same as red salmon. It is a medium sized fish with firm red flesh. It contains a significant amount of fish oil and is a good source of vitamins and minerals. This is the type usually sold as "Alaskan salmon."

Canned salmon is one the most nutrient dense of all supermarket foods. It is a dense source of amino acids, fatty acids, B vitamins, coenzymes, and minerals. Some individuals currently avoid eating it, largely due to concerns of fat content as well as the pollution aspect. Pollution is a legitimate concern, but the fat in salmon is a type which assists and nourishes body functions. However, virtually all foods are contaminated with chemicals, and starving to death is not an option, nor is living on lettuce and broccoli. The fact is virtually all foods are contaminated with residues of toxic chemicals. In some cases, fruits and vegetables contain a higher percentage of toxic chemical residues than meat. Don't worry excessively about chemical contamination. Instead, fight it by taking extra doses of the nutrients which detoxify contaminants. Such nutrients include selenium, vitamin E, beta carotene, bioflavonoids, glutathione, vitamin C, riboflavin, and folic acid. Herbs which inactivate toxic chemicals and aid in their elimination include turmeric, ginger, garlic, onion, sour grape, oregano, basil, saffron, wild strawberry leaf, sage and rosemary. So, to help alleviate the problems of chemicals in the fish, liberally season it with spices and herbs. This aids in the inactivation and detoxification of chemical contaminants. Another method to minimize exposure is to buy fish from regions of reduced pollution. Thus, Alaskan salmon would be a superior choice versus Atlantic or fresh water salmon. Even so, all corners of the earth are polluted, and there is little which can be done about it.

Salmon may be regarded as the sort of nutritional cadillac of fish. For instance, it is inordinately rich in fish oils, which have dozens of physiological uses. In contrast, the more commonly consumed fish in family menus, such as haddock, cod, and perch, contain minimal amounts of these oils. Salmon is also highly dense in vitamins and is one of the few fish consistently listed near the top of the charts. Its impressive array of vitamins is noted by Ensminger, who places it as a top source of pantothenic acid, pyridoxine, niacin, vitamin B_{12}, vitamin D, and vitamin E. Few foods match its nutritional density.

Top Salmon Tips

1. Buy fresh salmon as often as possible. It is both tastier and richer in vitamins than the canned variety. However, canned salmon is a sufficient option, if the fresh is unavailable.
2. Be sure to wash fresh salmon prior to cooking. Supermarkets often dip fresh fish in solutions containing antibiotics and synthetic preservatives. Formaldehyde, the same substance used to preserve cadavers, is a common additive. Incredibly, although public outcry has reduced its usage, it is still used as a fish preservative. Rinsing removes the majority of chemical residues as well as noxious microbes. Better yet, buy the fish from stores which don't dip the fish in chemicals.
3. When preparing fresh salmon, baking, grilling, or poaching are ideal methods. Salmon contains plenty of oil, and there is no need to fry it. When baking salmon try smothering it in onions and garlic. These herbs help accelerate the digestion and absorption of the salmon oil.
4. Salmon should be consumed as a regular part of the diet. It is one of the most nutrient rich of all fish and contains the added benefit of the cardioprotective fish oils, which are found only in relatively few species of fish. Eat it at least once per week and preferably two or three times per week. Try to avoid fish from the Great Lakes, since they are highly toxic.
5. Salmon salad is an ideal means of serving this wonderful food. Such salads are essentially complete one dish meals, and, not only are they nutritious, but they are also incredibly convenient.
6. If you travel often, buy salmon while on the road. It is nutritious and filling and provides much needed anti-stress nutrients such as vitamins A, D, and E as well as niacin and potassium. When looking in the grocery store for a traveler's lunch, choose a small can of salmon. Smother the salmon with olives, baby onions, and/or capers, and enjoy a filling and nutritious entree without spending lots of money at a restaurant and without the risk of getting sick.

7. If eating canned salmon, be sure to reserve the juice or use it in the recipe. Or, drink it immediately. The juice is rich in valuable fatty acids and fat soluble vitamins such as vitamins A, D, and E.

Top Salmon Cures

1. Salmon is perhaps the best food for reversing cold sensitivity. This is because it contains a variety of oils which help insulate the body against cold. These oils also improve blood flow by decreasing sludging of the blood. Thus, salmon, as the Eskimos know full well, is an ideal winter survival food.

2. If you have a skin disorder in which the skin is inflamed, such as dermatitis, eczema, hives, rosacea, or psoriasis, the regular consumption of salmon is a necessity. Salmon oil fights inflammation and speeds the healing of damaged skin.

3. PMS and severe menstrual cramps readily respond to salmon. This is because the essential oils in it are highly active in reducing inflammation and irritation within the female organs. If you suffer from menstrual cramps, endometriosis, uterine fibroids, ovarian cysts, menstrual cramps, or PMS, eat salmon several times per week.

4. Arthritis meets it match with salmon. This is because salmon is rich in a variety of nutrients which help block inflammation in the joints. Furthermore, salmon is a top source of pantothenic acid, a vitamin which is required for normalizing the function of the glandular system. With arthritis, there is always an imbalance in glandular function, and the adrenal glands are particularly affected. Pantothenic acid is necessary for the normal function of these glands and assists in the production of cortisone, which is the body's natural defense against arthritis. In other words, if the individual fails to consume sufficient quantities of foods rich in pantothenic acid, the output of cortisone from the adrenal glands declines. This increases the risk for developing joint disease. Other excellent sources of pantothenic acid include rice fractions (the outer coating of brown rice), liver, nuts, eggs, and poultry.

5. Salmon provides oils which nourish the skin. In fact, researchers document how salmon oil helps reverse skin diseases, including psoriasis, eczema, and dermatitis. If you suffer from these diseases or if you have

"sick skin," eat salmon on a regular basis. You will probably improve quickly as a result of eating this nutrient dense food.

6. In the United States obesity has become a national epidemic. Contrary to popular belief, foods which are naturally rich in fat are safe additions to a weight loss program. While salmon is about 50% fat, it is entirely safe to eat when dieting. In fact, the natural oils in salmon help the body burn excess fat.

7. If you strictly avoid red meat, at least eat salmon. It is sort of the red meat of fish, and its red color is a reflection of the intensity of its nutrient content. In fact, the types of salmon with the most intense color are also the most nutritious. Pale pink salmon contains the least amount of essential nutrients.

Salt

The average individual would never think of salt as being a cure, but it is invaluable to our existence. Without salt, fatality would eventually result.

Salt, which is merely the elements sodium and chloride, is necessary for the function of every organ and cell in the body. Vital functions, such as blood flow, the pumping of the heart, hormone synthesis, nerve conduction, and hydration, are entirely dependent upon it.

In modern times salt has been maligned, but this was not always the case. Remember the saying "salt of the earth" or "he was worth his salt." These sayings reiterate the former status of salt: that of a valuable commodity. In fact, salt was so valuable in ancient times that it was regarded as being worth its weight in gold. Indeed, historians record that ancient traders plied the interior continents where salt was rare and were rewarded for it in gold. Furthermore, wars were fought to gain control of commodities such as salt.

The importance of salt was also understood in early America. A glimpse of this is evident from the Old West movies. Whenever the farmer or trader came to town for supplies, a bag of salt was a prerequisite. Native Americans valued it highly and vigorously traded for it. However, now, in our modern "sophistication" we seem to have rebelled against salt as a necessity. This is catastrophic.

Salt is required by the body for several critical functions. It is the major electrolyte of the blood, accounting for its osmotic pressure, meaning its ability to hold onto fluid. Put simply, salt helps keep the fluids in the body in their proper places. This function is absolutely essential, since, without sodium, the entire blood vessel system, including the heart, would collapse. It is the major substance accounting for cell membrane pumps, that is specialized cell components which drive critical nutrients into and out of cells. Salt helps regulate the output of fluid by the kidneys, preventing excessive fluid loss, and this is particularly crucial in times of fluid starvation. The production of certain adrenal hormones, notably aldosterone, is sodium dependent. Our nerve cells require sodium for the normal transmission of impulses. The brain is dependent upon it, for, without sodium and chloride, irritability, anxiety, depression, somnolence, confusion, and, ultimately, coma would result.

The best type of salt is crude unprocessed sea salt. This is because, in addition to sodium and chloride, natural sea salt is rich in iodine and magnesium, plus it contains hundreds of other "trace" minerals (see Appendix B).

Top Salt Tips

1. Be aware that table salt is not just salt. It contains added aluminum and sugar. The sugar is in the form of dextrose, and the aluminum is in the form of aluminum silicate. Sugar is added to enhance taste and also to make the salt addictive. The aluminum is used to make it slippery and prevent caking, so it will shake easily from the salt shaker.
2. Buy unprocessed salt with no additives, in other words, sea salt. One drawback is that some sea salt is processed to the degree that the iodine, as well as certain other critical trace minerals, are destroyed. If the sea salt is pure white, it is probably processed and deficient in iodine, unless it is fortified.
3. Pure unprocessed sea salt has a slightly darkened color and is never pure white. It is more of a grey color. The white color is unnatural and is the result of chemical bleaching. Sun-bleached salt will retain a slightly greyish color, the result of various minerals, including iodine. The point is pure white salt is chcmically bleached, and bleach destroys iodine, potassium, and other delicate minerals.

4. If the salt is low in iodine or if it is not iodized, it may be necessary to add iodine. Potassium iodide, a prescription item, can be ordered by your doctor. Simply add a few drops of potassium iodide to your sea salt and shake the bag. Let dry; you now have a type of natural iodized salt. The iodine is needed to boost thyroid function.

5. Be sure to use salt as a preservative whenever making canned or dried foods. Salt prevents microbial growth as a result of its osmotic powers, but, in contrast to synthetic preservatives such as BHA and BHT, it is non-toxic to human cells. While salt can kill microbes, its presence in a balanced amount encourages human cell metabolism and growth.

6. Use salt when cooking vegetable, meat, and starch dishes. It adds zest to the food, and the added taste gives vigor to the appetite. In other words, don't prepare the food salt free and rely only on the salt shaker.

7. Don't salt meat right away during cooking, because it makes meat tough. Add it toward the end of the cooking process.

Top Salt Cures

1. Fatigue may be a warning of sodium deficiency. Remember, it is possible to become deficient in sodium despite a reasonable intake. Sodium and chloride help stimulate the synthesis of anti-stress hormones from the adrenal glands. These hormones are needed for enhancing metabolism, maintaining circulation and boosting energy.

2. Low blood pressure is a warning of sodium deficiency. Sodium and chloride are the primary electrolytes of the blood, accounting for over 90% of the electrolyte content. The electrolytes are natural substances which help maintain normal circulatory volume. They exert other invaluable functions such as the control of pH and stomach acid synthesis.

3. Poor protein digestion is a signal of salt deficiency. This is because sodium and chloride are needed for the synthesis of stomach acid (i.e. hydro*chloric* acid); the activity of certain pancreatic enzymes are also dependent upon their presence. If you have a difficult time digesting heavy food, such as meat or eggs, try adding salt in the form of sea salt to the food.

4. Muscular weakness, muscle soreness, and leg cramps are all symptoms

of sodium deficiency. While these symptoms may also represent certain vitamin deficiencies, such as a lack of pantothenic acid, folic acid, or vitamin E, salt deficiency is a likely culprit. This is because tens of millions of Americans follow a low salt diet. Furthermore, numerous medications, such as diuretics, cortisone, prednisone, aspirin, and antacids, deplete sodium from the body. If your muscles are weak and/or spastic and no cause has been determined, be sure to have your doctor check your sodium levels, especially if you are taking numerous prescription medications.

5. Certain heart patients need salt. That's right, the latest evidence proves that salt is needed for normal cardiac function. Actually, this has been known for decades, but, because of the fad of a low salt diet, the critical role of sodium, as well as chloride, in cardiac function has been neglected. Profound proof of this was delineated by Dr. Alderman of New York's Albert Einstein University. Dr. Alderman discovered, quite by accident, that heart patients who had the lowest blood levels of sodium were 400% more likely to have heart attacks than those with normal levels. He reasoned that the heart patients were dying rapidly, because their blood pressures were bottoming out. Sodium is needed to maintain normal blood flow and volume, so that blood continuously perfuses the heart muscle. This means that in severe sodium deficiency the amount of blood reaching the heart muscle is critically insufficient. Incredibly, his cure was to infuse a saline solution by vein and add salt into the diet. It worked stupendously, and Dr. Alderman reversed the high rate of cardiac deaths—through "salt therapy."

6. Salt creates strength and energy. Both sodium and chloride are required for the function of a critical cellular system known as the *sodium pump*. This ionic transport system is found in every cell in the body. If this pump fails, fatigue and, ultimately, muscular collapse results. If you are exhausted, add salt to the diet. The boost in energy you will receive may be tremendous.

Sardines

This tiny fish has long been relished as a tasty health food. The Greeks were aware that sardines were good for vigor and vitality. Because of their health-enhancing properties, they have been relied upon as a major food in Mediterranean countries since ancient times.

Sardines are a top food source of several nutrients, but they are particularly rich in nucleic acids, fish oils, and minerals. A mere dozen sardines contains approximately 680 mg of calcium, which makes them more abundant in this mineral by weight than milk, yogurt, or cheese. A dozen sardines also gives a whopping 5 mg of iron, 800 mg of phosphorus, and 900 mg of potassium. The vitamin A content of sardines is considerable, and they offer approximately 350 I.U. per dozen. Sardines are relatively rich in B vitamins, with a can providing about 8 mg of niacin, 1.3 mg of pantothenic acid, 25 mcg of folic acid and, perhaps more importantly, 15 mcg of vitamin B_{12}. This critical nutrient is found in relatively few foods. With the exception of liver, sardines are a better source of B_{12} and folic acid than any other type of meat.

Top Sardine Tips

1. Don't buy sardines in added oil. The most commonly used oil is soybean oil, and this oil is refined and adulterated. Buy sardines packed in water or in their own natural oil. The latter are known as sardines packed in "sild," an European term for natural sardine oil.
2. Some sardines are packed in mustard or tomato sauce. These sauces are fine, but be sure to check the label for other undesirable additives such as sugar, MSG, wheat starch, and vegetable oil.
3. Sardines are easy to digest, so they are an ideal food for babies, toddlers, the elderly, or for individuals suffering from emaciation. Anyone who complains of difficulty digesting protein will find sardines to be among the most readily digested of all protein meals.
4. For those who are sensitive to odors the smell of sardines can be reduced by dousing them with vinegar. Add chopped parsley or watercress for further odor reduction. This will also help block any residual odor after eating. What's more, vinegar, parsley, and watercress aid in the digestion of the fats and proteins in the sardines.
5. For an innovative taste make a sardine salad. In a medium bowl dice two cans of sardines, add chopped onions, and minced garlic. Add vinegar and top with chopped parsley. This dish is rich in nucleic acids.

6. Don't worry if the oil free sardines you purchase appear to have oil in them after opening. This is the natural oil found in the flesh, which is liberated with time into the water pack. Sardines are mostly oil. Don't pour off the water pack, instead, eat it with the sardines.

Top Sardine Cures

1. Sardines are the ideal remedy for disorders of the nervous system. This is because they supply rich amounts of the nutrients necessary for enhancing the function of the nerves. These nerve calming and nourishing nutrients include calcium (it is one of the top sources of this nutrient), niacin, pyridoxine, fatty acids (fish oils), and nucleic acids (RNA and DNA). If you suffer from a mental or nervous disorder, eat sardines every day. You will notice an improvement shortly, probably within a week.

2. Sardines are a good food for cancer patients, especially those undergoing radiation or chemotherapy. Cancer patients desperately need essential oils, protein, and nucleic acids, and sardines supply all of these substances. Furthermore, chemotherapeutic agents and radiation destroy the nuclear material and oxidize protein, so these need to be supplied regularly in the diet to help the body rebuild its stores. Eat at least one can of sardines daily if you are undergoing toxic cancer therapy.

3. If you have diabetes, you should eat sardines. Free of sugar and carbohydrate, sardines are an ideal food for the diabetic. They supply large amounts of fish oils, niacin, and pyridoxine, all of which improve blood sugar control. Furthermore, researchers have discovered that the oil found in sardines assists the pancreas' ability to produce insulin. The regular consumption of sardines will likely lead to a decreased need for insulin or other blood sugar-lowering drugs.

4. If you wish to live a long time, eat sardines regularly. Several of my patients who have lived past ninety are regular sardine eaters. One gentlemen, well over 100 years old, was asked what contributed most to his long life. He confided that every day he consumed at least one can of sardines. This makes sense; sardines are the richest dietary source of anti-aging substances known as *nucleic acids*.

5. Cold extremities is a symptom which responds to the sardine prescription. This is because sardines are the richest dietary source of fish

oils, which improve blood flow to the extremities. Fish oils improve peripheral circulation by decreasing the degree of sludging of the blood. These oils accomplish this feat by inhibiting platelet aggregation and by decreasing the levels of sticky fats within the blood.

Shrimp

Seafood has generally been maligned, largely because of concerns of pollution and cholesterol. Both of these concerns are overrated. Pollution is a legitimate problem for all foods—animal and vegetable. For those who are concerned with the toxicity of the oceans, and, therefore, the shrimp, farm raised varieties are now available.

Eating shrimp should never be a concern for individuals watching their cholesterol or for heart patients. Shrimp contains little or no fat, and the type of cholesterol found within it fails to increase blood cholesterol; On the contrary, it helps normalize it. As noted by William Castelli, director of the Framingham Heart Study, shrimp is actually an ideal heart food.

Shrimp is one of the most nutrient dense of all foods. This seafood is a nutritional powerhouse, packing valuable quantities of protein, vitamins, and minerals. It is one of Nature's best sources of iodine, and a few shrimp daily provide well in excess of the minimum daily requirement. Shrimp is one of the finest sources of protein of any food and provides an easily digested type of protein. The fact is shrimp is essentially pure protein. It is also one of the top sources of selenium, which it concentrates from sea water, and it is an excellent source of naturally occurring sodium, which, again, arises from its watery environment. Shrimp also contains the highly touted fish oils, which may account for the fact that the regular consumption of shrimp actually helps reduce high cholesterol.

Top Shrimp Tips

1. Be sure to wash shrimp thoroughly before cooking. Rinse only with cold water. This rinsing removes germs and noxious chemicals as well as preservatives, which may be added to fresh shrimp by the shipper or grower.

2. Be sure to de-vein fresh shrimp before cooking. The vein contains bacteria and other wastes, which must be removed. Remove the veins with a knife and rinse the remainder.

3. Buy shrimp originating from the least polluted areas possible. Opt for shrimp from Alaska, Indonesia (i.e. prawns), or other areas of reduced pollution. A second option is to buy farm-raised shrimp, but they are less nutrient dense than wild shrimp. For instance, farm-raised shrimp are lower in iodine than ocean shrimp.

4. Eat shrimp as an appetizer. Make home-made shrimp sauce with lemon, tomato sauce, and horseradish. Serve shrimp with vegetable trays. This will add much needed protein to the vegetable appetizer and provide variety to make the vegetable tray more appealing.

5. Make shrimp based soups. This method of cooking is ideal for shrimp, because it preserves its critical nutrients. Iodine is water soluble and is lost in cooking water. Thus, shrimp soup is superior nutritionally than boiled shrimp.

6. If preparing unpeeled frozen shrimp, don't thaw it. That makes it slippery and difficult to peel, plus it gives bacteria a chance to grow. Instead, peel the shrimp frozen while running them under cold water.

7. If you like boiled shrimp, try them New Orleans style. Add a cajun spice mix to the boiling water, or make cajun shrimp sauce with plain boiled shrimp. This provides flavor, plus the spices stimulate the digestive juices, and the improved digestion increases the nutritional powers of the shrimp.

Top Shrimp Cures

1. If you are constantly cold or if you are sensitive to cold weather, drafts, or air conditioning, eat shrimp often. Try the various soup recipes in the recipe section. Shrimp soup is a powerful remedy for cold sensitivity. The iodine in shrimp empowers thyroid gland function. This gland is known descriptively as the "Master of Metabolism," meaning that it controls metabolic rate and, therefore, body temperature. Iodine feeds the thyroid gland, helping it produce thyroid hormone, the latter being made from iodine and various amino acids. Shrimp is the perfect thyroid supporting food, as it contains a plethora of amino acids along with the iodine.

2. If you have difficulty digesting protein or if you have a protein deficiency, shrimp is the ideal food. Shrimp is pure protein, and it is also perhaps the most readily digested of all seafood.

3. Be aware that allergy to shrimp is relatively common. If you are sensitive to seafood or iodine, eating shrimp may prove disastrous. Allergic reactions to shrimp may be manifested by rash, hives, itchy skin, difficulty breathing, headaches, and sinus problems.

4. Shrimp soup is an excellent remedy for poor digestion, excessive weight loss, and malabsorption. It provides much needed amino acids, which are necessary for building and repairing the immune defenses plus various vitamins and minerals in the broth. The medium of broth is the easiest means of absorbing the nutrients in the event of illness. Furthermore, shrimp broth is rich in iodine, one of Nature's most powerful antibiotics. Iodine is used by white blood cells as a cofactor for killing microbes, plus it possesses significant antifungal properties.

5. Shrimp is the ideal food for dieting, as it is low in calories and high in protein. Because it is high in protein, vitamins, and minerals, it helps satisfy the appetite. Contrary to popular belief, shrimp is low in fat and has no ill effects upon blood fats. In fact, regular consumption of shrimp helps normalize cholesterol and triglyceride levels. This effect is due to a cholesterol-like substance in shrimp which antagonizes blood cholesterol, plus shrimp is rich in iodine, which the body uses to accelerate fat combustion.

Spinach

Virtually everyone has eaten spinach with the intent of bettering health. True, many individuals eat it only because they have no other choice— remember that bland, soft, slimy spinach in the school lunch? Yet, when prepared properly, it is one of the tastiest of all vegetables. Spinach is more correctly categorized as an herb rather than a vegetable, which may explain its unusually valuable healing properties.

A native of Persia, spinach was introduced to the West during the 11th century; it was brought to Spain by Islamic traders, and from there it was popularized throughout Europe. Its name implies its origin, since spinach is a derivation of the Arabic term *isfanakh*. From Spain it quickly became popular in Southern Europe, where it grew readily.

Fresh spinach, is a powerhouse of nutrients. By weight it contains a greater amount of vitamin C than oranges and is one of the richest vegetable sources of vitamin A (as beta carotene). The vitamin A content is massive, with 100 gms providing nearly 10,000 I.U. of vitamin A. Spinach contains another type of carotenoid called *lutein*. While having no vitamin A activity researchers have found that lutein offers special anti-cancer actions and is particularly protective against lung and prostate cancer. Other research points to lutein's beneficial effects for vision.

Fresh or frozen spinach are the most beneficial nutritionally. Vitamin/mineral loss in canned spinach is extensive, with 70% or more of the nutrients lost. For instance, vitamin C losses in canned spinach may reach 80%. In some batches there may be no detectable vitamin C. Spinach can also be juiced, and it supplies the most nutritional benefit when combined with other vegetables such as carrots, beets, celery, parsley, and other green leafy vegetables.

Spinach is a top vegetable source of certain B vitamins. Incredibly, it is richer by weight in riboflavin than whole milk. One cup of raw spinach contains 190 mcg of folic acid; one cup of cooked, which equals four cups of raw leaves, provides well over the RDA for this B vitamin, illustrating that cooked vegetables may provide a higher concentration of nutrients than raw. Furthermore, spinach contains a considerable amount of protein compared to other dark green vegetables.

For a vegetable, spinach contains unusually large amounts of minerals. It is an excellent source of magnesium, in fact, it is one of the richest vegetable sources of this nutrient. A mere 100 grams contains nearly 90 mg of magnesium, which means a couple of large helpings of spinach could supply much of the minimum requirement. The calcium content is also considerable, with a cup containing around 95 mg. However, this calcium is largely unavailable to the body, as it is bound by oxalic acid, a substance which antagonizes calcium absorption. As is well known, spinach is rich in iron, but few people realize just how rich it is. A large helping (about 2 cups) of raw spinach supplies 6 mg of iron, which is one third of the minimum daily amount. That makes spinach the richest vegetable source of iron. Spinach is also relatively rich in potassium, sodium (in a natural form), and phosphorus.

Top Spinach Tips

1. Never boil spinach in large amounts of water. This type of cooking ruins its nutritional value and taste. Instead, steam it gently or cook it in a pan with a small amount of water just until it changes color.

2. Canned spinach has been depleted of the majority of its nutrients. If fresh spinach is unavailable, buy frozen spinach. Nutrient loss in frozen spinach is minimal. Frozen spinach is easier to use in some recipes such as quiche and other casserole type dishes.

3. Spinach should ideally be cooked with butter or perhaps in a cream sauce. The reason is that the fat aids in the absorption of the pigments, notably beta carotene and bioflavonoids. Furthermore, milk products contain calcium, which neutralizes the toxic effects of oxalic acid, a substance found in spinach in large quantities. Cooking also destroys much of the oxalic acid content. No wonder previous generations enjoyed spinach cooked in cream sauce and/or butter. Abandon fat paranoia and revive this luscious and nutritious recipe.

4. Oxalic acid, which is found in large quantities in spinach, especially raw spinach, may cause intestinal irritation. One way to neutralize it is to eat raw spinach with counteracting acids such as lemon juice or vinegar. On the positive side, oxalic acid usually only causes problems if large amounts of raw spinach are eaten. Symptoms of oxalic acid poisoning include stomach ache, gas, bloating, cramping, and diarrhea.

5. The leaves of spinach are highly nutritious, far more nutritious than ordinary lettuce. Be sure to add spinach leaves to salads as often as possible.

6. Be sure to wash spinach leaves ultra-thoroughly. Spinach is grown on sandy soil, and the leaves hold a considerable amount of dirt and dust.

7. Spinach is an ideal addition to egg, meat, and fish dishes. Add chopped spinach to an omelet, ground beef, or casseroles. It is particularly tasty when combined with melted cheese as in omelets, quiche, and casseroles.

8. Use spinach leaves as a type of "starchless" bread. Place a poached or turned-over egg in a large spinach leaf and eat it like a sandwich. The same can be done with sliced roast beef, chicken, or turkey. Add mustard or homemade mayonnaise for extra taste. This leafy sandwich is the ideal type for individuals watching their weight.

Top Spinach Cures

1. Spinach is a great hydrating food. This is because it is up to 93% water. Furthermore, it is rich in vitamins and minerals which combat the ill effects of heat, notably potassium, magnesium, vitamin C, pantothenic acid, and vitamin A. When the heat is intolerable, try a spinach salad consisting of spinach and lettuce leaves plus tomatoes and onions. Top with vinegar, olive oil, and salt.

2. If you were to analyze the food charts for calcium rich foods, you would probably rely upon spinach, since it is one of top vegetables on the list. However, its rich calcium supply is not available in a usable form. In fact, spinach contains a potentially toxic chemical, at least in respect to calcium metabolism, called oxalic acid. This acid destroys calcium. This means that spinach is a poor source of calcium. On the plus side, oxalic acid is partially destroyed by cooking, so some of the calcium may be rendered available when spinach is steamed or sautéed. Unfortunately, with raw spinach the absorption of calcium may be as low as 4%, which makes it essentially useless as a source of this mineral.

3. Anemia meets its match with spinach. A large serving contains an incredibly large amount of iron, about 7 milligrams. Plus, spinach is rich in vitamin C, which potentiates the absorption of iron. Spinach contains riboflavin, niacin, pyridoxine, and vitamin A, all of which are required for the manufacture of healthy red blood cells.

4. Certain diseases are associated with wasting of the tissues. Such diseases include diabetes, cancer, multiple sclerosis, ALS, muscular dystrophy, and myasthenia gravis. Spinach is an ideal food for these conditions. This is because it is a veritable nutritional power-plant of vitamins, minerals, and amino acids. Amino acids are needed to prevent muscular or tissue wasting. Incredibly, a large serving of spinach contains as much amino acid healing power as a helping of cottage cheese. For additional amino acid density add spinach to high protein foods such as cheese, egg, fish, and meat entrees.

5. Individuals with a history of kidney stones may need to eat spinach with caution. This is due to the oxalic acid content, a substance which may irritate the kidneys as well as precipitate stones. The fact is certain individuals have a tendency to form stones made from oxalic acid bound to minerals, known appropriately as oxalate stones. Other foods rich in oxalic acid include almonds, cashews, cocoa, rhubarb, and tea.

6. Spinach is an ideal food to consume for individuals suffering from lung disease. This is because spinach contains several nutrients which nourish the lungs, including vitamin A (as beta carotene), vitamin C, vitamin K, vitamin E, and magnesium.

Squash

It would be difficult to find a food easier to cook than squash. Available year round, pound for pound it is one of the most nourishing and cost effective of all foods. Squash is one of the top sources of beta carotene. It is also a good source of vitamin C, potassium, folic acid, and fiber.

It appears that the beta carotene in squash, that is cooked squash, is easier to absorb than the type found in carrots. It has been long known that antioxidants in foods, particularly beta carotene, vitamin E, and vitamin C, protect against cataract formation. Researchers from Harvard studied nurses over a 12 year period and found that those eating large amounts of beta carotene rich foods, particularly squash and sweet potatoes, were protected against cataract development. However, the carrot eaters were not protected—even large amounts of carrots failed to help. Thus, the researchers concluded there are other reasons for squash's superiority. Furthermore, while carrots are essentially devoid of vitamin C, a large helping of squash provides a reasonable supply, and squash is also rich in vitamin E, which is preventive against cataracts.

There are dozens of varieties of squash. The following are the most commonly available types:

a) acorn: this has a dark green rind. It is a convenient size for baking. It is relatively low in beta carotene, and its flavor is bland.

b) buttercup: this is similar in appearance to acorn squash, however, the dark green outer color is interrupted with light green streaks. It is sweet and gives more flavor than acorn squash.

c) butternut: this is a large tan-colored squash that is noted by a narrow neck and bulbous end. It is perhaps the most common variety available in supermarkets. Rich in beta carotene, it is ideal for baking and tastes sort of like sweet potatoes.

d) spaghetti: this is a football shaped squash with a light yellow exterior.

It is so named, because when it is baked the insides resemble spaghetti noodles. It is rich in beta carotene and mildly sweet in taste
e) yellow: this is more of a type of zucchini than a squash. When steamed or fried it exhibits a pleasantly sweet taste. Yellow squash is high in fiber and minerals and virtually devoid of beta carotene

Top Squash Tips

1. Squash is the ideal type of "bakery" food for assisting weight loss. In contrast to potatoes or bread it is relatively low in calories but is high in nutrients and fiber. Thus, it is very filling. Potatoes and sweet potatoes are higher in sugar and starch than squash and pumpkin are, therefore, more likely to cause weight gain. Squash is high in vitamins, minerals, fiber, and protein—everything good and nothing bad.
2. Cook squash with fat. Squash is rich in beta carotene, and fat aids in its absorption. Be sure to butter the squash or cook it in stir fry or casseroles containing meat, cheese, butter, or oil.
3. Use spaghetti squash instead of spaghetti noodles. Pour the meat sauce over strands of spaghetti squash. The squash "noodles" are far more nutritious than the flour noodles, plus, they are higher in fiber and lower in calories than regular noodles.
4. Don't add sugar to squash. This vegetable possesses its own natural sweetness. If you must sweeten it, add butter or coconut milk, both of which provide the natural sweetness of saturated fats. If desired, top with cinnamon, which also is naturally sweet.
5. Remember, squash is available throughout the year. Use it as a winter food for providing much needed vitamin A (as beta carotene), trace minerals, and vitamin C. Vitamin A and C needs are greatly increased during the winter months as a result of cold exposure.

Top Squash Cures

1. Squash is an excellent food for the health of the colon. This is because it is an excellent source of fiber, and the type of fiber it contains is gentle upon the gut. Plus, it is one of the most readily digested of all foods. Eat

squash regularly if you suffer from colitis, irritable bowel syndrome, Crohn's disease, or ulcerative colitis. Allergic intolerance to squash is relatively rare.

2. If you wish to lose weight, eat lots of squash. Because it is rich in fiber and nutrients, squash is extremely filling. Furthermore, it is lower in starch and calories than potatoes or pasta. Thus, eating fiber-rich squash helps the pounds come off, while eating potatoes and pasta tends to put the pounds on quickly.

3. Individuals suffering from heart disease and/or high blood pressure should habitually eat squash. This vegetable is supremely rich in potassium, which is ultra-important for circulatory health. The rich beta carotene content helps protect the heart and arteries from degenerating. In other words, the regular intake of squash helps prevent atherosclerosis as well as coronary artery disease.

4. Squash is the perfect vegetable for combating lung disorders, including asthma. Its high content of B vitamins, minerals, and beta carotene come to the aid of ailing lungs. In particular, the lungs have a high requirement for beta carotene, which is the premier antioxidant of the lung cells. Be sure to eat squash with dietary fats, because fat is necessary to provoke the absorption of the curative factors, the carotenoids.

5. If you want smooth blemish-free skin, eat plenty of squash. Both potassium and beta carotene are needed to keep skin cells healthy, and these are found in squash in dense amounts. Squash also contains special chemicals, which aid in keeping the skin moist, giving it a smooth texture, and preventing blemishes/infection. For a superior effect also eat the seeds, which are rich in essential fatty acids and zinc, both of which are needed for beautiful skin.

Strawberries

Strawberries are perhaps the most nutrient dense of all fruits. The reason for this density is rather obvious: they are ground hugging plants, and, therefore, they absorb tremendous quantities of nutrients from the soil. Like many other foods, such as milk, almonds, parsley, and lettuce, strawberries possess their own unique calming agent, which may be why strawberries and cream is such an intensely popular and craved dish.

While the majority of berries are fruit of the vine, strawberries are a receptacle of a flower, which bears the fruit on its surface. Over the millennia this fruit was gathered in the wild as a delicacy of the primitives. Perhaps its earliest use as a farmed fruit was in South America, where it was cultivated thousands of years ago. Strawberries were first grown in Europe in the 16th century, whereas in Chile, they had been cultivated centuries prior.

Strawberries are over 90% water, 1% protein, and are lower in sugar than most fruits, containing only about 7.4%. Compare that to oranges, which contain over 20% sugar. The tart taste of strawberries is due to the fact that they contain relatively large amounts (1%) of acidic compounds, notably malic acid, which is important for digestion and energy production.

Strawberries possess numerous curative chemicals. They are rich in bioflavonoids, which block inflammation and fight cancer. That red color of strawberries is not just for beauty; it is evidence of an invaluable array of natural chemicals, including bioflavonoids and ellagic acid. The main chemical responsible for the color is an anthocyanodin known as *pelargonidin 3-monoglucoside*. This chemical is a powerful anti-disease and anti-cancer substance. So, be sure to consume any strawberry juice residue down to the last drop, because the juice is super-rich in this substance. Strawberries are one of the top sources of vitamin C, containing a whopping 80+ mg per cup, which makes them richer per ounce than oranges or grapefruit. The extra vitamin C is invaluable as an aid for the immune system and is necessary for the maintenance of healthy skin, hair, nails, and joints. Strawberries are the main source of a newly discovered chemical called *ellagic acid*. This substance is a powerful antioxidant. It is even more powerful than beta carotene or vitamin E for blocking oxidative damage to the tissues. This may explain the U.S. Government finding that strawberries are superior to virtually any other food as a source of antioxidants. Furthermore, recent research documents that ellagic acid is an effective defender against cancer.

It is crucial to realize that only organically grown chemical free strawberries offer these benefits. Commercial strawberries are hopelessly contaminated with pesticides and herbicides. Recent government studies show that of all grocery store foods, strawberries are perhaps the most chemically contaminated. Thus, by eating commercially grown strawberries, the individual might actually instigate cancer.

Strawberry leaves are also rich in nutrients, containing a considerable amount of minerals as well as vitamin C. According to Gibbons strawberry leaves are richer in vitamin C than any other herb tested and are considerably richer per gram than the berries themselves. They are also an excellent source of minerals, particularly potassium and silicon. Only wild strawberry leaves can be relied upon as a dependable source of vitamin C. Furthermore, these leaves are chock-full of bioflavonoids, such as ellagic acid, containing far more than the berries themselves. Wild strawberry leaves are currently available as the key ingredient of Wild Power Tea.

Top Strawberry Tips

1. Preserve strawberries after purchasing by placing a wedge or two of lemon in the container. Strawberries tend to mold easily, and the essential oils in lemon help retard spoilage. Rinsing the strawberries in a dilute solution of vinegar may also retard mold growth. Or, for a more powerful anti-mold effect dip them in a solution of water plus a few drops of oil of oregano.
2. Strawberries go well with both fruit and vegetable salads. Surround or top salads with sliced strawberries. They add flavor, while enhancing visual appeal.
3. There is good news for fans of the old fashioned recipe of strawberries and cream. The cream helps liberate certain nutrients, such as lycopene, ellagic acid, and beta carotene, so they may be more readily absorbed. Also, add strawberries to full fat cottage cheese. They enhance the flavor and also provide vitamin C, which is lacking in milk products.
4. Don't store strawberries for prolonged periods, because they spoil rapidly. Eat them within 48 hours of purchase or, if purchasing a large batch, freeze any extra berries immediately.
5. Strawberries are relatively low in sugar and make an ideal snack for children and adults alike. They are also an ideal dessert, because they satisfy the sweet desire while improving digestion of a heavy meal.
6. Only organically grown strawberries can be relied upon as a curative food. Wild strawberries are of even greater value, but they are unavailable. Commercial strawberries are so utterly laced with pesticides

that the negative effects of the contaminants cancels any positive benefits of the berries. Demand that your grocer stock chemical free strawberries.

Top Strawberry Cures

1. Strawberries help brighten stained teeth. Native Americans used the juice of wild strawberries as a tooth whitener. Apparently, it is the red pigment, which is also found in commercial varieties, that exerts this effect.
2. Strawberries are a top aid for indigestion and are certainly superior to antacids for this purpose. Eat a handful of strawberries after meals for a tasty digestive tonic, and the heartburn/indigestion will generally be dissipated.
3. The warning signs of vitamin C deficiency include fatigue, irritability, memory loss, easy bruising, nose bleeds, sensitive skin, poor wound healing, bleeding gums, petechiae, and muscular weakness. Strawberries are an ideal anti-scurvy medicine and provide a greater amount of vitamin C per serving (one cup) than oranges or grapefruit. If you suffer from fatigue, whether mental or physical, or any of the cardinal symptoms of vitamin C deficiency, use strawberries as the vitamin C source of choice. They provide natural vitamin C, which is more biologically active, and, thus, more effective in combating illness than the synthetic variety. For an even more potent natural vitamin C punch, drink *Wild Power Tea*. One cup per day provides as much vitamin C as a pint of orange juice, plus it is super-rich in bioflavonoids, far richer than citrus juice.
4. Strawberries are the perfect fruit for individuals who are sensitive to sugar. This is because they are relatively low in sugar, containing less than 7% by weight. Oddly, lemons and limes, as well as grapefruit, despite their sour taste, contain a greater amount of sugar than strawberries. For diabetics and hypoglycemics who can tolerate fruit, strawberries are one of the top choices, as they are less likely to cause a disruption in blood sugar than bananas, oranges, apples, pears, grapes, etc.
5. Strawberries are a top fruit for fighting cancer. This is because they are rich in a variety of compounds proven to prevent or perhaps reverse this disease. These substances include beta carotene, vitamin C, bioflavonoids, and an extremely powerful cancer fighter known as ellagic acid. There is a word of caution: only organically grown strawberries are

244

dependable cancer fighters; commercially grown strawberries contain pesticide residues, which are themselves carcinogens.

That deep red color of strawberries explains their anti-cancer action. The strawberry pigments actually inhibit the growth of cancer cells and may even help the body destroy cancer. The leaves are the best source of the strawberry pigment, but only the wild leaves are a reliable source. If you have a family history of cancer or if you suffer from the disease, drink Wild Power Tea, 1 to 2 cups daily.

6. Strawberries are useful in bowel regulation. They help prevent both diarrhea and constipation. Individuals with sluggish bowels might try a tasty remedy: eating a large bowl of fresh strawberries in the morning is certain to stimulate digestive function.

7. Wild strawberry leaves have been used for thousands of years as a natural diuretic. If you suffer from sluggish kidneys, bloating, and/or water retention, use Wild Power Tea regularly. Drink at least 1 cup of tea daily. The more that you drink of this luscious tea the better will be your overall health.

Sweet potato

Sweet potatoes are, in reality, not potatoes. Native to the American tropics, they belong to the morning glory family and are actually the root of a flowering plant.

Sweet potatoes have as their greatest nutritional notoriety one important fact: they are incredibly rich in vitamin A. One sweet potato provides well over the minimal daily requirement of this invaluable vitamin in the form of beta carotene.

The term sweet potato is often confused with the term yam. This is an important misnomer, since the two are entirely different nutritionally and botanically. Yams are tubers, while sweet potatoes are the roots of a flower. Yams are indigenous to Africa, while sweet potatoes originate from the New World. Yams contain no vitamin A, not even a milligram. Fortunately, true yams are found in Africa, not in supermarkets. In fact, virtually all of the so-called yams in the supermarket are, in reality, sweet potatoes. The name change occurred in Louisiana during a marketing promotion of a certain type of sweet potato. Unfortunately, this name distinction has held ever since. The real difference is a result of the fact that there are two primary types of sweet potatoes. There is the hard moist fleshy variety, which is often elongated, and there is the usually shorter and softer dry-fleshy variety. The soft/elongated type is almost always identified in supermarkets as "yams," while the dry fleshy type is called sweet potato. To reiterate, both are sweet potatoes, and, therefore, both are rich in vitamin A. For years, I have informed people not to buy yams, because the nutritional textbooks list them as being devoid of vitamin A. I had no clue until I wrote this book that commercial yams are packed with vitamin A, because they are, indeed, sweet potatoes. My co-author and nutritionist, Judy Kay Gray, first made this never before published distinction.

While the vitamin A content is overwhelming, sweet potatoes contain good amounts of vitamin C, pyridoxine, folic acid, and biotin. A small sweet potato contains as much as 25 mg of vitamin C, which is nearly one half the RDA.

Sweet potatoes, being a type of root vegetable, are rich in minerals. They are superior to bananas as a potassium supplement, with one medium potato containing half the RDA. Depending upon the size a sweet potato may contain up to a milligram of manganese and .5 milligrams of copper. These minerals are needed to maintain healthy red blood cells. Manganese is useful for digesting and processing sugars, and perhaps this is why sweet potatoes are often well tolerated by individuals who are sugar sensitive. Sweet potatoes also contain significant amounts of calcium, phosphorus, magnesium, and iron.

A common worry about sweet potatoes is that they are fattening. This misconception is largely a result of their intensely sweet taste. It is assumed that they are a caloric time bomb. Shockingly, they are relatively low in calories; a 5 inch sweet potato contains merely 120 calories, about the same amount as a comparable white potato.

Top Sweet Potato Tips

1. Eat sweet potatoes with fatty foods. Adding butter to a baked sweet potato is the ideal prescription, since the butter aids in the absorption of beta carotene, which is fat soluble. Don't deny yourself the wonderful taste of butter on a freshly baked sweet potato and add it liberally, if

desired. If you are allergic to butter, add instead coconut fat or nut butter.

2. Add sweet potatoes to stir fry, but be sure to use oil in order to enhance beta carotene absorption. Use only cold pressed oils such as extra virgin olive, rice bran, avocado, or hazelnut oils and cook with very low heat.

3. Sweet potatoes are highly vulnerable to fungal rot. Don't buy sweet potatoes with soft spots or black blemishes, which are evidence of fungal growth. Don't merely cut out the spots and expect to remedy the problem. Once the rot begins, the entire potato is ruined, both in taste and nutrition. Furthermore, fungi produce potentially dangerous chemicals, which can cause a type of food poisoning. When it doubt, throw it out.

4. Don't over-cook sweet potatoes. They require only half the cooking time of regular potatoes. Over-cooking may destroy much of the vitamin A and vitamin C content.

5. Add sweet potatoes to soup as an alternative to pasta, noodles, or white potatoes. Alternatively, left over sweet potatoes may be pureed and used as a base for cream soups. Such soups provide invaluable amounts of vitamin A. To accelerate the vitamin A absorption, be sure to add real cream or butter. If you are allergic to cream, use extra virgin olive oil or coconut milk in the soup base.

6. Sweet potatoes make an ideal snack for hungry children. Simply cook them in a convection or regular oven until done. Serve hot topped with butter. Often, this will resolve a child's desire for sweets.

7. Don't add sugar to sweet potatoes; they are sweet enough. If you wish enhance the flavor, use sweet unsalted butter and spices such as cinnamon and nutmeg.

Top Sweet Potato Cures

1. Sweet potatoes are an ideal remedy for skin disorders, especially dry or flaky skin. This is because they are one of the richest sources of vitamin A (as beta carotene). If you suffer from dry skin or dermatitis, eat a sweet potato each day for two weeks, then eat one or two per week. What a tasty way to eradicate an illness.

2. Those suffering from weakened immunity must regularly consume sweet potatoes. The rich content of beta carotene provides immense vitamin A value, and this latter nutrient is critical to immunological

defenses. All immune proteins, such as immunoglobulins, albumin, enzymes, and interferon, require vitamin A for their synthesis. Vitamin A is also necessary for activating the thymus gland, which is the master gland of immunity.

3. If your skin is sensitive to sunlight, eat sweet potatoes several times per week. They are a top source of beta carotene. A single medium sweet potato contains five times the RDA for vitamin A (as beta carotene), and this amount could readily be destroyed by one day's exposure to sunlight. So when the sun is irradiating your skin, protect it by eating a sweet potato every day.

4. Sweet potatoes are a top remedy for the eyes. This is again because of the dense supply of vitamin A. The regular consumption of sweet potatoes offers protection against a wide range of eye disorders, including nearsightedness, farsightedness, cataracts, macular degeneration, and glaucoma. For prevention of these disorders, eat at least one sweet potato per week. If you suffer from a degenerative eye disease, eat a sweet potato per day for at least one month. This natural "megadose" of vitamin A will likely induce a significant improvement in the condition.

5. Sweet potatoes are an ideal food for individuals suffering from poor appetite and/or anorexia. They are readily digested, plus the vitamin A aids in the normalization of appetite. Vitamin A is required for the production of stomach acid and pancreatic enzymes, which are the primary secretions needed for the digestion of food. Furthermore, vitamin A is crucial for the maintenance of a healthy intestinal lining. The cellular lining of the stomach and intestines is the most rapidly growing tissue in the body. Every five to seven days these cells die and must be replenished. Vitamin A is required for this cellular regeneration.

6. Diseases of the intestines may be due to vitamin A deficiency. These diseases include colitis, Crohn's disease, diverticulitis, pancreatitis, gastritis, diarrhea, and/or constipation. In all of these instances it is necessary to consume vitamin A on a regular basis. Sweet potatoes provide a type of vitamin A that is readily absorbed, especially if the potatoes are eaten with fat. The fat instigates the release of fat digesting enzymes and bile, which promote the absorption of vitamin A (and beta carotene) into the blood and lymph. Without dietary fat, vitamin A absorption is nil.

Sweet potatoes are allowed on a low fat diet. However, what is the value of eating them if the vitamin A is lost in the stool? Yet, this dietary approach of avoiding all added fat in meals is regarded as health enhancing. Ironically, by inducing a vitamin A deficiency, the low fat diet does a greater degree of harm than perhaps if the individual followed a traditional diet containing uncensured amounts of fat.

Without vitamin A, cellular death is inevitable. Ultimately, death of the organism will occur. Vitamin A deficiency is the major cause of digestive diseases and diarrheal illness world wide and is a primary contributor to death in third world countries. What a travesty it is that we, in this world of convenience, might join the impoverished in their hapless state by forcibly inducing vitamin A deficiency through fad diets. Yet, this is precisely what is happening in America, since vitamin A deficiency has reached epidemic proportions, afflicting over 50% of the adult population. Children, teenagers, and the elderly are particularly vulnerable.

For Americans, the primary causes of vitamin A deficiency include:

low fat diet (the number one cause)
cholesterol lowering medicines
deep fried oils (contain substances which oxidize vitamin A)
inorganic iron (found in refined flour and rice products)
vegetarian or macrobiotic diets
hypothyroidism and diabetes
aspirin, Motrin, Naprosyn, or other antiinflammatory agents
long-term antibiotic therapy
acetaminophen abuse
alcoholism (moderate drinking also lowers vitamin A)

Tomatoes

While they are universally regarded as a vegetable, tomatoes are in reality the fruit of a vine. In fact, technically they are a type of berry. They became known as a vegetable as a result of legislation. Because of a tariff dispute in 1893, the Supreme Court declared the tomato to be a vegetable.

Tomatoes are one of God's greatest health foods. They originated in the Americas and were grown by Native Americans. They were brought to Europe in the 16th century by the Spaniards, who found them growing in Central and South America. Though it may be a surprise, tomatoes didn't originate in Italy or France.

Nutritionally, tomatoes are most notable for their rich content of vitamins C and A, although they are a good source of calcium, potassium, and iron. They are also one of those rare foods which contain a considerable amount of vitamin K. They are one of the best plant sources of folic acid. A large sun-ripened garden tomato may contain as much as 50% of the RDA for this vitamin.

On the negative side tomatoes may contain a significant amount of tryptamine, which is a type of highly reactive protein. Certain individuals, particularly migraine sufferers, may be highly sensitive to tryptamine, and this may account for the fact that tomatoes are reported as a cause of migraines.

Unfortunately, the majority of tomatoes in the supermarket are picked green. They are artificial ripened by exposing them to a gas, usually ethylene dioxide, which rapidly turns the outer skin to a red color; a sort of fake ripeness is induced. Yet, the insides haven't ripened on the vine, which means there is less sunlight induced nutrition. The vitamin C and bioflavonoid content of tomatoes is directly related to how much sunlight they receive. Some supermarket tomatoes may contain virtually no detectable vitamin C. There is even a considerable reduction in the beta carotene content of commercial tomatoes.

Let's assume for a moment that tomatoes are grown in a natural way, ripened by sunlight. On a weight basis they are one of the richest known sources of vitamin C and are richer in this nutrient than the majority of vegetables. A large ripe tomato may contain as much as 40 mg of vitamin C and nearly 1000 I.U. of vitamin A (as beta carotene). After accounting for water, tomatoes are mostly carbohydrate, yet, they contain a greater amount of protein than most fruits.

Historically, tomatoes have been acclaimed for their ability to aid gout, stop arthritis, diminish sinus congestion, correct impaired digestion, and lessen high blood pressure. Several reports illustrate how tomatoes, perhaps because of their rich vitamin C content, aid in curing the common cold. The best way to receive this cold-fighting power is to consume tomato concentrates, such as tomato sauce, paste, or juice. The juice is easy to consume with the sore throat, congestion, and/or low appetite typically seen with viral infection. The flavonoids, particularly lycopene, aid the immune system in battling the virus. Tomatoes are an excellent source of vitamin K. This makes them ideal for bleeding disorders such as nosebleeds, poor blood clotting, and ulcers.

In folk medicine it is believed that eating tomatoes is beneficial to the skin. This may be accounted for by the high content of vitamin C, flavonoids, and beta carotene. Tomatoes are an excellent food for individuals suffering from acne, boils, cysts, or other infections of the skin.

Tomatoes have been unduly blamed as a cause of arthritis. The arthritis connection has been attributed to the fact that tomatoes are related to nightshades, which are poisonous. However, while tomatoes are in the nightshade family, they contain no poisonous chemicals. Rather, they contain a wide variety of curative chemicals which enhance health. In fact, tomatoes are rich in a variety of natural chemicals, such as vitamin C, beta carotene, and bioflavonoids, which help prevent arthritis.

The arthritis/tomato connection was fostered largely upon hearsay. It arose mainly because of the personal experience of Dr. Norman Childers, who is not a physician but is a horticulturist. It is hearsay, because the theory generates from Foster personally. Dr. Foster had developed a debilitating form of arthritis and found that changing his diet improved his symptoms. The foods he eliminated included, among other things, the edible nightshades such as tomatoes. His joint symptoms and arthritis vanished. Although not a shred of research was performed, he disseminated his theory, and it became as if it was fact. Now, virtually every nutritionist attempts to cure arthritis by removing the nightshades from the diet despite the fact that tomatoes contain some of the most powerful anti-inflammation and anti-degenerative substances known. Eliminating tomatoes should only be done if a proven food intolerance or allergy exists. In my research, which was done with blood testing, less than 10% of individuals with arthritis were allergic to tomatoes. Allergy to other nightshades, particularly potatoes, was more common, but this was largely due to an intolerance to the starchy aspect of potatoes or perhaps the mold content rather than any poisonous effects inherent to potatoes.

Tomatoes contain an invaluable compound called *lycopene*. This substance, responsible for the red color of tomatoes, is closely allied to beta carotene, the latter being respected for its anti-cancer actions. However, compelling research published in the 1980s-90s shows that lycopene is significantly more effective in blocking cancer than beta carotene. Lycopene is a major deterrent to pancreatic cancer. Researchers measured lycopene levels in the blood of individuals with cancer and found that levels are far lower than normal. For individuals with a low blood level, the likelihood of developing pancreatic cancer jumps nearly 100%. In other words, low levels mean the individual is twice as likely to develop the disease. In fact, those with the lowest levels were five times more likely to develop pancreatic cancer than individuals with high levels. Low levels of lycopene are also associated with an increased risk of prostate cancer. Researchers from Harvard found that individuals who consumed the most tomato products had the lowest risk of prostate cancer. The fascinating part of this research was that the greatest benefit was seen with cooked tomato products such as tomato sauce. The researchers determined that lycopene, a fat soluble substance, must be consumed with fat for optimal absorption. This research indicates that the use of a strict low fat diet for prostate cancer is actually dangerous. So when you eat tomato sauce or cooked tomatoes, add extra virgin olive oil and/or ground beef; the added fat not only enhances taste, but it also increases lycopene absorption.

Lycopene is found in relatively few foods. In the American diet watermelon and tomatoes constitute the primary sources, although red sweet peppers and pink grapefruit contain a fair amount. Not all red foods contain it. For instance, there is little or none in raspberries or strawberries; their red color comes from other pigments. Other sources include rosehips, papaya, red guavas, and apricots.

Here is how to get the greatest benefits from lycopene:

1. Eat lycopene in food; don't rely on supplements
2. Eat raw tomatoes with fatty foods. Slice a tomato and surround with olives, feta cheese, or avocado. Drizzle with extra virgin olive oil.
3. Cook tomatoes with fat-rich foods. Add ground beef, cheese, olives, and/or olive oil to the recipe. For stewed tomatoes cook with added oil.
4. Cook red sweet peppers in a base of fat. Chop and add to hamburger dishes. Sauté in stir fry with added extra virgin olive oil or coconut milk. Add extra virgin olive oil to red pepper sauce.

5. Make a Lycopene Salad. Section and peel a whole red grapefruit; set aside. Dice one half red sweet pepper. Cut into slices one half medium avocado (for the fat). Slice or dice one half papaya. Place ingredients in bowl and gently mix. Top with a few cherry tomatoes. Drizzle with extra virgin olive oil, if desired.

There seems to be little doubt that lycopene is a cancer deterrent. Researchers at the University of Illinois at Chicago found that women with the highest levels of lycopene had the lowest risk, some five times lower, for developing cervical dysplasia. In a Hawaiian study tomato eaters cut their cancer risks dramatically, and the tomatoes worked better than synthetic vitamins. The researchers had expected that beta carotene pills would work equally as well. Yet, the food beat the vitamins. This is corroborated by Germany's Dr. Helmut Sies and Dr. Wilhelm Stahl, who determined that the tomato pigment was twice as powerful as beta carotene at preventing cancerous changes.

Top Tomato Tips

1. Tomatoes are the leading source of naturally occurring vitamin C in the average American's diet, largely because they are consumed so prolifically and also because tomatoes are found in several different forms. Tomatoes, tomato sauce, and tomato juice are a convenient way to get your vitamin C.
2. Never refrigerate tomatoes. Not only does it inhibit ripening, but it also damages the tomatoes' skin.
3. Don't waste time making home-made tomato sauce from commercial tomatoes. Buy instead canned tomato sauce. The tomatoes used in canning are ripe and are richer in nutrients, such as vitamin C and bioflavonoids, than are they commercial "fresh" tomatoes. Remember, fresh tomatoes are ripened artificially. Make homemade sauce only if using garden or farm fresh tomatoes. Ideally, consume tomato sauce made from organically raised tomatoes.
4. Use sun-dried tomatoes in sauces and casseroles. This is a convenient method for consuming vine-ripened tomatoes. Sun-dried tomatoes are richer in vitamin C than commercial tomatoes.
5. Avoid buying green or pale red tomatoes during winter. These tomatoes

are lower in nutrients than the summer batch of tomatoes. Instead, use canned tomato products and/or sun-dried tomatoes. Try an Italian or French market for a wide variety of imported tomato products. While imported tomatoes are not guaranteed organic, they are less likely to contain pesticide residues versus the supermarket varieties.

6. Don't just eat tomatoes raw. Use them frequently in cooking. Tomato sauce, diced tomatoes, whole canned tomatoes, fresh tomatoes, and sun dried tomatoes make excellent additions to most prepared dishes. Don't be afraid to cook tomatoes with added oil, because fat increases the absorption of the disease-fighting tomato pigments.

7. For children or adults who are always snacking, keep cherry tomatoes in the house continuously. They make a tasty, tart, and refreshing snack. Not only do they satisfy the appetite, but they also keep you healthy by helping curb the tendency to binge on junk foods.

Top Tomato Cures

1. If you have a cold, drink as much tomato juice as possible. Buy the juice in the can, since canning preserves the vitamin C from being oxidized by light. Drink 2 quarts per day until the cold is eradicated. For optimal effects add two tablespoons of extra virgin olive oil to each quart, since this aids in the absorption of the active ingredient.

2. If you are constipated, eat cherry tomatoes three times daily. Carefully clean about 20 cherry tomatoes, and eat the entire amount before or after breakfast, lunch, and dinner. Cherry tomatoes contain a greater amount of fiber than regular tomatoes, plus they contain a tonic which improves digestion and, therefore, bowel function.

3. If you are anemic, it isn't enough just to eat tomatoes. Tomatoes contain acids which draw iron from cast iron cookery. So, to gain the best anti-anemic punch cook tomatoes and tomato sauce in a cast iron pot or pan. The iron content of a single cup of tomato sauce jumps from 6 mg to 100 mg just by simmering it in the cast iron container. The tomato acids help deliver the iron into the blood where it is needed. Tomatoes are also rich in copper, which is also needed to build blood.

4. If your digestion is in disarray and you are constantly plagued with bloating, heartburn, and/or indigestion, cherry tomatoes may help. Eat a

handful of cherry tomatoes after each meal. Add them to salads. Snack on them between meals.

5. Fatigue may be quickly reversed by a large helping of fresh cherry tomatoes. Notice use of the term "fresh." Sun-ripened cherry tomatoes are supremely rich in vitamin C and bioflavonoids, which provide a tremendous boost to cellular energy.

6. If your skin is sensitive to sunlight or chemicals, try eating cherry tomatoes every day. Consume at least one pint per day. The rich content of vitamin C, bioflavonoids, and lycopene will decrease the sensitivity of the skin to sunlight and increase its ability to heal once it is damaged. Thus, the immune system of the skin will benefit greatly from the cherry tomato prescription. The prescription will also help block the development of wrinkles and age spots. Lycopene, which is found primarily in tomatoes, is more potent than vitamin E and beta carotene in fighting cell damage from toxicity. Whether that toxicity arises from sunlight, cigarette smoke, food additives, or toxic chemicals, lycopene helps fight the cellular danger. Currently, the best way to get it is by eating plenty of tomatoes (as well as watermelon).

Turnips

The turnip is one of the finest foods available to humankind. However, the problem seems to be that nobody knows what a turnip is, nor have the majority of people eaten turnips. I have purchased a lot of turnips, and it is interesting to observe the reaction of the check out clerk. Invariably, when the turnips are weighed, the question is "What is this" or "Are these turnips?" Obviously, the majority of Americans have never even seen turnips let alone eaten them. Perhaps they regard them as bland food or food for "poor folk." Or, perhaps they know what they are but think it is humorous to denigrate them. Yet, belittlement of turnips began long ago. The Romans used to pelt unpopular public figures with them. The French word for turnip means "flop." Ironically, the French make heavy use of the vegetable. They even make a sort of turnip sauerkraut and relish it highly. The dictionary lists alternative meanings for turnip as "a stupid person" or "blockhead."

Turnips were one of the most valued and commonly consumed of all vegetables during ancient times. They were first cultivated in the Near East some 4,000 years ago. The Greeks and Romans grew several varieties, many of which they developed. From Rome, turnips were taken to northern Europe, where they became exceptionally popular. There, peasants grew turnips as a staple. They were deemed as a sort of super-nutrition and were even used as a feed for cattle. As late as the 17th century they were consumed as the primary vegetable in Europe. The reason they are no longer a primary food is that they were displaced during the 18th century by potatoes and never regained their formerly lofty status. This is unfortunate, since turnips, while containing only one third the starch calories of potatoes, are richer in certain vitamins than their starchy adversary, notably vitamin C, folic acid, and zinc.

The turnip is a phenomenal disease fighter. Plus, it is inexpensive and rarely spoils.

Turnips are rich in vitamin C. In fact, by weight they are richer in vitamin C than tomatoes. One cup contains nearly 50 mg of vitamin C, which clearly places them in the same arena as a vitamin C source along with citrus fruit. They are an excellent source of folic acid, containing about 27 mcg per cup. If combined with an equal amount of turnip greens, the folic acid content of a large serving leaps to some 217 mcg. Obviously, the greens should be eaten with the turnips. They provide nutrients not found in significant amounts in the root, particularly vitamin A (as beta carotene), magnesium, vitamin E, thiamine, and riboflavin. The vitamin E content of turnip greens is considerable, and a mere 100 grams contains nearly 5 mg of naturally occurring vitamin E. That is an incredibly large amount for a vegetable. Fresh turnip greens contain massive amounts of vitamin A, vitamin K, vitamin C, and calcium plus a decent amount of iron. Their vitamin A content supercedes that of any other green vegetable, and, incredibly, when eaten fresh they may even overwhelm the more commonly touted vegetable vitamin A sources such as pumpkin, spinach, and sweet potatoes. A cup of raw turnip greens contains the beta carotene equivalent of 15,200 I.U. of vitamin A, nearly twice that found in spinach and over three times the amount found in pumpkin. Ideally, cook the greens immediately after purchase or use them in salads; they tend to spoil quickly.

Turnips contain unusually large amounts of selenium, and, if they are grown on selenium rich soil, they are one of the best sources of this mineral. Being a root, turnips and turnip greens are rich in a number of minerals, including potassium, iron, and phosphorus. A turnip a day is a sensible prescription for virtually anyone.

Top Turnip Tips

1. Don't overeat raw turnips. One or two raw turnips per day is plenty for good health. The reason moderation is prescribed is because turnips contain chemicals, known as goitrogens, which interfere with the function of the thyroid gland. Goitrogens block the metabolism of iodine, a nutrient required for thyroid function. If you eat raw turnips, always salt them with iodized salt or, preferably, sea salt. If you have a history of a severe thyroid problem, cook the turnips. Heat inactivates the goitrogens.
2. Add turnips to your daily cooking. They make an excellent addition to soups, stir fry, and casseroles. Use turnips in soups and casseroles as a less starchy and fattening replacement for potatoes.
3. Select medium-sized or small turnips. These younger turnips are usually sweeter tasting and more tender than the larger variety.
4. Before buying be sure the turnips are firm; softness is abnormal and a sign of spoiling. Avoid turnips which are shriveled.
5. Turnips make an excellent substitute for potatoes. They may be used in an equivalent manner. If a recipe calls for 6 potatoes, you may use 3 potatoes and 3 turnips. This provides a wider array of nutrients than just from the potatoes alone, plus the starch content of the meal will be reduced significantly.
6. Use turnips often on vegetable trays. They make an invaluable addition, because they provide potentially missing nutrients such as selenium and sulfur. Simply slice the turnips like large, thick potato chips and dip in cheese, bean, or salsa dips.

Top Turnip Cures

1. Respiratory infections, including sinusitis, bronchitis, and colds/flu, may be a warning sign of nutritional deficiencies, notably selenium, sulfur, vitamin C, and riboflavin. A deficiency of naturally occurring sulfur weakens immunity, making the individual vulnerable to allergic reactions and infection. Turnips are supremely rich in sulfur compounds. Sulfur compounds act as natural antiseptics. Furthermore, they exert direct effects upon the mucous membranes of the lungs and sinuses, enhancing their capacity to combat infections and allergic reactions. If you suffer

from allergies, sinus problems, lung disorders, or various infections, the regular consumption of sulfur rich foods, such as turnips, radishes, and mustard greens, might provide significant relief. Furthermore, turnips are rich in selenium, a mineral which enhances immunity and improves the anti-allergy response. Selenium deficiency leads to increased vulnerability to allergic sinusitis, and rhinitis as well as sinus/bronchial infections. In particular, a lack of selenium leaves the body open for attack by fungi. Selenium is also a cancer fighter. Recent research shows that the regular intake of selenium reduces the risk of cancer by as much as 50%. A daily ration of turnips, rich in selenium, is an ideal supermarket remedy for sinus or bronchial relief and infections of all types.

2. Turnips are one of Nature's most effective digestive aids and rarely cause allergic reactions or digestive upset. If you are plagued with indigestion or heartburn, eat one or two raw turnips and usually the symptoms will disappear. Consider eating turnips for breakfast—they are a tremendous digestive stimulant.

3. Turnips are a cancer fighter. They contain a variety of sulfur compounds and indoles, which not only strengthen the defenses against cancer but also help the immune system fight cancer once it strikes. If there is a family history of cancer, eat a turnip or two daily. While there is no guarantee, it is an inexpensive and tasty means of defense. With one of three individuals contracting cancer at some point during his/her lifetime, every effort must be made to enhance the natural defenses. This is a major reason to include turnips in the diet.

4. Turnips are an excellent tonic for the kidneys. If you have a history of sluggish kidneys or chronic kidney infections, eat at least 2 raw turnips every day. Turnip juice is an extremely valuable remedy for the kidneys and is a cure for kidney stones. Be sure to also juice the tops. To dissolve or prevent kidney stones, drink one cup of turnip/turnip top juice daily for one week. Thereafter, drink one or two cups per week.

5. Turnips are one of the best vegetables for strengthening the ailing heart. Whether heart disease, high blood pressure, enlarged heart, cardiac arrhythmia, or hardening of the arteries, all respond to the daily consumption of turnips. This is because turnips provide valuable heart nourishing minerals, notably selenium and sulfur. Both selenium and sulfur protect the heart from degeneration and also block the degeneration of the arterial walls.

6. If you suffer from irritable bowel syndrome, cook turnips with their tops and consume them regularly. This recipe is exceptionally rich in three nutrients—calcium, vitamin A, and sulfur—which are needed to heal the colon and settle the nerves. Turnips are high in vitamin C, and this is required for strengthening the mucous membranes of the colon wall.

7. Raw turnips are extremely low in starch and contribute very few calories. They are an ideal vegetable for dieting. Eat sliced turnips between meals for a tasty and nutritious weight loss snack. Sprinkle with salt, if desired.

8. Turnips help calm the nerves. This is because they are rich in calcium, and this mineral is a nervous system sedative. The type of calcium found in turnips is readily absorbed. Make a nerve calming soup using beef or chicken broth as a base along with large quantities of calcium rich vegetables: chopped turnips, turnip greens, carrots, parsley, and broccoli.

Vinegar

The seemingly lowly vinegar may indeed be the most perfect food. If Dr. Jarvis were still alive, the country doctor and author of *Folk Medicine*, he would agree wholeheartedly. It was Dr. Jarvis who first awoke America to the immense value of this medicinal food. However, vinegar has an ancient history. It has been utilized to preserve food since the beginning of human history. Hippocrates dispensed various types of vinegar for his patients. The Prophet Muhammad was also a fan of vinegar and first informed the world about its medicinal powers, touting it as a tonic for good health and long life. Jarvis confirmed the Prophet's findings when he observed that vinegar is Nature's most potent potassium supplement, since it concentrates the naturally occurring potassium, as well as other minerals, from vegetation. Other authors note that certain vinegars, such as red wine, apple cider, grape, and balsamic, are essentially bioflavonoid supplements, since these nutrients are also concentrated from the tonnage of vegetation used in making vinegar.

Jarvis, an M.D., was perhaps the first physician in modern times to dispense vinegar as a medicinal source of potassium. Located in Vermont, Dr. Jarvis became famous for his successful use of vinegar, as well as other potassium rich foods, for the treatment of disease. His interest in vinegar was provoked in part by the fact that in Vermont the soils are potassium-poor, and, therefore, potassium deficiency is common there, both in humans and animals. Researching this further he determined that the lower than normal height and weight of Vermont residents, as well as their dairy cattle, was directly related to potassium deficiency. In his book he notes how simply adding apple cider vinegar to the rations of dairy cattle lead to increased weight and height plus improved hair coat. Calves born to the vinegar-fed cows were stronger than usual and possessed great resistance to disease. In humans the results are similar. Unless the potassium deficiency is repaired, growth stagnates, there is failure to thrive, and the resistance to disease diminishes. The hair, skin, and nails are usually in poor health; the hair lacks luster and strength, the complexion is pale, and the fingernails are brittle or soft. Jarvis lists the warning signs of potassium deficiency as follows: hair loss, lack of hair luster, tooth decay, calluses on the feet/hands, slow growing fingernails, toenails, soft fingernails, and brittle fingernails. Other warning signs include persistent fatigue, depression, irritability, acne, constipation, muscle cramps, muscular twitching, edema, poor circulation, joint pain, irregular heartbeat, and thickened skin.

As he describes the functions of potassium Jarvis observes that the meat of cows fed potassium is exceptionally tender. From this fact he makes a brilliant presumption. Potassium, says Jarvis, functions to keep the tissues "soft and pliable," and, in this respect, it is a powerful substance for diminishing the aging process.

Because of its rich supplies of potassium, vinegar is a useful dispensation for a wide range of diseases, including heart disease, high blood pressure, chronic headaches, arthritis, obesity, chronic fatigue, asthma, depression, and diabetes. Yet, there is another major reason for prescribing vinegar: its antiseptic powers. Jarvis describes this in a curious way. He recommends visual proof: the earthworm. Place a worm on a hard surface and douse it with vinegar. After writhing in pain it dies instantly. For those lacking the interest in third grade research perhaps it is sufficient to accept this fact: vinegar's acidic components not only inhibit microbial growth but are also capable of killing microbes outright. This fact breeds a panorama of usages for vinegar: for fighting food poisoning, treating intestinal infections, resolving sore throats, curing lung infections, eradicating skin infections, obliterating the common cold and much more. Indeed, Jarvis utilized it successfully for all of these infections and held hundreds of cases of cures in his files to prove vinegar's efficacy.

Vinegar is produced from the fermentation of fruit or grain sugar. The sugar is fermented by yeasts to alcohol, and the alcohol is converted by bacteria to acetic acid. This acid is what gives the vinegar a sour taste and is responsible for its acidic pH. Alcohol is toxic, while acetic acid is entirely safe for human consumption. Acetic acid is the active ingredient of vinegar and largely accounts for it therapeutic powers.

In the past, that is previous to the 1970s, the term vinegar meant exclusively cider vinegar. This was mostly because for the majority of the 20th century, cider vinegar was the only type commonly available in America. Fortunately, supermarkets now contain a wide variety of vinegars, including apple cider, malt, rice, wine, grape, and balsamic vinegars. Darker colored vinegars may be more nutritious, as they contain a larger quantity of bioflavonoids. The dark color may also be due to residues of tannin, which arises from the lining of wooden casks in which the vinegar is produced. Tannin is valuable, since it is a natural antibiotic and antifungal agent.

Top Vinegar Tips

1. It is best to keep open bottles of vinegar refrigerated. This is to prevent the formation of "mother," which is the regrowing of the culture, i.e. mold. If vinegar has visible mold, heat it and this will sterilize it. If the mold is on the surface, it may be poured or scooped off.
2. Keep in mind that vinegar will often mold more readily if it contains added herbs and fruit. If you are mold sensitive, buy pure vinegar without added plant matter. However, the addition of garlic cloves, raw onion, oregano, tarragon, and thyme will help keep the vinegar sterile. These substances possess antiseptic powers and help prevent fungal growth.
3. There are a variety of excellent vinegars. My favorite is balsamic vinegar. This dark vinegar is exceptionally rich in various health enhancing natural chemicals, including bioflavonoids. The rich taste of balsamic vinegar gives evidence to its corresponding richness in

nutrients. It makes an excellent condiment for salads, soup, and stir fry, and it enlivens the taste of meat, especially when added during cooking.
4. Vinegar is a superb tenderizer. Add it to meat dishes, or marinate the meat overnight in a combination of vinegar and spices. Vinegar and the juice of a kiwi fruit will tenderize even the toughest cuts of meat.
5. Always drizzle salads with vinegar. It adds taste and improves digestion. It helps inactivate bacteria or parasites and, thus, helps prevent food poisoning, which may result from contaminated vegetables. Finally, if it is a high grade raw vinegar, it greatly adds to the nutritional value of the salad, providing dense amounts of potassium and bioflavonoids. The darker the color is of the vinegar the greater is its bioflavonoid content.
6. Vinegar is an excellent condiment for any fried food. Perhaps it is instinctive that the English love to eat vinegar with fish n' chips, since vinegar greatly aids in the digestion of heavy fats.

Top Vinegar Cures

1. When dining, always consume vinegar. Add it to salads, soups, or pour it over meat and fish dishes. Drink it straight or add it to water. Vinegar is a valuable remedy for preventing food poisoning, and dining is the most common mode of transmission. Eating restaurant food while traveling abroad notoriously leads to diarrheal diseases. For instance, imagine the disastrous scenario of being on a cruise ship during a food poisoning epidemic; the individual could become severely ill with no where to turn and no doctor to be found. It can and does happen every day. The wise individual will habitually consume vinegar with every restaurant meal. Vinegar may not be effective once the infection sets in, but it can help prevent it from occurring. If severe food poisoning strikes use oil of oregano as the front-line remedy (see the Oregano section).
2. Vinegar is an aid to immunity in the event of allergy, toxicity, or infection. It helps acidify the blood, which inhibits the growth of virtually all microbes. It exerts direct antibiotic powers, plus, it stimulates immune cells to kill invaders. If you have a weakened immune system, use vinegar regularly; consume at least one tablespoon daily.
3. For sore throat or tonsillitis, gargle and/or rinse with vinegar and salt. Add one tablespoon of vinegar and a half teaspoon of salt to 4 to 6 ounces

of water; gargle and rinse at least four times daily. The pain should be diminished within 24 hours.

4. Vinegar is an excellent cure for dandruff. Rinse the hair with two tablespoons of apple cider or rice vinegar; leave on hair for at least 12 hours. Repeat at least three times weekly until dandruff is resolved.

5. If you suffer from dry or itchy skin, try a vinegar bath. Simply add a cup of vinegar to a tub of hot water; soak in the tub for at least one hour. Repeat three times weekly until the skin condition improves.

6. Vinegar's rich potassium content makes it an ideal food for individuals with heart disorders, because more potassium in the diet means a healthier heart. If you have heart disease, consume at least two tablespoons of unprocessed vinegar on a daily basis. The vinegar prescription is especially important in the event of a low blood potassium level.

Watercress

This dark green leafy vegetable has been long considered to possess exceptional medicinal value. A cruciferous vegetable and member of the mustard family, it is a close relative of broccoli, cauliflower, kale, and cabbage. Its relationship botanically to mustard explains its tart flavor.

As indicated by its name, watercress is water loving. It grows naturally near the edges of streams and lakes. Most of the watercress available commercially is produced in hot or green houses.

Watercress is exceptionally dense in nutrients. Incredibly, one cup of packed watercress contains as much calcium as a cup of milk. This makes it one of the finest vegetable sources of calcium. It is also exceptionally rich in vitamin C and is an excellent source of beta carotene. As a rule dark greens are excellent sources of vitamin C and watercress is exceptionally rich. A good sized helping, such as a half of a bunch, easily provides the minimum daily requirement. The top sources in the dark greens are few, notably watercress, kale, mustard greens, and turnip greens. More commonly consumed vegetables, such as romaine lettuce, tomatoes, Brussels sprouts and cabbage, are listed as only "good" vitamin C sources. This means that watercress should be a staple on the menu, especially in the winter, when vitamin C consumption from fruit typically declines. In many respects, watercress should be regarded as a vitamin C supplement. Currently, its usage is minimal, in fact, the majority of Americans have never eaten it. This is unfortunate, since watercress is one of the most readily digested, nutritious, and therapeutically valuable foods known.

There is much need to utilize watercress in the diet. One major reason is that it is a life-saving and unique vitamin C source. Currently, nearly one half of the vitamin C supply in North America comes from citrus fruit and tomatoes. However, if watercress accrues the place in the diet it deserves, this ratio could change; a large bunch provides well over the minimum requirement. Keep in mind that watercress is far richer on a per weight basis in vitamin C than citrus fruits or tomatoes. Plus, it is more readily digested and rarely causes allergic intolerance, a dilemma which is relatively common with citrus fruits as well as tomatoes.

This tangy food is one of the most nutritionally complete of all vegetable foods. The fact is watercress is one of the few vegetables which could, by itself, promote sustenance. In one study performed on growing boys the addition of watercress alone to the diet stimulated growth and development almost as much as milk.

While watercress is nearly 90% water its density of nutrients remains high. The plant contains massive amounts of beta carotene. Watercress is a top source of calcium, vitamin C, potassium, and folic acid. It also contains a fair amount of vitamin E. Watercress is one of the few vegetables containing significant amounts of riboflavin. Incredibly, an equal weight of watercress contains a greater amount of riboflavin than an equal amount of sardines or oatmeal.

The immense nutritional value of watercress was first delineated in the 1920s by Dr. Mann, whose research described the positive effects of watercress consumption on children. Dr. Mann attempted to prove whether the addition of key foods to a typical nutritious diet would enhance the physical or mental strength of school children. He regarded milk and dark green leafy vegetables to be nutrient-dense; Dr. Mann described them as "protective foods." The gist of his research is as follows: the children were divided into several groups; a control group received the standard diet, another the diet plus a pint of milk or a ration of butter, another the diet plus a few teaspoons of sugar, yet another the diet plus a ration of watercress. The milk fed children exhibited superiority, both physically and mentally, but so did those fed watercress, which placed a close second. The point is that watercress was able to duplicate some of the same physiological benefits in growing children who were fed milk. This is a significant finding. Just think of the benefits children would derive if both fresh whole milk and watercress were regularly included in the diet.

Watercress juice is essentially a natural calcium supplement, offering large amounts of a type of calcium which is readily absorbed. According to the U.S. Department of Agriculture calcium accounts for .79 percent of the weight of watercress juice and that is a substantial density, considering that the vast majority of this plant consists of water. Depending upon where and how it is grown the calcium content may exceed 1%, making watercress juice a type of vegetable milk. For creating a more nutritionally complete vegetable milk add one half avocado to a cup of watercress juice; blend in blender, adding cold water until it develops the consistency of milk. Although lacking vitamin D and riboflavin, this mixture is perhaps the most easily digested and nourishing of all types of "imitation" milk. Indeed, watercress alone was used early in this century as a sort of milk substitute. As discussed in Sherman's *Essentials of Nutrition* researchers in the 1930s sought to determine if the vegetable could sustain growth. They found that when watercress was regularly added to the diet of children their growth and development was enhanced and they fared better both in physique and intellect than those failing to receive the vegetable.

Top Watercress Tips

1. Always wash watercress thoroughly. Don't just do a fast rinse. Really wash it under cold running water. This is because, depending upon where it is grown, it may carry parasites as well as bacteria. However, watercress which is grown in greenhouses will ordinarily be free of contamination. At any rate, thorough washing will remove any residues of microbes. Soaking watercress in a surfactant will help remove both chemicals and microbes. It has become sort of a fad to soak vegetables in oxidizing agents such as chlorine bleach and hydrogen peroxide. Don't soak vegetables or fruit in such compounds, as this will destroy the

nutritional value, plus they are toxic. Bleach and bleach fumes don't belong in the kitchen. If you are concerned regarding microbial contamination, consider using a natural antiseptic when soaking vegetables. Oil of oregano is safe for soaking vegetables. It destroys noxious microbes without harming the nutritional value of the food. Add merely one drop per quart of cold water. Oil of Oregano by North American Herb & Spice may be ordered by calling (800) 243-5242.

2. Watercress, especially if pureed, lends itself extremely well to soups. Use it in any soup recipe, especially creamed soups.

3. Watercress is a tangy vegetable. It adds zest to rather ordinary recipes such as casseroles, tossed salads, and stir fry. Chop fresh watercress and add it to soups, salads, and casseroles to create an invigorating taste. When cooking, add it at the end, and cook for just a moment.

4. Watercress juice is both tasty and nutritious. It is a superb source of calcium and a top source of vitamin C. Be sure to drink it immediately to maximize the nutritional potency. Vitamin C is readily lost from freshly juiced greens. Up to 50% may be lost in a matter of days. If more is produced than can be consumed, be sure to cover and refrigerate as soon as possible. Store in a container which blocks light, for instance, a milk carton or dark colored bottle.

5. Use watercress as a garnish for meat dishes, but be liberal with the portion. In Europe watercress is commonly served with meat, especially wild game. Europeans seem to know instinctively that watercress aids in the digestion of meat. The reason is that it is rich in enzymes and sulfur compounds. Furthermore, it acts as a tonic for the stomach, increasing the flow of stomach acid as well as other digestive juices.

6. Rather than using it as an occasional garnish and salad ingredient, use watercress as a staple food. Eat large helpings of it on salads, and add it liberally to soup and stir fry. Prepare salads with watercress as the base and top with tomatoes, onions, carrots, etc. Make watercress a part of the weekly or, preferably, daily menu.

Top Watercress Cures

1. In the case of failure to thrive in children or inappropriate weight loss adding watercress in the diet is a must. It should be consumed daily in

large amounts, as much as a bunch or two per day. A ration of watercress juice should also be consumed. One cup of watercress juice per day usually suffices, although in extreme cases of failure to thrive or emaciation as much as three cups may be necessary. The juice should be consumed daily until noticeable gains are made in weight, appetite, and physical prowess. Once the condition is resolved, the juice may be drunk once or twice per week for maintenance. If milk is tolerated, this should also be consumed, as it contains nutrients that the watercress juice cannot provide, and the two work in unison. For cow's milk intolerance try acidophilus milk or buttermilk. Or, use goat's milk, which is the most readily digested type of milk (short of human milk).

Watercress is invaluable as a source of body building nourishment, because the nutrients within it are readily digested and absorbed. Watercress provides invaluable stores of calcium and magnesium, which are required for rebuilding muscle mass. It is a tonic for digestion and, thus, it aids in the digestion of other foods. Ideally, it is necessary to achieve the highest dosage of nutrients possible, and this means the watercress must be juiced. Drink at least one cup of juice daily with meals. Additionally, use watercress as often as possible in menus.

2. If you suffer from leg cramps, drink watercress juice. Juice and drink two bunches of watercress every day until the cramps cease. Watercress is a dense source of calcium and magnesium, both of which are needed for calming the nerves that control the muscles. Leg or foot cramps are usually eliminated when the calcium and magnesium levels in the muscle and nerve cells are normalized. Other nutritional causes of leg cramps include deficiencies of folic acid, vitamin D, vitamin E, and pantothenic acid.

3. Watercress is the ideal vegetable for enhancing the health of the skin. It is rich in sulfur, which aids in the growth of healthy skin cells and prevents aging of the skin. Watercress is also high in vitamin C and beta carotene, both of which are needed to prevent aging of the skin as well as skin infections. If you have a history of a skin disorder, such as acne, eczema, psoriasis, dermatitis, or wrinkling, watercress should be a common addition to the menu.

4. Watercress combats fatigue. It contains natural chemicals which boost both physical and mental energy. It performs this function by accelerating the metabolic rate. Watercress is rich in B vitamins and magnesium, which augment energy and enhance metabolism.

5. Watercress helps fight depression. This may be partly due to its rich mineral content; magnesium, calcium, and potassium, are all found in it in dense amounts, and all of these minerals soothe the nerves. Eat a watercress salad every day and regularly add it to soups if you suffer from depression, anxiety, mood swings, panic attacks, apathy, or irritability.

6. Watercress is an ideal food for fighting and, particularly, for preventing hair loss. If there is a history in the family of balding, eat watercress on a daily basis. If you have a juicer, drink one cup of watercress juice at least twice weekly. Watercress is rich in sulfur, which is needed for the growth and maintenance of hair.

7. Fighting or preventing cancer is on the minds of most Americans and for good reason. Currently, approximately one in three Americans will develop cancer at some point during their life-times. Watercress is an ideal food to incorporate in the cancer prevention plan. It contains sulfated compounds which aggressively block the development of cancer. In the event of cancer, drink two cups of watercress juice daily. However, don't do this forever. Watercress contains substances which may interfere with thyroid gland function, and constant consumption could induce a mild hypothyroid state. As always, use moderation as a rule. However, mild hypothyroidism is a minor concern compared to cancer. In other words, if you do have cancer, eat the watercress, and drink the juice as often as possible.

8. If you suffer from depression, eat watercress often. Herbalists use it for combating depression and anxiety; its positive effects are likely due to its rich content of calcium and magnesium, which are nerve sedatives.

Watermelon

Watermelon is an invaluable source of nutrition world wide. In some cultures watermelon is essentially a staple. To some degree the melon serves this purpose in certain Southern states, where it becomes the primary summer fruit. Interestingly, while everyone regards watermelon as a fruit there may be some doubt about this. It was surprising to read that Otto Carque, in his book *Rational Diet*, published in 1926, lists melons within his chapter on vegetables. This makes sense, since melons grow from vines, and vines yield vegetables, while trees (and shrubs) yield fruits. Although Carque never specified melons as vegetables, yet, upon giving it thought, I realized he was correct in principle. Melons belong to the gourd family and are the "vegetable" of ground-hugging vines. Therefore, they are indeed technically vegetables, although the closest description found in current nutritional textbooks is that they are "the fruit of a vine." However, Ensminger acknowledges that watermelons, rather than being related to fruit, are a relative of "pumpkin, squash,...and cucumber", all of which are vegetables.

The ancient Egyptians were the first people known to cultivate watermelons, although this melon almost assuredly originated in tropical Africa, where to this day they may be found growing wild. From Egypt, melons were disseminated to the Middle East, where they have been a staple food for untold centuries. In fact, they are a reliably nourishing element of the dessert diet, and dozens of varieties of melons are found growing in Egypt, Ethiopia, Palestine, Syria, Persia, Turkey, Jordan and the Arabian peninsula.

Watermelon contains unique compounds, yet to be identified, which dramatically increase urine flow. These substances help normalize blood pressure. Watermelon also contains a type of coolant, which is useful for combating heat exhaustion. Second only to tomato, watermelon is a top source of lycopene, a substance which has been determined to prevent cancer. Lycopene is the pigment responsible for watermelon's reddish color. The color is especially vivid in sun ripened organic watermelons, and this is a sign of exceptionally rich lycopene content.

Watermelon is a good source of vitamin C, beta carotene, folic acid, and biotin. For minerals it is highest in potassium and magnesium.

Watermelon is approximately 93% water. The water content is invaluable, and watermelon provides a highly active form of this fluid, which is efficiently utilized by the body. It is rich in the electrolyte, potassium, which aids in the transport of water from the intestines into the blood. Sodium, the other electrolyte, is also needed for water transport but is available only in a minute amount. By salting watermelon it not only seems to taste sweeter, but it also provides a better balance of electrolytes.

Watermelon is a superior cure for dehydration, even more so than plain water. It is most effective for rehydration when salted. As a thirst quencher it is infinitely better than juice or sports drinks.

Top Watermelon Tips

1. Buying a watermelon is a futile endeavor unless you know how to select a ripe one. There is nothing worse than buying an unripe melon. Here are some simple rules that will allow you to enjoy the best tasting watermelon in the bunch:

a) the key technique is to *sound* the melon. Hit it with the middle knuckle, much like a doctor thumping an abdomen. If the melon resounds with a dull noise, like a thud, it is ripe. If it is resonate or sharp, it is too green. The thud sounds like hitting the leather heel of an old shoe.

b) Ripe melons reveal themselves partly by their bottoms. If the underside is yellow or creamy colored, it is probably ripe. If it is green or greenish-white, it is probably unripe.

c) Look also at the end where the vine met the melon. If the vine remnant is shriveled, brown, and crusty, it is probably ripe. If it is green and thick, it may well be unripe.

2. Eat the watermelon seeds, shell and all. It is guaranteed that a watermelon won't grow in your abdomen. Watermelon seeds are rich in a variety of nutrients, particularly amino acids and fatty acids plus vitamin E, potassium, and phosphorus. They provide immense fuel value for the creation of cellular energy, as they are rich in digestible fatty acids. Furthermore, watermelon seeds contain a substance which helps eradicate intestinal parasites. To optimize absorption of the curative substances it is essential that they be thoroughly chewed, because the coarse outer seed cannot be digested and the nutrients will be wasted.

3. Use watermelon primarily as a summer food. It is one of the most alkaline types of food and is a poor winter food. During winter months the natural production of acid in the stomach often decreases, and this may cause an imbalance in acid-base chemistry. Since the body often becomes more alkaline in pH during the winter, it is wise to eat acid forming foods and avoid alkaline forming foods. Acid forming foods include meat, eggs, cheese, milk, yogurt, fish, almonds, pistachios, pecans and peanuts. Alkaline forming foods include melons, citrus fruits, grains, beans, and vegetables. Perhaps this is partly why individuals living in the upper regions of the Northern hemisphere have traditionally relied upon such foods as beef, wild game, fish, milk, cheese, and eggs as primary foodstuffs for the winter, eating vegetables and fruit only sparingly. While

vitamin C deficiency needs to be corrected (and this can be accomplished by taking herbal teas, especially Wild Power Tea), the acid food diet is a more nutrient dense and cold protective one than is a diet of fruits, vegetables, and grains. Furthermore, acid foods help keep the body pH within the normal range, and even mild fluctuations in pH lead to ill health. The point is use watermelon primarily as a hot weather food.

4. Watermelon makes an ideal breakfast food and is readily digested and highly refreshing. Eat it with high protein food such as steak, ground beef/turkey patty, or eggs. The protein provides an acidic reaction, which helps offset the alkaline reaction of the watermelon. So have a wedge of watermelon with your eggs in the morning. The two work as a team, and together they create a tremendously nutritious and energizing breakfast.

5. Carefully inspect the watermelon before buying to ensure there are no bruises. Often, the bruising occurs on the ends. Bruising rapidly leads to spoiling of the fruit. Remember, watermelons are transported to supermarkets by the truck load and are often handled roughly. A bruised melon means a bad tasting or rotten melon.

6. Don't accept a bad melon unconditionally. If you find it is sour or unripe, take it back and select a different one or get a refund. Most supermarkets are happy to assist customers in returns. Grocers should supply top grade food and they are liable for inferior produce. If you have difficulty making a selection, ask for help. There is usually someone available who can choose a good ripe melon and plug it or cut it open for your satisfaction. Always wash the outside before cutting.

Top Watermelon Cures

1. Watermelon is a natural diuretic. Obviously, anyone who has eaten large amounts of it knows how well it works. It is the ideal food for combating water retention regardless of the cause. If you tend to retain water, the consumption of watermelon will usually help.

2. Watermelon is an ideal food for the sick and infirm. It is readily digested and provides simple sugars, which are valuable for providing fuel. It is an excellent source of potassium, which is available in a form that is readily absorbed. It is an ideal food in the event of poor appetite resulting from sickness, drug therapy, cold, flu, or cancer.

3. Watermelon seeds kill parasites, especially worms. Be sure to eat the seeds whenever possible, and it is important to chew them thoroughly, because the outer shell is indigestible. It is the inner white meat which exhibits the anti-parasitic action.

4. If you are sensitive to heat and/or if you have a history of heat exhaustion or heat stroke, it is life-saving to eat watermelon. It is the top anti-heat food and acts to dramatically increase heat tolerance. No wonder it is so commonly eaten in the deep South as a refreshing summer food. Southerners seem to know instinctively that by eating watermelon they are able to better handle the sweltering summer heat and humidity. The fact is watermelon is the best possible food to eat in the event of heat-induced illnesses. Individuals who develop any type of sickness from the heat, even heat exhaustion, should eat large amounts of watermelon and salt it liberally. It is far superior as a heat defeating cure than any sports drink, in fact, the synthetic sugar found in sodas and sports drinks only exacerbate the problem.

Watermelon provides much needed potassium and vitamin C, which is readily lost in the sweat as a result of heat exposure. Since sodium and chloride are lost in vast amounts during sweating, the watermelon should be salted freely; preferably, use sea salt. If you cannot handle hot humid weather, eat watermelon every day and be sure to salt it. Your tolerance for defeating the heat will improve dramatically.

5. If there is a history of heart disease or heart rhythm disturbances, such as atrial fibrillation, tachycardia, and palpitations, watermelon may be an important dietary addition. It is rich in naturally occurring potassium, containing considerably more of this critical mineral than traditional sources such as bananas and orange juice. Plus, the type of potassium it contains is quickly absorbed into the bloodstream. Furthermore, watermelon's natural diuretics help decrease the pressure on the heart by stimulating the kidneys to remove excess water from the tissues. This at least partially explains why primitive societies in which watermelon is a regular part of the diet rarely suffer from heart disease.

6. Mitral valve prolapse may also be caused by a buildup of fluid in the body, plus it is associated with a deficiency of minerals such as potassium and magnesium. If you have this condition, eat watermelon on a regular basis, since this melon supplies naturally occurring potassium and natural diuretics, both of which help take the pressure off the heart valves.

7. Watermelon is an excellent digestive aid. If you suffer from indigestion eat a wedge of watermelon with meals. The high content of water and potassium stimulate digestive juices and ease elimination. Thus, watermelon may be helpful for alleviating constipation.

8. If you are trying to lose weight, watermelon is a perfect food. It is very filling, full of fiber, and rich in nutrients. Best of all, despite its sweet taste there are only 7 calories per ounce.

Wild Rice

Wild rice is a hidden nutritional treasure on the supermarket shelves. Unfortunately, only a small percentage of Americans have ever purchased it. True, a few grains of wild rice are found in certain commercial rice products or in rice pilaf served at restaurants, but there is not enough in such products to make a nutritional difference. The fact is the majority of Americans have never eaten pure wild rice as a separate serving. However, this was not always the case. Native Americans thrived on a diet rich in wild rice. For certain tribes it was the staple food, providing much needed protein, complex carbohydrates, vitamins, and minerals. Plentiful in the Northern and Eastern United States, wild rice became a primary food for settlers, who relied upon its fuel calories to carry them through the long winters. The Natives rarely used it as a separate dish, as we do with commercial rice, but, instead, cooked it with meat and vegetables. Apparently, the settlers made a wilderness soup from a combination of wild rice and wild blueberries, which certainly must have been a nutrient packed and tasty dish.

Wild rice is botanically neither rice nor grain. It is a seed of a water-grass known as *Zizania aquatic*. It is one of the few foods in the supermarket which may be regarded as a sort of wild, organic food.

Virtually all Americans could use a greater amount of fiber in the diet. Wild rice offers a type of fiber known as soluble fiber. This type of fiber is more gentle upon the digestive tract than any other type and is certainly superior in this regard to grain fiber. Plus, soluble fiber is the most effective type for helping normalize cholesterol and triglyceride levels. Recently, researchers have documented how soluble fiber serves as a type of fuel for bacteria living in the colon. Thus, a steady consumption of wild rice could help stimulate the growth of beneficial bacteria. Wild rice is an excellent source of soluble fiber.

Wild rice is one of the most digestible of all foods. Allergic reactions to it are exceedingly rare, and this may be one of the reasons it is so well tolerated by individuals with food sensitivities. .

Wild rice is a richer source of certain nutrients, notably niacin, phosphorus, and iron, than commercial brown rice. Plus, it is usually chemical-free, while commercial brown rice is commonly contaminated with pesticide residues. The fact is it contains more than twice the niacin content of brown rice, offering a whopping 7 mg per cup of cooked rice. It is several times richer in riboflavin than brown rice and is one of the few starchy foods high in this nutrient. It also is rich in an excellent type of highly digestible starch and is a far superior source of starch compared to commercial whole grains such as barley, wheat, corn, and rye. As a general rule if you had to select a starch for the menu, wild rice would be the number one choice. The protein content of wild rice is considerable, with one cup of cooked rice containing over six grams.

Top Wild Rice Tips

1. Get accustomed to eating wild rice "straight"; don't always mix it with other types of rice. It is important to achieve the richest nutritional density possible. Unfortunately, many grocers demand top dollar for a small box of wild rice, and, often, it is commercially raised and not wild at all.

2. Make heavy use of wild rice as a new found starch. Use it instead of potatoes, bread, or beans. It is one of the most nutritious and tasty of all types of starches. It supercedes virtually all other starchy foods in fiber and mineral content. If you are a "starchoholic," try displacing breads, pasta, and potatoes with a serving of wild rice. Your palate may well find it irresistible, and, while potatoes need not become a thing of the past, at least there will be greater nutritional variety in the menu by making wild rice a staple.

3. Use pure wild rice instead of white rice and even brown rice. It is more readily digested than any type of commercial rice, plus it is less likely to be contaminated with chemicals. Furthermore, wild rice is richer in protein and minerals than commercial or organic rice. Wild rice is meant to be eaten as a whole food, not as a garnish.

4. Add wild rice to all bakery recipes, including pancakes, waffles, bread, buns, and cookies. It lends itself well to bakery, providing much needed fiber, B vitamins, and minerals. Wild rice flour can be prepared by grinding the rice seeds, and this may be used to fortify any flour.

5. Wild rice tastes excellent with spices. Cook it with garlic and onion powder or add freshly chopped garlic and onions. Try it with a sprinkling of curry powder or add a bit of cayenne. Accentuate wild rice by cooking it with a dehydrated vegetable mix, or add freshly chopped vegetables such as carrots, red sweet peppers, zucchini, and celery. Cook it in a base of beef or chicken broth. Dust it with chopped parsley. Wild rice is one of the easiest of all foods to manipulate, and it lends itself to virtually any herb, spice, or vegetable.

Top Wild Rice Cures

1. For reversing digestive disturbances, including heartburn, spastic colon, and constipation, eat wild rice on a daily basis. The fiber in wild rice gently increases the bulk of the stool. Be sure to drink plenty of fluids, or the extra fiber can't help.

2. If your immune system is feeble, eat wild rice on a daily basis. Consume it as a starch portion instead of regular rice, brown rice, pasta or potatoes. It is richer in nutrients than any of these starches, plus it contains fibers which enhance the growth of the bowel's healthy bacteria.

3. If you are sick and cannot hold down food or if you have a poor appetite, try eating wild rice broth. In essence, this is a starch soup made from wild rice. Simply boil a cup of salted wild rice until it becomes completely soft. Drink the broth and retain the rice. Pour a few cups of water over the retained rice and re-cook. Continue this process until the sickness or diarrhea is cured. Wild rice broth is the ideal nutriment and electrolyte cure for diarrhea and far supercedes commercially available remedies such as Gatorade or Pedialyte.

4. If you have constant heartburn or indigestion, eat wild rice at least twice daily. Have it as a side dish for lunch, and cook it as a main dish for supper. Wild rice contains starch and fiber, which absorbs excess acid. Plus, the rich supply of vitamins and minerals improves digestion, and this leads to a decrease in heartburn, indigestion, and gas.

5. If you have a child who cannot or will not eat decent food, try feeding

him/her wild rice on a daily basis. This can be accomplished by adding the wild rice into the child's favorite soup or casserole. Get your children to eat wild rice instead of other less healthy starches such as bread, instant potatoes, and pasta. The benefits will be immense: within one month the child's appetite will be vigorous and the health will improve dramatically. 6. If you suffer from irritable bowel syndrome, constipation, diverticulitis, or Crohn's disease, you need a greater amount of fiber in your diet. Wild rice provides vast amounts of a type of bulk known as soluble fiber. This type of fiber is gentle on the digestive tract, plus it may be digested readily. In other words, the nutrients in the fiber are utilized, which is not the case with insoluble types of fiber such as wheat bran. It is important to note that doctors frequently recommend against eating fiber for patients with diverticulitis. Yet, this disease is directly due to a lack of fiber. Diverticulitis is a disease in which the colon develops weak pockets within its walls. The weakened pockets arise as a result of straining on the stool, which is caused by a lack of fiber and an excess of refined foods such as sugar, white rice, and white flour. While certain types of fiber should be avoided by diverticulitis patients, particularly coarse wheat, rye, or corn bran, soft and soluble types of fiber, such as the type in wild rice, should be consumed. Other types of soluble fiber include oat bran and brown rice bran.

Yogurt

Virtually everyone knows that yogurt is a curative food. In some societies it is regarded as more of a medicine than a food. For instance, in Bulgaria yogurt is well known for its ability to fight diarrhea and yeast infections. Yet, there is a negative side to it: food allergy. A significant percentage of Americans are allergic to milk products, and yogurt is no exception. If an individual is allergic to cow's milk, goat or sheep yogurt may be well tolerated as an alternative.

Researchers have documented how yogurt improves digestion, fights infection, improves bone density, prevents degenerative disease, and, perhaps, extends life. These actions are readily understood as a result of its nutrient profile. Yogurt is a nutritional powerhouse, packing rich amounts of amino acids, minerals, and B vitamins, particularly folic acid, pantothenic acid, pyridoxine, and riboflavin. It's fat soluble vitamins include vitamin A, vitamin D, and vitamin K. Yogurt contains a high density of calcium, and the type of calcium in it is readily absorbed. It is one of the best sources of enzymes, and the reason it is so high in them is because of the fermentation process through which it is made. When bacteria ferment the milk into yogurt they produce massive amounts of enzymes. The enzymes remain active as long as the yogurt is not heated excessively. Yet, there is perhaps another reason for yogurt's health giving properties: its digestibility—it is the most easily digested of all solid foods. Certainly, this fact is related to its rich content of enzymes. It is also related to the fact that yogurt is a predigested food—the bacteria act upon the milk, breaking it down into simpler molecules, which are readily absorbed. This is important, because digestion is a strenuous process consuming large amounts of energy. In contrast to other solid foods, yogurt places few demands upon the energy stores of the body and, in fact, provides enzymes which enhance digestion of other foods. Yogurt provides energy and vigor in a degree matched by few other foods.

Yogurt is perhaps best known as a source of bacteria—the useful, valuable bacteria known as Lactobacillus. It may contain several species of Lactobacilli, notably bifidus, bulgaricus, thermopholus, and acidophilus. These bacteria are essential for human existence and are indigenous inhabitants of a healthy intestinal tract. Normally, they are found by the billions in the body, the vast majority being located in the lower bowel. Yogurt is the top dietary source of these bacteria, and a cup of it, if made from healthy culture, contains uncountable millions of these microbes.

The microbes found in yogurt are of immense value to our bodies. The energy we derive from our food is largely produced as a result of the workings of the beneficial bacterial regiments. The bacteria act as microscopic factories, producing vitamins, amino acids, and enzymes, which the cells of our bodies utilize. Their numbers in the body are mind-boggling; there are a greater number of microbes in a single individual's intestines than there are humans on this earth. As can be readily imagined, it is critical to have the correct type of bacteria—too many of the wrong type could quickly poison you. This is because the obnoxious bacteria produce a wide range of poisonous compounds and fail to synthesize the

277

valuable ones. The result of their overgrowth is fatigue, mental disturbances, weakened immunity, and, ultimately, outright disease.

Hundreds of scientific studies document that yogurt produces a wide range of beneficial effects, including augmentation of immunity, prevention of cancerous changes, acceleration of cellular energy, enhanced digestion, increased enzyme activity, and reduction of cholesterol levels. This plethora of effects is certainly related to the nutritional content of yogurt but is also a consequence of the Lactobacillus content. Researchers have discovered that the organism itself, even without the yogurt, produces many if not all of these effects.

As described by Kathleen Hunter in *Health Foods and Herbs*, yogurt has been used to successfully reverse the toxic effects upon the gut that typically occur as a result of antibiotic therapy. Certainly, this is due to its content of helpful acidophilus bacteria, which are destroyed by antibiotics. Yet, it is also likely the result of yogurt's ability to repair damage to the intestinal walls. Hunter also notes that yogurt has been used extensively world wide as a remedy for stomach ulcers. As reported by numerous researchers the regular consumption of yogurt appears to prevent the formation of stomach and duodenal ulcers. The fact is such ulcers are rare in civilizations wherein yogurt is a staple food. Recently, it has been discovered that stomach and duodenal ulcers are caused largely by infection. The culprit is a curly shaped bacteria known as *Helicobacter pylori*. When the immunity is weakened this bacteria may readily attach to the inner linings of the stomach, causing tissue damage and, ultimately, ulcers. The fact that infection causes ulcers certainly lends credence to the yogurt cure, since the natural acidophilus bacteria are the body's defense against pathogens such as Helicobacter.

One of the most fascinating effects of yogurt's "good" microbes is their ability to produce antibiotics. Undoubtedly, these antibiotics are more gentle on the body than the prescription type. Furthermore, in contrast to prescription antibiotics, the naturally produced antibiotics are highly effective in improving the health of the body. The primary function of these Lactobacilli-produced antibiotics is to inhibit the growth of noxious microbes and in some cases kill the bad organisms outright. According to Russian researchers publishing in *Mikrobiologiya* the Lactobacillus-produced antibiotics are capable of inhibiting the growth of difficult to kill microbes such as Salmonella, E. coli, and

278

Shigella. Furthermore, the acidophilus antibiotics are particularly valuable for inhibiting the growth of yeasts and other fungi. Other researchers have determined that healthy bacteria aid in the production of hydrogen peroxide, as well as peroxidase enzymes, both of which outright destroy toxic microbes. Even viruses are not immune to the antiseptic powers of the healthy bacteria. Dr. Mayer, publishing in the *Journal of Physical Medicine and Rehabilitation*, noted that the tough to disable Herpes virus was controlled, if not destroyed, by bifidobacteria, a microbe found in fermented milk.

There has been a great deal of negative press regarding milk products. There is nothing inherently wrong with them, although some individuals may be allergic to milk products. In the latter case it would be appropriate to avoid them. However, if no allergy exists they represent one of the most nutrient dense of all foods. Milk products are the richest food source of calcium, and they are a top source of protein and fat soluble vitamins. Indeed, few other foods contain this combination of dense supplies of calcium, fat soluble vitamins, and protein. However, there is one major problem with milk besides allergy, and that is what is added to the milk. It is a travesty that various synthetic substances are either fed to cows or injected within them, as such chemicals eventually are deposited within the meat and milk. Chemical residues which may be found in milk include various drugs and agricultural chemicals, particularly antibiotics, pesticides, fungicides, herbicides, and hormones. After the DES debacle of the 1970s public concern over the cancer causing effects of hormones led to a reduction in the use of synthetic hormones in cattle. However, the restraints have again been removed: enter bovine growth hormone (BGH). Produced by Monsanto Corporation, a chemical company, bovine growth hormone is used strictly for the purpose of inducing cows to make more milk. Residues of the chemical are found in the milk of treated cows. It is important to realize that Bovine Growth Hormone has never been proven to be safe for human consumption. Despite this fact it has been legalized for use in milk cows since 1993.

Some dairies have opted against using BGH. Support these dairies by buying their milk products. The way to determine if the dairy uses BGH is to request this information in writing.

Top Yogurt Tips

1. Never buy low fat yogurt. Buy instead the full fat variety. In order to make low fat yogurt the milk must be heavily processed. As always, it is important to consume food as close to its natural state as possible. Milk naturally contains fat. That fat is a valuable fuel, plus it is loaded with nutrients, particularly fat soluble vitamins such as vitamins A and D. Plus, the whole fat variety tastes better. Why deny yourself a good thing?

2. Avoid sweetened yogurt, and buy the plain variety instead. Make your own fruit mixes. Put the yogurt in a blender with fresh fruit and a bit of honey, if desired. Blend it fresh, without the sugar or NutraSweet. It is important to note that refined sugar destroys the health benefits of yogurt for several reasons. Sugar interferes with calcium absorption and metabolism, and one of the main reasons to eat yogurt is because it is rich in calcium. Sugar also disrupts the balance of bacteria in the intestines, encouraging the growth of yeasts and harmful bacteria. In contrast, raw honey kills noxious bacteria, while enhancing the growth of the beneficial ones.

3. Eat yogurt as a high protein snack. Buy plain whole fat yogurt, and keep it in the refrigerator at home and work for a convenient and refreshing snack. It will halt hunger spells that normally drive the individual to eat junk food. If you don't have a refrigerator, yogurt will keep for awhile, but don't chance it any longer than 12 hours.

4. Prepare your own yogurt whenever possible. Make it from fresh whole milk. Whole goat's milk makes a luscious yogurt, which is readily digested and exceptionally nutritious.

5. Use yogurt in sauces and as a base for meat recipes. It makes an excellent addition to casseroles. Yogurt packs a phenomenal taste when heated in food and imparts a sour taste that rivals lemon and lime. This is especially useful for individuals who are allergic to citrus fruits.

6. Don't just add fruit to yogurt. Make yogurt based salads. Add various herbs and vegetables. Yogurt lends itself wonderfully to cucumbers, turnips, parsley, and cilantro. Spices also blend well in yogurt, and the fats in yogurt help liberate the volatile oils in the spices.

7. Pour yogurt over brown or wild rice. It imparts a luscious flavor and makes the meal more nutritionally complete. Rice is mostly starch and yogurt is mostly protein and fat. Both rice and yogurt provide a plethora of B vitamins.

8. Avoid eating frozen yogurt; it has little or no active cultures. According to Jean Carper in *Food-Your Miracle Medicine* researchers testing various brands of frozen yogurt found all to be devoid of active enzymes, the latter being a marker of the nutritional quality of yogurt.

9. The curative powers of yogurt are dependent upon the quality of the milk from which it is made. Ideally, the milk should be free of all contaminants. The presence of synthetic chemicals, such as bovine growth hormone, pesticides, herbicides, and antibiotics, certainly detracts from the health benefits native within milk. For making yogurt the milk should be fresh, and whole milk should be used instead of reduced fat or skim milk.

10. Cook with yogurt. It may be used as a replacement in any recipe calling for cream or milk. Add yogurt to rice, vegetable, or meat dishes. Add the yogurt at the very end of the cooking process as a sort of topping. Use yogurt on baked potatoes instead of sour cream.

Goat's milk is the finest type of milk to use for making yogurt. Goats tend to be more free of disease than cattle, plus the milk is the most digestible type available short of human milk.

11. One reason yogurt is a useful source of calcium is because it is acidic. Calcium is readily absorbed only in an acid environment. To increase acidity try adding lemon, lime, sour grape or vinegar to the yogurt. They provide a lively taste and the acids accelerate calcium absorption.

Top Yogurt Cures

1. Yogurt is a beauty aid, both inside and outside of the body. For a skin tonic apply a paste of yogurt on the face and let it sit for at least two hours, then rinse. Do this every day for a week to improve complexion and reverse blemishes.

2. Yogurt is an ideal food for individuals suffering from impaired digestion, colon disorders, or stomach diseases. It is a highly effective digestive tonic, and enhances the natural appetite. For weight loss and/or malabsorption, eat one quart of yogurt daily (or every other day) for two or three months. The weight should gradually normalize and the malabsorption should be cured. After this, eat a cup or two of yogurt three times per week If you are allergic to cow's milk, try this therapy with

goat's milk yogurt. However, be aware that some individuals cannot tolerate any type of milk product. In this instance, mix the yogurt with raw honey; this may dramatically improve the tolerance and cause the yogurt to be assimilated without ill effect. Individuals suffering from gastritis, colitis, diverticulitis, ulcers, and malabsorption should incorporate yogurt regularly into the diet.

3. If you have a chronic tendency for loose stools, yogurt is an inexpensive, simple, and effective remedy. Tests performed at the University of Minnesota document how yogurt helps destroy the noxious microbes that cause diarrhea. Other researchers have determined that the regular consumption of yogurt tremendously reduces the risk for contracting diarrhea. This is no modern discovery. Eli Metnikoff, the modern discoverer of the health benefits of yogurt, performed the ultimate scientific trial on yogurt. After drinking yogurt for several weeks, he drank a dose of cholera organisms. Horrifying as it appears, Metnikoff never got the disease and suffered not so much as one bout of diarrhea. He attributed this protective effect entirely to the yogurt, which he drank by the quart. For optimal anti-diarrheal action mix honey with the yogurt, about 3 tablespoons for every cup.

4. If you must take antibiotics, be sure to eat plenty of yogurt during the course of treatment. Yogurt supplies the healthy acidophilus bacteria, which are rapidly destroyed by antibiotics. Eat a minimum of two cups of yogurt every day during treatment and a cup per day for at least one week after treatment is ceased.

5. Yogurt boosts immunity, so it is an ideal food for those suffering from any immune defect. The problem is that many individuals with immune defects also suffer from food allergies, and allergies to milk products are often top on the list. However, for those who are free of sensitivity yogurt effectively increases immunoglobulin formation, white blood cell killing power, and interferon synthesis. In particular, it accelerates the synthesis of an antibody known as *secretory IgA*, which protects the gut from toxic reactions and infection. Of note is the fact that eating yogurt may boost interferon levels by as much as 500%. However, if you are allergic to it, eating it could aggravate the immune deficiency.

One way to combat milk allergy is to consume antiseptic herbs. In particular, wild oregano is exceptionally valuable as an anti-allergy tonic. For instance, my ability to tolerate milk products, to which I am allergic, improved dramatically after the regular intake of oil of oregano as well as wild oregano herb (as in Oregamax). The fact is I developed a severe deficiency of riboflavin as a result of following a strict milk-free diet for many years (milk products are the main source of riboflavin in human nutrition). Now I can eat nutritionally valuable milk products, such as whole milk, yogurt, and cheese, without ill effects, thanks to the wild oregano.

6. Yogurt can be an anti-cancer aid. Researchers at Kraft General Foods found that when commercial yogurt was fed to mice, it dramatically reduced cancer rates. In other words, mice fed yogurt were more likely to defeat cancer, while those not fed yogurt were more likely to die. Apparently, yogurt accelerated the cancer killing powers of the mices' white blood cells. Fresh homemade yogurt from an active culture would be the best yogurt for fighting or preventing cancer. The fresher the yogurt is the richer it will be in cancer-fighting enzymes.

7. If you suffer from low blood calcium and/or calcium malabsorption or if you have osteoporosis, you must eat yogurt. Yogurt contains a rich supply of calcium plus acids, such as lactic and acetic acid, which provoke efficient calcium absorption. Researchers have proven that eating yogurt boosts blood levels of calcium. Adding a small amount of raw honey to the yogurt stimulates calcium absorption.

Calcium may be difficult to absorb depending upon the source. Calcium supplements often contain forms of calcium which are poorly absorbed. Examples are oyster shell calcium, which is virtually impossible to absorb, rock (in the form of dolomite or calcium phosphate), and bone meal. All of these forms require an acid environment before the calcium is liberated. That means that the stomach must be functioning optimally, that is it must produce large amounts of stomach acid to render the calcium soluble. Aging is associated with a significant decline in stomach acid production, and the typical calcium supplements are often poorly tolerated and/or absorbed in the elderly. The fact is the calcium in these supplements is poorly absorbed compared to the calcium in yogurt. Yogurt is also a good source of vitamin K, which is necessary for strengthening the bones. Furthermore, the yogurt bacteria boost the body's vitamin K stores by synthesizing it in the gut. Vitamin K is needed for the formation of the type of protein in bone which makes it flexible and strong. This protein is known medically as *osteocalcin*.

8. Yogurt might help you live longer. In Russia and Bulgaria the longest lived people are regular consumers of yogurt. Bulgaria, the top yogurt producer, boasts a greater number of centenarians than any other region in the world. These centenarians consume yogurt on a daily basis—by the quart. Bulgarian type yogurts are especially delicious.

9. Yogurt may help reverse depression and/or anxiety. This is because it is a good source of B vitamins and contains a considerable amount of the nerve calming amino acid tryptophan. If the yogurt is rich in healthy bacteria, regular consumption will help increase the body's stores of B vitamins through intestinal synthesis. The result will be calmer nerves and improved mood.

10. For women, yogurt is an effective suppository for reversing vaginal inflammation and infection. Researchers document how yogurt administered intravaginally was more effective than antibiotics in curing yeast as well as bacterial infections. It not only kills the noxious microbes but it also helps reestablish the level of healthy acidophilus bacteria within the vagina. The numbers decline dramatically as the result of the ingestion of antibiotics. The yogurt applications diminish the typical annoying symptoms of vaginitis, including pain, odor, burning upon urination, inflammation, and itching.

11. Unsweetened yogurt is a common breakfast food in many countries of the world. It is frequently combined with fresh fruit, honey, grape syrup, and/or cereal. It improves digestion and bowel function, and constipation is elimitated.

Appendix A: Ordering Information for Nutritional Supplements

The following is a list of nutritional supplements mentioned in this book. All of these products are produced from the highest quality materials available and are free of chemicals, additives, and preservatives. No irradiation or fumigation is used for the spices.

Product Name	Ingredients
Agonex	Hibiscus, garlic, wild strawberry leaves, coriander seed, onion powder, basil, ginger
HerbSorb	Fenugreek, cumin, black caraway, coriander, cardamom
Hercules Strength	wild rosemary, Rhus cariaria, wild oregano, wild sage
Nutri-Sense	whole grain rice fractions, rice bran, flax, lecithin, sour grape, natural vitamin E
Oregamax	crushed wild oregano, Rhus cariaria, garlic, onion
Red Sour Grape	sour grape powder
Red Grape Syrup	whole red grapes, oregano oil
Royal Kick	freeze dried royal jelly, pantothenic acid, acerola cherry
WildPower Tea	wild strawberry leaves, wild hibiscus flowers, wild borage flowers
Oil of Cumin	extra virgin olive oil, cumin oil
Oil of Fennel	extra virgin olive oil, fennel oil
Oil of Oregano	extra virgin olive oil, wild oregano oil
Oil of Rosemary	extra virgin olive oil, rosemary oil

All products may be ordered by calling 1-800-243-5242. For a free information packet describing these products and a price list send a self-addressed envelope stamped with $1.28 (four first class stamps) to:

North American Herb & Spice Co.
P.O. Box 4885 • Buffalo Grove, IL 60089
To order immediately call **1-800-243-5242.**

Visit our WebSite: www.drcass.com

Appendix B: Gourmet Foods Mentioned in the Supermarket Cures

Numerous foods are mentioned in this book which may be difficult to find in the marketplace. Furthermore, there is great need for a source of chemical-free foods. The following is a list of the various unique food products mentioned in this book. The list includes foods/spices which may be difficult to find in the typical supermarket.

Dry roasted almonds
Unsulfured apricots
Dried cilantro leaves
Coriander seed powder
Cumin seeds
Dill weed
Fennel seeds
Dry roasted filberts
Filbert flour
Filbert oil
Red grape syrup
Red grape vinegar (no sulfites, not from wine)
Red pepper sauce (from hot peppers)
Red sweet pepper sauce
Raw honey
Extra virgin olive oil (fresh, guaranteed)

Organic oat bran cereal
Pickled oregano
Oregano bunches (whole plant)
Orega-Salt
Crude, unbleached sea salt
Organic canned pumpkin
Wild organic rosemary
Organic chunky tomato sauce
Organic sun dried tomatoes
Pickled turnips
Wild rice

For information about ordering the above items send a self-addressed stamped envelope to:

Gourmet Natural Foods
P.O. Box 855
Lincolnshire, IL 60069-0855

This company specializes in unique, delicious, nutritious, chemical free foods.

Appendix C: Top Sources of Nutrients as found in the Cures

This chart lists the five best sources of nutrients found in the Cures. The selections were made by two criteria: total density of the nutrient plus bioavailability, that is how readily the nutrient is absorbed from the food. Eat these vitamin/mineral rich foods to get the nutrients you need on a daily basis. Remember, food is the best source of nutrients.

Vitamins	Top Five Supermarket Sources
Vitamin A	sardines, salmon, eggs, yogurt, beef
Vitamin B$_{12}$	eggs, sardines, salmon, beef, yogurt
Vitamin C	cilantro, parsley, kiwi, strawberries (esp. wild strawberry leaves), grapefruit
Vitamin D	salmon, sardines, eggs, whole milk yogurt, beef
Vitamin E	almonds, filberts, unrefined olive oil, peanuts, salmon
Vitamin K	turnip greens, broccoli, cabbage, spinach, watercress
Beta carotene	sweet potatoes, parsley, pumpkin, apricots, spinach
Biotin	Royal Kick, rice bran, eggs, peanut butter, sardines
Choline	eggs, cabbage, rice bran, turnips, oat bran
Folic acid	eggs, beef, chicken, spinach, parsley
Inositol	rice bran, beef, chicken, oat bran, almonds
Niacin	rice bran, peanuts, chicken, beef, salmon
Pantothenic acid	Royal Kick, eggs, rice bran, peanut butter, salmon
Pyridoxine	rice bran, salmon, brown rice, beef, avocados
Riboflavin	Royal Kick, eggs, almonds, turnip greens, yogurt
Thiamine	rice bran, oat bran, Royal Kick, eggs, peanut butter

Minerals	Top Five Supermarket Sources
Calcium	basil, dill weed, oregano, rosemary, sardines
Chloride	sea salt, shrimp, sardines, salmon, oregano
Chromium	eggs, beef, rice bran, grapes, chicken
Cobalt	salmon, eggs, sardines, chicken, beef
Copper.	beef, chicken, almonds, filberts, peanuts
Fluorine	sardines, salmon, shrimp, sea salt, artichokes

Minerals	Top Five Supermarket Sources
Iodine	sardines, salmon, oregano, sea salt, artichokes
Iron	cumin, beef, parsley, eggs,
Magnesium	cilantro, dill weed, basil, fennel seed, rice bran
Manganese	rice bran, cloves, ginger, brown rice, peanuts
Phosphorus	pumpkin/squash seeds, rice bran, beef, sardines, eggs
Potassium	coriander/cilantro, basil, parsley, apricots, avocados
Selenium	vinegar, turnips, garlic, oats, eggs
Silica	strawberry leaves, rice bran, oat bran, beef, chicken
Sulfur	beef, chicken, yogurt, eggs, rice bran
Zinc	oregano, beef, peanut butter, eggs, chicken

Misc. Nutrients	Top Five Supermarket Sources
Amino acids	beef, chicken, peanuts, almonds, sardines
Carnitine	beef, chicken, salmon, sardines, avocados
Cholesterol	eggs, beef, chicken, salmon, shrimp
Coenzyme Q-10	beef (esp. hearts), salmon, sardines, garlic, avocados
Hydrogen	beef, chicken, salmon, sardines, yogurt
Lecithin	eggs, almonds, filberts, peanut butter, rice bran
Linoleic acid	pumpkin seeds, peanuts, almonds, filberts, eggs
Lycopene	tomato, watermelon, red pepper, grapefruit, apricot
Omega-3 fats	sardines, salmon, shrimp, rice bran, oat bran

Appendix D: Top Nutrients for the Supermarket Cures

This chart is a reversal of the information in Appendix B. Use this chart to select foods to get the vitamins and minerals you need. To discover your specific nutrient needs for virtually every vitamin and mineral known see Dr. Ingram's *Self-Test Nutrition Guide*. The following is a list of the key nutrients found in each of the supermarket cures. Other nutrients exist in good amounts, but these have been specifically selected because of their high density.

Supermarket Cures   Key Nutrients

Almonds ....magnesium, calcium, vitamin E, riboflavin
Apricots ....beta carotene, iron, potassium
Artichokes ....folic acid, cynarin, iodine, sodium
Avocados ....pyridoxine, fuel, vitamin E, carnitine, potassium
Basil......................calcium, magnesium, potassium
Beef ....iron, amino acids, carnitine, phosphorus
Beets ....betaine and potassium
Blueberries..............flavonoids and manganese
Broccoli ....vitamin C, folic acid, beta carotene, calcium
Cabbage ....vitamin C, vitamin U, sulfur, selenium, vitamin K
Cantaloupe..............vitamin C, potassium, beta carotene, folic acid
Chicken ....protein, niacin, thiamine, pyridoxine
Cilantro ....vitamin C, essential oils, potassium
Coriander seed........potassium, essential oils,
Cumin ....iron, potassium, magnesium, phosphorus
Dill.......................potassium, calcium, magnesium
Eggplant.................fiber, potassium, mucilage
Eggs ....amino acids, lecithin, zinc, vitamin $B_{12,}$ pantothenic acid
Fennel ....potassium, magnesium, calcium
Filberts..................vitamin E, potassium, calcium, fuel
Garlic ....sulfur, selenium, volatile oils
Ginger ....vitamin C, enzymes, manganese
Grapes (as sour grape) ....potassium, resveratrol, manganese, chromium
Grapefruit ....vitamin C, pectin, folic acid, bioflavonoids

Honey ....edible sugars, organic acids, potassium
Royal Jelly..............pantothenic acid, riboflavin, biotin, niacin, steroids
Horseradish ....enzymes and vitamin C
Kiwi......................folic acid, fiber, vitamin C, vitamin E
Oat bran.................thiamine, fiber, vitamin E, iron, phosphorus
Olive/Olive oil........fuel, beta carotene, vitamin E
Onion.....................sulfur and vitamin C
Oregano ....calcium, iron, niacin, essential oils
Papaya ....vitamin C, folic acid, enzymes, beta carotene
Parsley ....magnesium, vitamin C, folic acid,
                         chlorophyll, beta carotene
Peanut butter ....thiamine, niacin, pyridoxine, protein
Red sweet pepper....vitamin C, potassium, lycopene, beta carotene
Pumpkin..................beta carotene and potassium
Radishes.................selenium, sulfur, water
Rice bran ....magnesium, niacin, thiamine, choline, pantothenic acid
Rosemary...............calcium, iodine, sodium, vitamin C, essential oils
Sage ....calcium, magnesium, potassium, iron, beta carotene,
                         essential oils
Salmon...................fish oils, iodine, vitamin D, vitamin E
Salt.........................sodium and iodine
Sardines ....protein, fish oils, vitamin D, calcium
Shrimp ....protein, iodine, sodium
Spinach ....beta carotene, vitamin E, vitamin K, iron, riboflavin
Squash ....beta carotene, potassium, fiber
Strawberries...........ellagic acid, vitamin C, carotenoids
Sweet potato ....beta carotene, vitamin E
Tomatoes ....vitamin K, lycopene, vitamin C
Turnips...................sulfur, selenium, vitamin C
Turnip greens.........beta carotene, calcium, vitamin C, folic acid
Vinegar ....flavonoids, potassium, acetic acid
Watercress ....vitamin C, calcium, water, beta carotene, sulfur
Watermelon ....potassium, vitamin C, lycopene, water
Wild rice ....niacin, phosphorus, starch, iron
Yogurt ....calcium, amino acids, Lactobacillus

Appendix E: Common Illnesses and their Top Supermarket Cures

There are inherent dangers in today's world. Every day individuals are faced with potential health disasters. The possible health problems which might strike are innumerable; some are chronic illnesses and some may surface suddenly. The problem is the individual has no idea what to do if a sudden illness develops or if he/she is plagued with symptoms. The point is you need to know what to take to resolve the problem. The following is a list of diseases and symptoms not covered in the first chapter. Emphasis is on everyday ailments which may strike at any moment. This chart will help the individual rapidly identify the needed remedies.

Note that oregano oil and/or Oregamax along with rosemary and cumin oil are listed under virtually every condition. Indeed, these natural substances are highly versatile and, obviously, are effective universally. One reason oregano oil is so versatile is because a great majority of illnesses are caused by infection. Oregano oil is the top natural antiseptic available. It is also anti-pain and ant-inflammatory. Rosemary oil is highly active as a regenerative substance in a variety of organ systems and is particularly helpful for the nervous, digestive, and respiratory systems. Cumin is immensely valuable as an antioxidant, plus it is highly active in assisting the function of the digestive tract, particularly the liver and pancreas. Furthermore, selections were made for quick acting, effective substances. If such substances are going to be effective, they should produce results within a reasonable period of time, for instance, a day, a few days, or a week. Chronic conditions may take longer. Give it whatever time it takes. Your immune system governs the rate of healing.

It must be emphasized that only the edible essential oils may be used therapeutically. Typically, aromatherapy-type oils are not screened for edibility. The following advice applies only to the use of oils derived from certified natural sources free of chemical contaminants and from the correct medicinal species. Edible essential oils are produced by North American Herb & Spice Company (see Appendix A). As always for any serious/life-threatening disease see a physician immediately.

Condition	Top Supermarket Cures
Abscess	oregano oil, onion (raw), garlic (raw)
Acne	oregano herb (Oregamax), oregano oil, sage
Adrenal insufficiency	royal jelly (as Royal Kick), rosemary oil, salt
Age spots	oregano oil, cumin seed/oil, Royal Kick
AIDS	oregano oil, Oregamax, rosemary oil
Anxiety	rosemary oil, cumin oil, Royal Kick
Arthritis	oregano oil, almonds, papaya
Athlete's foot	oregano oil, Oregamax, rosemary oil
Attention deficit	rosemary oil, Hercules Strength, Royal Kick
Autism	Oregamax, oregano oil, rosemary oil
Back pain	oregano oil, almonds, papaya
Bad breath	rosemary oil, oregano oil, parsley
Bedsores	honey, oregano oil, Royal Kick
Bed wetting	WildPower Tea, sour grape, Oregamax
Bell's palsy	oregano oil, rosemary oil, Royal Kick
Bee sting	oregano oil, cumin oil, honey
Bladder infection	oregano oil, sage, sour grape
Blood clots	salmon, papaya, kiwi
Blood poisoning	oregano oil, cumin oil, Oregamax
Bloodshot eyes	Royal Kick, egg yolks, rosemary
Boils	honey, oregano oil, Oregamax
Bone pain	oregano oil, rosemary oil, almonds
Bone spurs	oregano oil, papaya, salmon
Brittle hair	beef, chicken, Nutri-Sense
Brittle nails	beef, chicken, Nutri-Sense
Bronchitis	honey, oregano oil, rosemary oil
Bruxism	Royal Kick, rosemary herb/oil, sage
Burns	oregano oil, rosemary oil, onion juice
Bursitis	oregano oil, rosemary oil, Royal Kick
Canker sores	oregano oil, rosemary oil, Royal Kick
Carpal tunnel syndrome	oregano oil, rosemary oil, Nutri-Sense
Cat bites	oregano oil, honey, onion (raw)
Cataract	oregano oil, rosemary oil, cumin oil
Chicken pox	oregano oil, rosemary oil, Oregamax
Coarse hair	shrimp, sardines, Nutri-Sense

Coated tongue ....oregano oil, Oregamax, rosemary
Cold extremities ....salmon/sardines, rosemary oil, oregano oil
Cold sores ....oregano oil, rosemary oil, Oregamax
Colds ....oregano oil, garlic, onion,
Constipation............Oregamax, HerbSorb, Nutri-Sense
Corns/calluses ....oregano oil, rosemary oil, honey
Cough ....Oregamax, oregano oil, rosemary oil
Cravings for sweets..beef/chicken, Nutri-Sense, salt
Crohn's disease ......rosemary oil, oregano oil, Oregamax
Croup.....................oregano oil, rosemary oil, honey
Cryptosporidium ....oregano oil, cumin oil, Oregamax
Cytomegalovirus ....oregano oil, Oregamax, rosemary oil
Cuts ....oregano oil, rosemary oil, honey
Cystic breasts..........oregano oil, cumin seed/oil, salmon
Dandruff ....oregano oil, cumin oil, rosemary oil
Depression..............rosemary oil, cumin oil, Royal Kick
Dermatitis ....salmon, oregano oil, rosemary oil
Diaper rash ....oregano oil (diluted), rosemary oil, honey
Diabetes.................HerbSorb, cumin oil, Oregamax
Diarrhea.................oregano oil, cumin oil, HerbSorb
Diverticulitis ....rosemary oil, oregano oil, eggplant
Dizziness ....rosemary herb/oil, Royal Kick, salt
Dog bites ....honey, oregano oil, cumin oil
Dry eye syndrome ..Nutri-Sense, sardines, salmon
Dry mouth ....Oregamax, cilantro, basil
Dry skin.................salmon, oregano oil, Royal Kick
E. coli....................oregano oil, HerbSorb, cumin oil
Ear ache.................oregano oil, rosemary oil, ginger
Easy bruising..........sour grape, rosemary, kiwi
Eczema ....oregano oil, Royal Kick, rosemary
Edema ....Wild Power Tea, horseradish, fennel oil
Emphysema............oregano oil, cilantro, rosemary herb/oil
Encephalitis ....oregano oil, cumin oil, Oregamax
Endometriosis ....rosemary oil/herb, oregano oil, salmon
Esophagitis ....papaya, rosemary herb/oil, ginger

Condition	Top Supermarket Cures
Exercise intolerance	salt, Hercules Strength, Royal Kick
Fatigue	Royal Kick, Hercules Strength, salt
Fever	oregano oil, Oregamax, Wild Power Tea
Food poisoning	honey, oregano oil, HerbSorb
Flu	oregano oil, garlic, onion
Flukes	oregano oil, garlic, cumin oil
Gallstones	cumin oil, rosemary oil, radishes
Gas	fennel oil, cumin oil, rosemary oil
Gastritis	fennel oil, oregano oil, rosemary oil
Geographic tongue	Nutri-Sense, beef, chicken (dark meat)
Giardia	oregano oil, Oregamax, garlic (raw)
Glaucoma	Royal Kick, rosemary oil, sage
Goiter	shrimp, Oregamax, salt (iodine-rich)
Gout	oregano oil, rosemary oil, Wild Power Tea
Grey hair	sage, rosemary oil, Royal Kick
Gum disease	oregano oil, sage, parsley (fresh)
Hayfever	oregano oil, Oregamax, Royal Kick
Headaches	Wild Power Tea, oregano oil, Royal Kick
Hearing loss	Royal Kick, oregano oil, cumin seed/oil
Heartburn	fennel oil, HerbSorb, kiwi
Heat intolerance	Royal Kick, rosemary herb/oil, sea salt
Heavy periods	cumin seed/oil, oregano oil, sour grape
Hemorrhoids	kiwi/papaya, rosemary oil, fennel seed/oil
Hepatitis	oregano oil, cumin oil, HerbSorb
Herpes	oregano oil, Oregamax, Royal Kick
Hiatal hernia	kiwi/papaya, rosemary oil, HerbSorb
High blood pressure	garlic, onion, rosemary
High blood sugar	cumin, garlic, oregano
High cholesterol	Rice bran/Nutri-Sense, garlic, cumin oil
High triglycerides	salmon, sardines, garlic
Hip pain	oregano oil, rosemary oil, almonds
Histoplasmosis	oregano oil, Oregamax, garlic
Hives	Royal Kick, oregano oil, rosemary
Hookworm	fennel oil, cumin oil, oregano oil
Hot flashes	sage, fennel oil, Royal Kick

Condition	Top Supermarket Cures
Hyperthyroidism	salmon, Royal Kick, Oregamax
Hypothyroidism	shrimp, salmon, salt (iodized)
Impetigo	honey, oregano oil, Oregamax
Impotence	cumin oil, Hercules Strength, rosemary oil
Insomnia	rosemary oil, Royal Kick, almonds
Iritis	oregano oil, Oregamax, rosemary oil
Itchy skin	oregano oil, Royal Kick, rosemary oil
Jaundice	oregano oil, cumin oil, HerbSorb
Joint stiffness	oregano oil, rosemary oil, Royal Kick
Kidney stones	sour grape, fennel oil, Hercules Strength
Knee pain	oregano oil, rosemary oil, kiwi
Lack of smell	beef liver, rosemary oil, cumin oil
Lack of thirst	salt, beef, royal jelly (Royal Kick)
poisoning	garlic, cumin herb/oil, WildPower Tea
Leg cramps	almonds, Royal Kick, Nutri-Sense
Lethargy	Royal Kick, Oregamax, salt
Low blood pressure	salt, royal jelly (Royal Kick), rosemary oil
Low blood sugar	Royal Kick, HerbSorb, Nutri-Sense
Lupus	Royal Kick, oregano oil, cumin oil
Lyme disease	oregano oil, Oregamax, Hercules Strength
Macular degeneration	blueberries, fennel seed/oil, rosemary
Malaria	oregano oil, Oregamax, garlic
Mastoiditis	oregano oil, garlic, Oregamax
Memory loss	rosemary oil, Hercules Strength, cumin oil
Meniere's syndrome	Royal Kick, salmon, rosemary herb/oil
Meningitis	oregano oil, Oregamax, garlic (raw)
Menstrual cramps	fatty fish, oregano oil, kiwi
Mercury poisoning	garlic, onions, cumin herb/oil
Mitral valve prolapse	sour grape, avocado, almonds
Moles	turnips/radishes, cumin oil, oregano oil
Mononucleosis	oregano oil, Oregamax, cumin oil
Mood swings	Royal Kick, beef, Nutri-Sense
Multiple sclerosis	eggs, oregano oil, Royal Kick
Muscle weakness	Royal Kick, Hercules Strength, salt
Muscular dystrophy	beef, cumin oil, rosemary herb/oil

Condition	Top Supermarket Cures
Nasal polyps	oregano oil, Oregamax, salmon
Nearsightedness	fennel oil, cumin oil, blueberries
Neck pain	oregano oil, papaya, rosemary oil
Nephritis	Wild Power Tea, oregano oil, sour grape
Nervousness	rosemary herb/oil, Royal Kick, Nutri-Sense
Nuclear irradiation	rosemary oil, oregano oil, garlic, cumin oil
Neuritis	oregano oil, Nutri-Sense, salmon
Neuropathy	Nutri-Sense, oregano oil, almonds
Noise sensitivity	Royal Kick, rosemary oil, salt
Nosebleeds	sour grape, kiwi, red onions
Numbness	Nutri-Sense, oregano oil, Royal Kick
Obesity	cumin, fennel, HerbSorb
Pernicious anemia	beef, egg yolks, cumin oil
Photophobia	blueberries, sour grape, Hercules Strength
Pinworms	fennel oil, cumin oil, oregano oil
Plaque	oregano oil, sage, Oregamax
Pneumonia	oregano oil, rosemary oil, garlic
Poison ivy	oregano oil, rosemary oil, Royal Kick
Poor appetite	cabbage, Nutri-Sense, beef
Poor breast milk	fennel oil, cumin oil, Nutri-Sense
Post nasal drip	oregano oil, Oregamax, rosemary oil
Prostate problems	cumin oil, tomatoes, Wild Power Tea
Psoriasis	oregano oil, Oregamax, rosemary oil
Puncture wounds	honey, oregano oil, garlic
Receding gums	beef, yogurt, garlic
Restless leg syndrome	rosemary oil, Hercules Strength, Royal Kick
Ringworm	oregano oil, Oregamax, garlic
Rosacea	oregano oil, garlic, yogurt,
Runny nose	oregano oil, Royal Kick, rosemary herb/oil
Salmonella	oregano oil, cumin oil, garlic (raw)
Sarcoidosis	oregano oil, Oregamax, HerbSorb
Scabies	oregano oil, garlic, rosemary oil
Sciatica	oregano oil, almonds, rosemary oil
Scleroderma	oregano oil, Oregamax, HerbSorb
Seborrhea	oregano oil, cumin oil, rosemary oil

Condition	Top Supermarket Cures
Shigella	oregano oil, Oregamax, HerbSorb
Shingles	oregano oil, Royal Kick, rosemary herb/oil
Sinusitis	oregano oil, rosemary oil, sage
Seizures	avocado, beef, Nutri-Sense
Skin tags	oregano oil, rosemary oil, cumin seed/oil
Sleep apnea	Royal Kick, rosemary oil, Nutri-Sense
Sleep walking	Nutri-Sense, Royal Kick, rosemary
Sore throat	honey, vinegar, oregano oil
Sour stomach	rosemary oil, fennel oil, cilantro
Spider bites	oregano oil, cumin oil, Royal Kick
Sprains	oregano oil, papaya, kiwi
Split ends	salmon, beef, sardines
Staph	honey, oregano oil, Oregamax
Sties	Oregamax, sage, oregano oil
Stomach ache	ginger, kiwi fruit, fennel
Stomach ulcer	cabbage juice, fennel oil, cumin seed/oil
Stunted growth	beef (liver), Nutri-Sense, eggs
Sunburn	rosemary oil, oregano oil, honey
Sweaty feet	oregano oil, Royal Kick, rosemary oil/herb
Swollen hands/feet	Wild Power Tea, fennel oil, dill
Tapeworm	oregano oil, cumin oil, garlic (raw)
Tendonitis	oregano oil, salmon, rosemary
Tinnitis	salmon, oregano oil, rosemary herb/oil
Tonsillitis	oregano oil, Oregamax, honey
Toothache	oregano oil, sage, rosemary oil
Tremors	Royal Kick, rosemary herb/oil, salmon
Trigeminal neuralgia	rosemary herb/oil, oregano oil,
Tuberculosis	oregano oil, garlic (raw), rosemary oil
Ulcerations	honey, oregano oil, rosemary herb/oil
Ulcerative colitis	oregano oil/herb, fennel oil, rosemary oil
Urethritis	oregano oil, fennel oil, Wild Power Tea
Uterine fibroids	oregano oil, rosemary oil, Royal Kick
Vaginitis	oregano oil (diluted), rosemary oil, honey
Varicose veins	sour grape, kiwi fruit, rosemary oil
Venomous bites	oregano oil, cumin oil, HerbSorb

Condition	Top Supermarket Cures
Warts	oregano oil, Oregamax, cumin oil
Water retention	fennel, wild strawberry leaves, rosemary oil
Weight loss (too thin)	Nutri-Sense, salmon, sardines
Wound infection	honey, oregano oil, rosemary oil
Wrinkles	rosemary herb/oil, cumin oil,
Yeast infection	oregano oil, cumin oil, Oregamax

Bibliography

Alfthan, G., et al. 1997. Plasma homocysteine and cardiovascular disease mortality. *The Lancet.* 349:397.

Angier, B. 1978. *Field Guide to Medicinal Wild Plants.* Harrisburg, PA: Stackpole Books.

Aqel, M. B. 1991. Relaxant effect of the volatile oil of Rosmarinus officinalis on tracheal smooth muscle. *Journal of Ethnopharmacology.* 33:57-62.

Baily, E.H.S. 1914. *Source Chemistry and Use of Food Products.* Philadelphia: Blakiston's Son & Co.

Bianchini, F. and F. Corbetta. 1976. *The Complete Book of Fruits and Vegetables.* New York: Crown Publ.

Bogert, L. J. 1949. *Good Nutrition for Everybody.* Chicago: Chicago University Press.

Bogert, L. J. 1955. *Nutrition and Physical Fitness.* Philadelphia: W.B. Saunders.

Bourne, G.H. and G.W. Kidder. 1953. *Biochemistry and Physiology of Nutrition.* New York: Holt.

Boxer, A. 1984. *The Encyclopedia of Herbs, Spices, and Flavorings.* New York: Crown Publ.

Braverman, E. 1987. *The Healing Nutrients Within.* New Canaan, CT: Keats Publ.

Brown, P., Preece, M.A., and R.G. Will. 1992. "Friendly fire" in medicine: hormones, homografts, and Creutzfeld-Jakob disease. *Lancet.* 340:24-27.

Castleman, M. 1991. *The Healing Herbs.* Emmaus, PA: Rodale Press.

Collins, P. J., et al. 1975. Inhibition of C. albicans by lactobacilli and lactobacillic fermented dairy products. *FEMS Micro. Rev.* 46:343.

Conner, D.E. and L.R. Beuchat. 1984. Effects of essential oils from plants on growth of food spoilage yeasts. *J. Food Sci.* 49:429.

Coles, B. and B. Ketterer. 1990. The role of glutathione and glutathione transferases in chemical carcinogenisis. *Critical Reviews of Biochemistry and Molecular Biology.* 25:47-70.

Cooper, L.F., et al. 1953. *Nutrition in Health and Disease.* 12th ed. Lippincott.

Duke, J.A. 1985. CRC *Handbook of Medicinal Herbs.* Boca Raton, FL:CRC Press, Inc.

The editors. 1988. Clinical observations on the wound healing properties of honey. *British Journal of Surgery.* 75(7): 679-81.

Ensminger, A.H., et al. 1983. *Food and Nutrition Encyclopedia.* Vol 1 & 2. Clovis, CA: Pegus Press.

Fallon, Sally. 1995. *Nourishing Traditions.* San Diego: ProMotion Publishing.

Flagg, E. W., et al. 1994. Dietary glutathione intake and the risk of oral and pharyngeal cancer. *Amer. J. Epidem.* 139:453.

Francheschi, S., et al. 1994. Tomatoes and the risk of digestive cancers. *Int. J. Cancer.* 59:181.

Fredericks, Carlton. *Eating Right for You.* New York: Grosset and Dunlap.

Giovannucci, E., et al. 1995. Intake of carotenoids and retinol in relation to prostate cancer risk. *J. Natl Cancer Inst.* 87:1767.

Gilliland, S. E. and M. K. Speck. 1977. Antagonistic action of Lactobacillus acidophilus toward intestinal and food-borne pathogens in associative cultures. *J. Food. Product.* 40:830.

Gregerson, J. 1992. *The Good Earth.* Vancouver: Whitecap Books.

Grieve, M. 1992. *A Modern Herbal.* London: Dorsett Press.

Griffin, H. C. 1979. The role of selenium in the chemoprevention of cancer. *Adv. Cancer. Res.* 29:419-442.

Grobstein, C. (chairman). 1982. *Diet, Nutrition, and Cancer.* Washington, D.C.: National Academy of Sciences.

Habeeb, V.T. (ed). 1966. *American Home All-Purpose Cookbook.* New York: M. Evans and Co.

Havsteen, B. 1983. Flavonoids, a class of natural products of high pharmacological potency. *Biochem. Pharm.* 32:1141.

Hollowell, J., et al. 1968. Homocystinuria as affected by pyridoxine, folic acid, and vitamin B_{12}. *Proc. Soc. Exp. Biol. Med.* 129:327.

Ingram, Cass. 1994. *Self-Test Nutrition Guide.* Buffalo Grove, IL: Knowledge House.

Ingram, Cass. 1997. *The Cure is in the Cupboard: How to Use Oregano for Better Health.* Buffalo Grove, IL: Knowledge House.

Inatani, R., et al. 1982. Antioxidant effect of the constituents of rosemary and their derivatives. *Agric. Biol. Chem.* 47:521-528.

Issam Bou-Holaigah, P. C., et al. The relationship between neurally mediated hypotention and the chronic fatigue syndrome. 274:961.

Jacobs, M.B. 1944. *The Chemistry and Technology of Food and Food Products.* New York: Interscience Publ., Inc.

Jacoby, W. B. 1978. The glutathione S-transferases: A group of multifunctional detoxification proteins. *Adv. Enzymol. Relat. Areas Mol. Biol.* 46:383.

Jarvis, D. C. 1958. *Folk Medicine.* Fawcett Crest Books.

Kadans, J.M. 1973. *Encyclopedia of Fruits, Vegetables, Nuts, and Seeds.* West Nyack: Parker Publ. Co.

Kaul, T. N., et al. 1985. Anti-viral effect of flavonoids on human viruses. *J. Med. Virol..* 15:71-79.

Keller, K. 1992. *Adverse Effects of Herbal Drugs.* (PAGM De Smet, ed). Berlin: Springer-Verlag.

Khan, L. and M. S. Bamji. 1983. Tissue carnitine deficiency due to dietary lysine deficiency: triglyceride accumulation and concomitant impairment in fatty acid oxidation. *J. Nutr.* 109:24-31.

Kim, Young-In. 1996. Can fish oil maintain Crohn's disease in remission? *Nutr. Rev.* 54:248.

Klein, Maggie Blyth. 1994. *The Feast of the Olive.* San Francisco: Chronicle Books.

Kowalchik, C. and W.H. Hylton (ed). 1987. *Rodale's Illustrated Encyclopedia of Herbs*. Emmaus, PA: Rodale Press.

Lindlahr, V.H. 1941.*The Lindlahr Vitamin Cookbook*. New York: National Nutrition Society.

Margen, S. (ed). 1992. *The Wellness Encyclopedia of Food and Nutrition*. New York: Rebus.

Martin, E.A. 1965. *Nutrition in Action*. New York: Hotl, Rinehart, and Winston.

McCarron, D. A. 1997. Role of adequeate dietary calcium intake in the prevention and management of salt-sensitive hypertension. *Amer. J. Clin. Nutr.* 65(Suppl):712-716.

Mindell, E. 1994. *Earl Mindell's Food as Medicine*. New York: Simon and Schuster.

Murray, M. and J. Pizzorno. 1991. *Encyclopedia of Natural Medicine*. Rocklin, CA: Prima Publishing.

Navarro, M. C., et al. 1992. Free radical scavenger and antihepatotoxic activity of *Rosmarinus tomentosus*. *Plant Medic*a. 59:312.

Norman, J. *Nuts*. New York: Bantam Books.

Platt, K. 1926. *Food: Its Use and Abuse*. London: Faber and Gwyer, Ltd (Scientific Press).

Pluyer, et al. 1987. Destruction of aflatoxins on peanuts by oven-roasting and microwave-roasting. *Journal of Food Protection*. Vol 50:504.

Potterton, D. 1983. *Culpeper's Color Herbal*. New York: Sterling Publ. Co., Inc.

Pusiner, S.B., et al. 1992. *Prion Diseases in Humans and Animals*. London: Ellis Horwood.

Proudfit, F. T. and C. H. Robinson. 1961. *Normal and Therapeutic Nutrition*. New York: Macmillan Co.

Pruthi, J.S. 1980. *Spices and Condiments: Chemistry, Microbiology, Technology*. New York: Academic Press.

Riccio, D. 1992. *Superfoods*. New York: Warner.

Roberts, G.W. 1995. Creutzfeld-Jakob disease and bovine spongiform encephalopathy: any connection? *British Medical Journal*. Nov 25, pp. 1419.

Rose, Mary Swartz. 1932. *A Laboratory Handbook for Dietetics*. New York: Macmillan.

Rosenburg, E. and P. Belew. 1982. Microbial factors in psoriasis. *Arch. Derm.* 118:1434-44.

Scholar, E., et al. 1988. Effects of diets enriched in cabbage and collards on metastasis of BALB/c mammary carcinoma (meeting abstract). *P. Amer. Assoc. Ca.* 29:149.

Schroeder, H.A. 1973. *The Trace Elements and Man*. Old Greenwich, CT: Devin Adair Co.

Schulick, Paul. 1993. *Common Spice or Wonder Drug? Ginger*. Brattleboro, VT: Herbal Free Press.

Schwanitz, F. 1966. *The Origin of Cultivated Plants*. Cambridge, MA: Harvard University Press.

Shah, A.H., Qureshi, S., and A.M. Ageel. 1991. Toxicity Studies in mice of ethanol extracts of *Foeniculum vulgare* fruit and *Ruta chalepensis* aerial parts. *Journal of Ethnopharmacology*. 34:167-172.

Shelef, L.A. 1983. Antimicrobial effects of spices. *J. Food Safety*. 6:29

Sherman, H.C. 1963. *Essentials of Nutrition*. 4th ed. New York: Macmillan & Co.

Shils, M.E., Olson, J.A., and M. Shike (eds). 1994. *Modern Nutrition in Health and Disease*. Philadelphia: Lea & Febiger.

Shug, A. L., et al. 1982. The distribution and role of carnitine in the mammalian brain. *Life Sci.* 31:2869.

Sivam, G. P., et al. 1997. In vitro susceptibility to garlic (*Allim sativum*) extract. *Nutrition and Cancer*. 27:118.

Sounin, L. 1952. *Magic in Herbs*. New York: M. Barrows & Co.

Stahl, Wilhelm and Helmut Sies. 1996. Lycopene: a biologically important carotenoid for humans? *Arch. Biochem. Biophysics*. 336(1):001.

Staessen, J. A., et al. 1997. Salt and blood pressure in community-based intervention trials. *Amer. J. Clin. Nutr.* 65:661.

Sturtevant, E.L.1972. *Edible Plants of the World*. Edited by U.P. Hedrick, New York: Dover Publ.

Subrahmanyam, M. 1991. Topical application of honey in treatment of burns. *British Journal of Surgery*. 78:479-8.

Svendsen, A.B. and J.J.C. Scheffer (eds). 1985. *Essential Oils and Aromatic Plants*. Dordrecht: Martinus Nijhoff/Dr. W. Junk Publ.

Taintu, D.R. and A.T. Grenis. 1993. *Spices and Seasonings: A Food Technology Handbook*. New York: VCH Publ.

Tannahil, R. 1973. *Food in History*. New York: Stein and Day.

Tisserand, R.B. 1977. *The Art of Aromatherapy*. Rochester, VT: Destiny Books.

Vietmeyer, N.D. 1987. The Captivating Kiwifruit. *National Geographic*; May.

Tanira, M.O.M., et al. 1996. Pharmacological and toxicological investigations on Foeniculum vulgare dried fruit extract in experimental animals. *Phytotherapy Research* 10:33-36.

Valnet, Jean. 1989. *The Practice of Aromatherapy*. Rochester, VT: Healing Arts Press.

Van Den Broucke, C. O. and J. A. Lemli. 1982. Antispasmodic activity of *Origanum compactum*. *Planta Medica*. 45:188-190.

Wang, H., et al. 1996. Total antioxidant capacity of fruits. *J. Agric. Food Chem.* 44:701-705.

Wardlaw, G.M. and P.M. Insel. 1990. *Perspectives in Nutrition*. St. Louis: Times Mirror/ Mosby College Publ.

White, L. 1966. *The Good Egg*. New York: Paperback Library.

Will, R.G. 1993. Epidemiology of Creutzfeld-Jakob disease. *Br. Med. Bull.* 49:960.

Youngken, H.W. 1943. *Textbook of Pharmacognosy*. Blakiston, PA.

Index

Anxiety, 61, 63, 74, 110, 114-115, 134, 228, 268, 283, 292

Apiol, 197

Appetite, 62-63, 67, 80, 99, 103, 106-107, 125, 143, 165, 170, 174, 180, 186, 197, 200, 203, 215, 229, 235, 248, 251, 254, 267, 271, 275, 281, 296

excessive, 80

Apricots, 44, 55-59, 158, 214, 252, 286-289

Arabic physicians, 221

Arsenic poisoning, 43

Arthritis, 2, 6, 8, 29-30, 34, 43, 60, 72, 119-120, 147, 158, 167, 171-172, 182, 196-197, 204, 216-217, 226, 250-251, 260, 292

Artichokes, 29, 33, 41, 59-64, 287-289

Aspirin, 30, 38, 54-55, 147, 149, 196, 219, 230, 249

Asthma, 2, 6, 15, 34-36, 69, 141, 183, 192, 216, 220, 241, 260

Atherosclerosis, 19, 54, 241

Athlete's foot, 191, 292

Attention deficit disorder, 16, 33-34, 52

Autism, 292

Avocado, 13, 21, 24-25, 29, 35, 39, 41, 46-47, 58, 64-68, 78, 81, 93, 102, 139, 210, 247, 252-253, 265, 287-289, 295, 297

B

B vitamins, 6, 21-22, 27, 29, 32-37, 41, 43-44, 47-48, 80, 84, 89, 106-107, 118, 125-126, 135, 201-203, 212-215, 224, 231, 236, 241, 267, 274, 276, 280, 283

see also individual B vitamins

Babylonians, 185

Back pain, 172, 292

Bad breath, 217-218, 292

Baldness, 127

Baser, Dr. H., 186

Basil, 4-5, 39, 69-72, 224, 287-289, 293

Bed wetting, 292

Bedsores, 292

Bee sting, 193, 292

Beef, 21, 24, 29, 33, 35-36, 39, 43-44, 47-48, 70, 73-81, 129, 166-168, 182, 188-189, 200, 218, 237, 252, 259, 270-271, 274, 287-289, 292-297

Beef liver, 80, 295, 297

Beet greens, 82, 166

Beets, 44, 81-85, 110, 289

Bell's palsy, 292

Berries, 35, 38, 41, 44, 72, 79, 82, 86-91, 131, 147, 153, 160, 185, 187-194, 218, 222-224, 234, 242-245, 266, 269-270, 272-276, 280, 282, 285-287, 290, 298-299, 323

wild, 86-89, 243

Beta carotene, 20-22, 24-26, 32, 37, 55-59, 61, 67, 89, 92-94, 100-103, 142, 155, 170, 181-182, 195-196, 198, 204-206, 209, 211, 223-224, 236-237, 239-248, 250-253, 255-256, 263-264, 267, 269, 287, 289-290

Betaine, 44, 82-85, 289

Bifidobacteria, 278

Bioflavonoids, 29, 31, 36, 48, 87, 89, 91, 94-95, 97-98, 103, 147-148, 152-155, 157-159, 182, 185, 209, 224, 237, 242-244, 250-251, 253, 255, 259, 261-262, 289

see also Flavonoids

Biotin, 32, 52, 55, 60, 65, 73, 100, 104, 118, 123, 125-126, 135, 161, 212, 246, 287, 290

Biotrition Laboratory, 30

Bites, 69, 136, 141, 186, 193, 220, 292-293, 297

Black caraway, 106, 111, 151, 285

Bladder infection, 292

Bloating, 39, 41, 97-98, 126, 143, 146, 191, 196, 199, 237, 245, 254

Blood clots, 54, 95, 149, 183, 196, 292

Blood poisoning, 17, 292

Blood vessels, 88, 95, 125, 135, 153, 157, 159, 205, 228

Bloodshot eyes, 292

Blueberries, 86-90, 153, 166, 273, 289, 295-296

Boils, 159, 165, 251, 292

Bone pain, 292

Bone spurs, 292

Boron, 29, 51

Bovine growth hormone, 279-280

Bowel, 6, 16, 25, 37, 39-41, 48, 63, 72, 81, 97, 120, 130, 158, 171, 175, 184-185, 199, 217, 241, 245, 254, 259, 275, 277

see also Colon; Intestines

Brain, 5-6, 12, 15, 31-32, 34-35, 63, 74-77, 84, 87-88, 114, 116, 137, 177, 212, 216, 218-220, 228, 303

Braverman, Dr. Eric, 21, 209

Brazil nuts, 42, 201, 221

Breast cancer, 15, 100, 142, 148, 207

Breasts, 15, 25, 100, 104, 134, 138, 142, 148, 207, 293, 296

see also Fibrocystic breast disease

Brewer's yeast, 161

British Journal of Surgery, 160, 163, 300, 304

British pharmacopoeia, 216

British physicians, 136

Brittle hair, 50, 292

Brittle nails, 50, 67, 292

Broccoli, 21-23, 26, 29, 33, 35, 48, 52, 91-95, 110, 198, 224, 259, 263, 287, 289

Bronchitis, 6, 16, 103, 158, 183, 192, 204, 217, 220, 223, 257, 292

Bruising, 89, 95, 153, 155, 159, 197, 244, 271, 293

Brussels sprouts, 22, 95, 110, 181, 263

Bruxism, 292

Burns, 127, 140, 163-165, 219, 292, 304

Bursitis, 6, 292

C

Cabbage, 22, 26, 83, 91, 95-100, 110, 166, 181, 263, 287, 289, 296-297, 303

Cabbage juice, 97-100, 297

Cachexia, 99

Caffeine, 33, 125, 141

Calcium, 8, 12, 21-22, 25, 29, 31-36, 43, 47-49, 51, 53-55, 60, 69, 91-92, 94-96, 104-105, 124, 126, 129, 131, 133-135, 150-151, 155, 175, 187, 198, 204-205, 216, 221-222, 231-232, 236-238, 246, 250, 256, 259, 263-268, 276, 279-281, 283, 287, 289-290, 302

Calf liver, 80

Cancer, 2, 7-8, 12, 15-16, 22-26, 43-44, 52-54, 56, 59, 85, 91, 94, 97, 99-100, 105, 108, 118, 120, 127, 138, 142, 148, 151, 153-154, 166, 168, 177, 184, 193, 204, 206-207, 209-211, 217, 220, 232,

E

E. coli, 16, 75, 78, 137, 160, 187, 278, 293

Ear ache, 82, 103, 192, 293

Easy bruising, 95, 153, 155, 159, 244, 293

Ebola, 16

Economic Botany, 112

Eczema, 16, 39, 50, 97, 169, 190, 204-205, 226, 267, 293

Edema, 95, 217, 260, 293

Eggplant, 118-120, 210, 289, 293

Eggs, 9, 11, 13-14, 20, 23-24, 29, 31, 33, 36, 41, 43-44, 46-47, 49, 52, 61, 65, 67, 73-74, 84-85, 90, 107, 119, 121-128, 132, 138-139, 161, 168, 170, 173-174, 176, 188, 195, 200, 226, 229, 237-238, 270-271, 287-289, 292, 295-297, 304

Egyptians, ancient, 3, 112, 115, 135-136, 160, 180, 269

Electrolytes, 46, 77, 163, 228-229, 275

Ellagic acid, 150, 152, 242-244, 290

Emphysema, 15, 204, 220, 293

Encephalitis, 293

Encyclopedia, 69, 194, 216, 299-302

Energy, 1-2, 21, 24, 34, 45-46, 49, 54, 64, 67-68, 71, 73, 80, 99, 103, 107, 110-112, 125, 135, 149, 157, 161, 165, 173, 178-179, 187, 193, 203, 210, 212, 214, 229-230, 242, 255, 267, 270, 277, 322

lack of, 45, 71, 80, 135, 166

Ensminger's Food and Nutrition, 69

Enzymes, 22-23, 25-27, 31, 36, 40-41, 48, 52, 79, 91, 97, 114, 132-133, 136, 139, 143, 147, 160, 163, 166-172, 179, 194-197, 210-212, 217, 229, 248, 266, 276-278, 280, 283, 289-290, 323

Epstein-Barr, 16

Esophagitis, 6, 97, 293

Essential fatty acids, 12, 27, 32, 34-35, 44, 50, 65, 129, 212, 214-215, 241

Estrogen, 51, 100, 128, 161, 322

F

Facial pores, 50

Farsightedness, 88, 90, 248

Fatigue, 16, 39, 45-48, 54, 61, 63, 107, 110, 112, 115, 126, 132, 142, 148, 157, 166, 173-174, 179, 193, 197, 203, 210-211, 213-215, 217, 229-230, 244, 255, 260, 267, 277, 294, 301

Fatty fish, 5-6, 20-21, 25, 74, 85, 90, 167, 232, 295

Fennel, 4-5, 41, 43, 90, 128-131, 285-286, 288-289, 293-298

Fennel oil, 41, 43, 128-131, 285, 293-298

Fenugreek, 106, 111, 115, 151, 285

Fever, 146, 197, 294

Fibrocystic breast disease, 134

Fibromyalgia, 16, 39, 45, 47-48, 158, 171-172

Filbert flour, 133-134, 286

Filbert oil, 132-134, 286

Filberts, 21, 25, 35, 42-44, 48, 102, 131-135, 201, 286-289

Fingernail fungus, 193

Fish, 3, 5-6, 14, 20-22, 24-25, 29, 31, 35, 37, 41, 48, 67, 73-74, 79, 81, 83-85, 90, 94, 107, 116, 129, 138-139, 144, 167, 193, 210, 223-225, 227, 230-233, 237-238, 262, 270, 290, 295, 301

Fish oils, 22, 29, 31, 35, 37, 41, 48, 67, 167, 223-225, 231-233, 290

Flavonoids, 8, 18, 22, 47-48, 148-150, 152, 189, 214, 219, 251, 289-290, 301

Flu, 2, 16, 99, 106, 136, 146, 183, 189-190, 195, 208, 211, 223, 257, 271, 294

Fluoride, 222

Fluorine, 287

Folic acid, 19-20, 22, 25, 29, 31-33, 35-36, 40-41, 44, 48-49, 51, 60, 62-63, 65, 73-74, 80, 82, 91, 94, 98, 100, 102-103, 118, 123, 125-126, 135, 154-155, 158, 170, 181, 195, 198, 201, 204-205, 211-212, 224, 230-231, 236, 239, 246, 250, 256, 264, 267, 276, 287, 289-290, 301

Folts, Dr. John, 149

Food allergy, 6-7, 30, 36, 40-41, 47-48, 56, 59, 80, 180, 185, 214, 251, 276, 282, 322

see also Allergies; Allergic reactions

Food and Nutrition Encyclopedia, 69, 300, 302

Food Intolerance Test, 30, 48

Food poisoning, 34, 75, 78, 101, 140, 182, 195, 222, 247, 260, 262, 294

Formaldehyde, 225

Fungal infection, 28, 37-38, 45, 140, 149, 151, 191-193

see also Candidiasis; Yeast infection

G

Galen, 3, 159, 197

Gallstones, 82, 184, 294

Garlic, 3-5, 9, 21-23, 26, 29, 39-40, 47, 61, 66, 79, 106, 113, 116, 119, 123, 135-142, 156, 180, 189, 207, 224-225, 261, 274, 285, 288-289, 292-297, 303, 322-323

Gas, 39, 41, 72, 96-98, 112, 126, 129-130, 139, 143, 191-192, 196, 199, 217, 237, 250, 275, 294

Gastritis, 6, 16, 97, 206, 248, 281, 294

Genital infection, 114

Geographic tongue, 294

Germanium, 138, 142, 150

Giardia, 16, 45, 137, 187, 294

Ginger, 4, 9, 36, 40-41, 48, 72, 79, 143-147, 157, 224, 288-289, 293, 297, 303

Glaucoma, 2, 248, 294

Glutathione, 23, 91, 113, 115, 224, 300-301

Glutathione S-transferase, 114, 219, 301

Goiter, 294

Goitrogens, 52, 92, 94, 100, 202, 257

Gout, 250, 294

Grape juice, 152

Gray, Judy Kay, M.S., 1, 322-324

Greeks, ancient, 3, 82, 95, 108, 112, 119, 143, 159, 176, 185-186, 197, 216, 220, 230, 255

Grey hair, 294

Grieve's Modern Herbal, 112

Gum disease, 222, 294

Gums, 95, 192, 244, 296

Guyton's textbook of physiology, 20, 68

H

Hair, 5, 50, 67, 104, 127, 142, 169, 180, 183, 218-219, 242, 260, 263, 268, 292, 294

Hair loss, 50, 67, 142, 180, 260, 268

Hantavirus, 16

Hardening of the arteries, 19, 28, 54, 95, 126, 183, 204, 219, 258

Hayfever, 294

Hazelnut oil, 53, 93, 132-134
  see also Filbert oil
Hazelnuts, 67, 131, 247
  see also Filberts
HDL, 22, 50-51, 65, 123, 138
Headache, 2, 7, 30, 54-55, 61, 63, 71-72,
  82, 110, 143, 145, 174, 186, 201, 216,
  219, 235, 260, 294, 322, 324
Healing Nutrients Within, 21, 299
Hearing loss, 294
Heart attacks, 20, 54, 68, 95, 149, 158,
  230
Heart disease, 12, 15, 18-21, 28, 56, 65,
  68, 102, 112, 117, 120-122, 126, 134,
  136-138, 148-149, 151, 157, 177, 183,
  199, 204-205, 217, 219, 241, 258, 260,
  263, 272, 322
Heartburn, 59, 126, 143, 145, 168, 171,
  174, 186, 196, 199, 206, 219, 244, 254,
  258, 275, 294
Heat exhaustion, 146, 269, 271-272
Heat intolerance, 294
Heat stroke, 146, 271
Heavy metals, 23, 142
Heavy periods, 294
Hebrews, 108
Hemoglobin, 80
Hemorrhoids, 40, 95, 120, 148, 153, 155,
  294
Hepatitis, 16, 43, 79, 97, 184, 294
Herbicides, 19, 23, 139, 152, 242, 279-
  280
Herbivore, 75
HerbSorb, 106, 111, 113-115, 151, 285,
  293-297
Hercules Strength, 218-220, 222-223,
  285, 292, 294-296

Herpes, 16, 278, 294
Hiatal hernia, 16, 294
High blood pressure, 5, 28, 67, 102, 117-
  118, 126, 135, 141, 148, 153-154, 200,
  216, 241, 250, 258, 260, 294
High blood sugar, 106, 294
Hip pain, 172, 294
Histoplasmosis, 16, 294
Hives, 39, 169, 226, 235, 294
Homocysteine, 126, 299
Honey, 3, 13, 27, 41, 57, 59, 118, 141,
  146, 153, 157, 159-165, 168-169, 174,
  191, 195, 222, 279-283, 286, 290, 292-
  298, 300, 304, 322-323
Hookworm, 130, 294
Hormones, 30, 42, 45-46, 78, 94, 104,
  114, 127-128, 136, 161, 165, 180, 215,
  227-229, 234, 279-280, 299
Horseradish, 26, 31, 36, 40-41, 166-169,
  234, 290, 293
Hot flashes, 115, 294
Hydrochloric acid, 76, 229
Hydrogen ions, 73
Hydrogenated oils, 21, 47, 61, 173, 201
Hypertension, 117, 134, 137, 302
  see also High blood pressure
Hyperthyroidism, 295
Hypochlorhydria, 43
Hypoglycemia, 52, 62, 81, 90, 115
Hypothyroidism, 249, 268, 295

I
Ibn Baytar, 3
Immunoglobulins, 248
Impetigo, 295
Impotence, 112, 114, 134, 295

313

Myasthenia gravis, 126, 238
Mycobacteria, 137
Myelin sheath, 125-126

N
Nail fungus, 193
Nails, 39, 50, 55, 67, 104, 242, 260, 292
    brittle, 50, 55, 67, 260, 292
Nasal polyps, 296
Native Americans, 86, 203, 227, 244,
    250, 273
Nausea, 2, 72, 143, 173
Nearsightedness, 88, 90, 248, 296
Neck pain, 296
Neuropathy, 111, 126, 296
Neutropenia, 37
New England Journal of Medicine, 17, 20
Niacin, 19, 25, 32, 44, 52, 55, 60, 65, 73-
    74, 80, 87, 104, 106, 108, 126, 133,
    135, 173, 175-176, 187, 201, 203, 212,
    214-215, 225, 231-232, 238, 273, 287,
    289-290
    see also Vitamin B$_3$
Night blindness, 87-88, 90
Nightmares, 115
Nitrosamines, 23
North American Herb & Spice Company,
    41. 114. 129, 131, 190, 194, 218, 219,
    266, 291
Nose bleeds, 95, 153, 155, 244
Nosocomial infections, 38
Nuclear irradiation, 23, 37, 296
Nucleic acids, 231-232
Numbness, 110-111, 143, 296
NutraSweet, 155, 279
Nutri-Sense, 29, 35, 44, 84, 89, 164-165,
    174-176, 212-215, 285, 292-298

O
Oat bran, 89, 172-176, 212, 276, 286-288,
    290
Oatmeal, 172-176, 264
Obesity, 52, 80, 107, 125, 128, 227, 260,
    296
Olive oil, 3, 12, 21-22, 28, 36, 50, 53, 61,
    64, 66, 68, 70-71, 79, 83, 85, 93, 106,
    112, 116, 119, 132-133, 138-139, 166,
    176-180, 188, 190, 195, 200, 208, 212,
    217, 238, 247, 252-254, 285-287, 290
Olives, 3, 12-13, 21-22, 24, 28, 36, 47,
    50, 53, 61, 64, 66, 68, 70-71, 79, 81,
    83, 85, 93, 106, 112, 116, 119, 122,
    132-133, 138-139, 166, 176-180, 188,
    190, 195, 200, 208, 212, 217, 225, 238,
    247, 252-254, 285-287, 290, 301
Omega-3-fatty acids, 212-213, 288
Onion, 4, 40, 66, 106, 113, 180-184, 189,
    198, 207-208, 224, 261, 274, 285, 290,
    292-294, 322-323
Oregamax, 188-193, 282, 285, 291-298
Oregano, 4-5, 9, 29, 31, 36, 38, 40-41, 44,
    47-48, 79, 101-102, 164, 179, 185-194,
    202, 224, 243, 261-262, 266, 282, 285-
    288, 290-298, 301, 322-324
Oregano oil, 31, 38, 79, 101-102, 164,
    179, 186-194, 202, 243, 262, 266, 282,
    285, 291-298, 323
Osler, Dr. William, 146-147
Ovarian cysts, 117, 134, 226
Oxalic acid, 236-238
Oxygen, 7, 18, 22, 54, 88, 124, 134, 184,
    205, 219

315

P

Pancreatitis, 16, 97, 99, 248

Panic attacks, 16, 42, 74, 115, 268

Pantothenic acid, 19-20, 32, 36-37, 41-42, 47, 73-74, 80, 84, 104, 135, 161-162, 165, 176, 201, 203, 212, 214-215, 225-226, 230-231, 238, 267, 276, 285, 287, 289-290

Papain, 196-197

Papaya, 26, 31, 41, 79, 102, 153, 171, 194-197, 252-253, 290, 292-294, 296-297, 322

Paralysis, 126

Parsley, 31, 69, 108, 110, 112, 119, 128, 139, 184, 197-200, 231, 241, 259, 274, 280, 287-288, 290, 292, 294

Pauling, Linus, 74

Peanut butter, 43, 46-47, 90, 200-203, 287-288, 290

Peanuts, 25, 35-36, 43, 200-203, 270, 287-288, 302

Peripheral neuropathy, 126

Pernicious anemia, 296

Peroxidase, 23, 168, 278

Pesticides, 19, 23, 34, 57, 78, 139, 144, 148, 150, 152, 156, 159, 173, 242-243, 245, 254, 273, 279-280

Phenol, 188

Phosphatidylethanolamine, 114

Phospholipids, 5, 8, 33, 44, 47, 114, 122

Phosphorus, 49, 51, 60, 65, 73, 82, 96, 104, 107, 123, 129, 131, 133-134, 151, 173, 204-205, 211, 216, 231, 236, 246, 256, 270, 273, 288-290

Photophobia, 296

Physician's Desk Reference, 21

Phytotherapy Research, 113, 304

Pinworms, 16, 137, 296

Pituitary, 50, 177

Plague, 15, 127, 135-136, 146

Planta Medica, 217, 304

Plaque, 63, 296

PMS, 39, 50, 117, 226

Pneumonia, 16, 103, 165, 183, 220, 296

Poison ivy, 140, 169, 296

Pollen, 160, 162

Poor appetite, 99, 186, 200, 215, 248, 271, 275, 296

Post nasal drip, 296

Potassium, 6, 8, 19, 21-22, 27, 29, 31-35, 37, 42-43, 48-49, 51, 57, 60, 65, 69, 73, 77, 82, 91, 94, 96, 100-103, 109-111, 116-118, 126, 129, 131, 134-135, 148-151, 155, 157, 170-171, 181, 194, 198-201, 204-205, 209-211, 216, 222, 225, 228-229, 231, 236, 238-239, 241, 243, 246, 250, 256, 259-260, 262-264, 268-272, 288-290

Prednisone, 230

Proanthocyanidins, 148, 152

Progesterone, 161

Propolis, 159-160

Protease inhibitor, 52

Proteus, 29, 137, 160

Prozac, 34, 38-39

Psoriasis, 16, 39, 50, 97, 171, 190, 205, 226, 267, 296, 303

Psychosis, 217

Pumpkin, 203-206, 256, 269, 286-288, 290

Pycnogenol, 31, 150-151

Pyorrhea, 192

Sinus, 39, 169, 185, 192, 207, 220, 235, 250, 258

Sinusitis, 6, 183, 192, 220, 257-258, 297

Skin, 7, 12, 15-16, 21, 25, 28, 34, 37, 39, 50, 58, 67, 69, 80, 83, 101, 104-105, 111-112, 114-115, 132, 138, 140, 142-144, 148, 151, 158-160, 163, 170-171, 173, 180, 190-193, 195, 204-205, 215, 218, 220, 223, 226-227, 235, 241-242, 244, 247-248, 250-251, 253, 255, 260-261, 263, 267, 281, 293, 295, 297, 322
dry, 16, 39, 50, 53, 58, 67, 82, 84, 133, 173, 201-202, 229, 246-247, 263, 286, 293
oily, 16, 50, 224

Skin cancer, 15, 204, 220

Skin diseases, 28, 67, 226

Skin infection, 16, 34, 50, 69, 160, 191, 192, 251, 261, 267

Sodium, 8, 46-47, 77, 106, 216, 227-230, 233, 236, 272, 289-290
see also Salt

Sodium chloride, 46, 77, 227-230, 272

Solomon, King, 159

Sore throat, 2, 103, 192-193, 195, 216, 222, 251, 262, 297

Sour grape, 22, 31, 36, 47-48, 149-154, 224, 281, 285, 289, 292-297
see also Red Sour Grape

Soy, 13, 23, 25, 81, 84

Spinach, 44, 52, 110, 132, 235-239, 256, 287, 290

Spinal cord, 74-75, 126, 137

Sprains, 297

Squash, 35, 53, 106, 139, 239-241, 269, 288, 290

Staph, 29, 97, 137, 160, 190, 297

Steroids, 5, 42, 105, 128, 161, 196, 290
see also Cortisone

Stomach acid, 43, 76, 143, 229, 237, 248, 266, 270, 283

Strawberries, 79, 153, 170, 214, 241-245, 252, 287, 290

Strawberry leaves, 72, 243, 245, 285, 287-288, 298

Strep, 29, 137, 160, 190

Stress, 18, 38-40, 42, 56, 61, 120, 137, 155, 157, 174, 195, 216, 220

Sugar, 6-7, 14, 27-28, 32-35, 38-39, 41, 42, 52, 54, 57, 60-63, 67, 74, 80-83, 85-87, 89-90, 101-102, 106-107, 111, 115, 125, 135, 141-142, 147-157, 160, 163, 165, 169, 173-174, 176, 178-180, 184, 194-195, 199, 202-203, 213, 228, 231-232, 240, 242-247, 261, 264, 272, 276, 279-280, 294-295, 322
refined, 6, 14, 21, 24, 27-28, 32-34, 36, 42, 61, 80-81, 84, 141, 173, 178, 191, 199, 231, 249, 276, 279

Sulfites, 33-34, 47, 56, 216, 286

Sulfones, 18, 94

Sulforaphane, 22, 91

Sulfur, 7, 12, 21, 23, 31, 40, 47, 51, 73, 94, 96, 124, 136, 142, 169, 181, 207, 257-259, 266-268, 288-290

Superoxide dismutase, 23

Sweet potatoes, 26, 35, 37, 53, 132, 239-240, 245-249, 256, 287, 290

T

Talmud, 136

Tannic acid, 189

Tapeworms, 16, 43, 45, 137, 297

Taurine, 74

Testicular cancer, 15
Testicular glands, 50
Testosterone, 128, 161
Thalassemia, 43
Thalassemia, 43
Thiamine, 19-20, 32, 40, 55, 62-63, 65,
    73-74, 84, 104, 106, 108, 123, 125,
    135, 172, 175-176, 201, 203, 212, 214-
    215, 256, 287, 289-290
Thyme oil, 194
Thymol, 192
Thyroid gland, 12, 27, 100, 177, 202,
    212, 234, 257, 268
Thyroid hormone, 234
Tierra, Michael, 216
Toenail fungus, 193
Tomatoes, 7, 26, 69-71, 90, 105, 110,
    113-114, 165, 181, 188, 199-200, 210,
    231, 234, 238, 249-256, 263-264, 266,
    269, 286, 288, 290, 296, 300
Toothaches, 82, 136, 192, 297
Trichomonas, 16, 137
Tryptophan, 74, 173, 175-176, 201, 283
Tuberculosis, 16, 136-137, 159, 186, 297
Turnips, 23, 26, 52, 91, 255-259, 263,
    280, 286-288, 290, 295
Tyrosine, 74

U-V
Ulcerations, 28, 159, 297
Ulcerative colitis, 16, 40, 43, 95, 120,
    171, 241, 297
Uterine fibroids, 226, 297
Vaginitis, 284, 297
Valnet, Dr. Jean, 216-217, 220, 304
Varicose veins, 95, 155, 297
Vasco da Gama, 143

Vasculitis, 6, 95
Venomous bites, 69, 136, 141, 186, 297
Vinegar, 22, 33, 43, 61, 66, 70, 79, 83-84,
    97, 112, 116, 119, 127, 141, 164, 166,
    168, 178, 195, 199-200, 208, 210, 231,
    237-238, 243, 259-263, 281, 286, 288,
    290, 297, 322-323
Visual purple, 87-89
Vitamins. *See individual vitamins*
Vitamin A, 2-9, 11-47, 49-283, 285-287,
    289, 291, 299-304, 322-323
Vitamin B, 6, 16, 21-22, 27, 29, 32-37,
    41, 43-44, 47-48, 55, 78, 80, 84, 86, 89,
    104, 106-107, 118, 125-126, 133, 135,
    137, 140, 152, 173, 201-203, 205, 210,
    212-215, 224, 228, 231, 236, 239, 241,
    267, 270, 274, 276, 280, 283, 286, 289,
    299-302, 304
    see also B vitamins
Vitamin B$_2$, 32, 51
    see also Riboflavin
Vitamin B$_5$, 32, 51
    see also Pantothenic acid
Vitamin B$_6$, 6, 32, 51, 65, 102, 104, 135
    see also Pyridoxine
Vitamin B$_{12}$, 20, 32, 44, 62, 73-75, 80,
    104, 123, 212, 225, 231, 287, 289, 301
Vitamin C, 6, 16, 19-22, 27, 29, 31-36,
    41-42, 44, 48, 51, 55, 57, 78, 82, 86-88,
    91, 93-95, 97-101, 103, 108, 140, 147,
    149, 154-159, 162, 166-167, 170-171,
    181-182, 194-196, 198, 204, 206, 209-
    211, 214, 221, 223-224, 236, 238-240,
    242-244, 246-247, 250-251, 253-257,
    259, 263-264, 266-267, 269-270, 272,
    287, 289-290, 299-304

Books by Dr. Cass Ingram and Judy Kay Gray, M.S.

#1 How to Eat Right and Live Longer (new edition, January, 1998) **$21.95**
320 pages, 6 x 9 inch softback ISBN 0911119229
You need to know how to eat right: at home, in restaurants, while traveling: this book gives you exact guidance. Learn how to improve your health quickly—just by changing the way you shop, eat, and dine. The food tastes better than ever; includes over 100 recipes.

#2 Self-Test Nutrition Guide $17.95
320 pages, 5 ½ x 8 ½ inch softback ISBN 0911119507
Everyone is nutritionally deficient. Test yourself for deficiencies from vitamin A to Zinc. Also, test yourself for syndromes such as rapid aging, adrenal burn-out, thyroid problems, estrogen imbalance, blood sugar disturbances, parasites, fungus, and liver dysfunction. Corrective recommendations included.

#3 The Cure is in the Cupboard: Oregano for Better Health $17.95
170 pages, 5 ½ x 8 ½ inch softback ISBN 0911119744
Oregano can help you regain your health and then keep you healthy. This is what saved Dr. Ingram's life. Learn how to use oregano and its essential oil for fighting infection and eliminating pain. Combat skin disorders, injuries, and dental problems. Particularly valuable for fungal disorders.

#4 How to Survive Disasters with Natural Medicines $13.95
140 pages, 5 ½ x 8 ½ inch softback ISBN 0911119442
Honey, vinegar, garlic, onion, papaya, and dozens of other remedies save your life in big or everyday disasters. Combat radiation/toxic chemical exposure, parasitic infection, bacteria, viruses, and water contamination with natural medicines. Specific protocols included.

#5 Killed On Contact: How to Use Tea Tree Oil, Natural Antiseptic $11.95
120 pages, 5 ½ x 8 ½ inch softback ISBN 0911119493
Tea tree oil is a natural antiseptic with unique properties good for anyone's medicine chest. Learn its versatile uses. Information valuable for travelers, wilderness buffs, fishermen, athletes, and parents.

#6 Who Needs Headaches (How to Reverse Migraines)   **$17.95**
170 pages, 6 x 9 inch softback ISBN 0911119329
Migraines and other chronic headaches are reversible. Find out the main causes (food allergy and hormonal disturbances) and how to correct them. Nutritional recommendations and remedies included.

#7 Supermarket Remedies $34.95
330 pages, 6 x 9 inch hardback ISBN 091119647
Reverse health problems simply with food. Learn about a supermarket juice that reverses heart disease and cancer, a vegetable that eliminates depression, a protein for energy, a berry for poor vision, a fruit which lowers cholesterol, a spice that kills germs, etc. Use supermarket remedies for all kinds of illnesses.

Cassette Tapes and Programs

#1 The How to Eat Right Series $39.95
3 tapes   Total time: 3 hours
Different from the book, includes tapes on the following subjects: (1) How to Eat Right at Home, while Traveling, or in Restaurants (2) Disease Prevention (3) Is our Water Safe? (4) Preventing Aging.

#2 The Survivor's Nutritional Pharmacy $29.95
3 tapes Total time: 1 1/2 hours
Learn exactly how to survive major disasters and everyday injuries that could threaten your health and life. Simple and inexpensive remedies such as honey, vinegar, garlic, onion and enzymes are life-saving.

#3 How to Use Oregano for Common Illnesses $9.95
1 tape   Total time: 1 hour, with Judy Kay Gray, M.S.
A must supplement containing information not found in the book; includes specific protocols for dozens of illnesses and diseases plus case histories. Learn hundreds of uses for wild oregano oil and herb—*from the Doctor himself.*

#4 Professional/Advanced Series: $89.85*
The Warning Signs of Nutritional Deficiency (manual and tapes)
4 tapes   T otal time: 4 hrs   Manual: 100 pages, with Judy Kay Gray, M.S.
Master Dr. Ingram's knowledge about nutritional deficiency and natural medicine. Find out how to discern your specific deficiencies; become proficient at spotting nutritional deficiencies in others. Includes life-saving information on the treatment of disease with nutritional medicine. **Become an expert.**

*Normal price for this program is $129.95. Save $40.00 when you order it from this book.

Supermarket Cures via Computer: **drcass.com**

Visit Dr. Cass Ingram on the Internet. Our website provides visuals and information about books and natural products. Simply type:

www.drcass.com

Order Form

Item	Quantity	Amount
Books by Dr. Cass Ingram and Judy Kay Gray, M.S.		
Book #1 How to Eat Right and Live Longer	_____	_____
Book #2 Self-Test Nutrition Guide	_____	_____
Book #3 The Cure is in the Cupboard	_____	_____
Book #4 How to Survive Disasters	_____	_____
Book #5 Killed On Contact	_____	_____
Book #6 Who Needs Headaches	_____	_____
Book #7 Supermarket Remedies	_____	_____
Tapes and Programs		
Tape #1 The How to Eat Right Series	_____	_____
Tape #2 Survivor's Nutritional Pharmacy	_____	_____
Tape #3 How to Use Oregano for Common Illnesses	_____	_____
Tape #4 Professional Series (tapes and manual)	_____	_____
Sub-Total		_____
Sales Tax (if any)		_____
Shipping*		_____
TOTAL		_____

* *Shipping Charges:* $4.00 for single orders - add $1.00 for each additional item. Payment by check, money order, or credit card.

Make checks payable to:
AICM • P.O. Box 4885 • Buffalo Grove, Illinois 60089
Phone: (800) 243-5242

Use the following for VISA, Mastercard or American Express orders:

Credit Card # _____ Exp. Date _____

Signature _____

Name _____

Address _____

City _____ State_____ Zip_____

Order Form

Item	Quantity	Amount
Books by Dr. Cass Ingram and Judy Kay Gray, M.S.		
Book #1 How to Eat Right and Live Longer	_____	_____
Book #2 Self-Test Nutrition Guide	_____	_____
Book #3 The Cure is in the Cupboard	_____	_____
Book #4 How to Survive Disasters	_____	_____
Book #5 Killed On Contact	_____	_____
Book #6 Who Needs Headaches	_____	_____
Book #7 Supermarket Remedies	_____	_____
Tapes and Programs		
Tape #1 The How to Eat Right Series	_____	_____
Tape #2 Survivor's Nutritional Pharmacy	_____	_____
Tape #3 How to Use Oregano for Common Illnesses	_____	_____
Tape #4 Professional Series (tapes and manual)	_____	_____
Sub-Total		_____
Sales Tax (if any)		_____
Shipping*		_____
TOTAL		_____

* *Shipping Charges:* $4.00 for single orders - add $1.00 for each
   additional item. Payment by check, money order, or credit card.

Make checks payable to:
   **AICM • P.O. Box 4885 • Buffalo Grove, Illinois 60089
   Phone: (800) 243-5242**

Use the following for VISA, Mastercard or American Express orders:

Credit Card # _____ Exp. Date _____

Signature _____

Name _____

Address _____

City _____ State_____ Zip_____